HANDBOOK OF GERONTOLOGY

Janny Lee

ALLIED HEALTH PRESS

Handbook of Gerontology

Author: **Janny Lee**

Allied Health Press
4164 Lakeshore Road
Burlington ON L7L 1A4
Canada
www.alliedhealthpress.com
Email: orders@arclereducation.com

ISBN: 978-1-77956-243-2

ABOUT THE AUTHOR

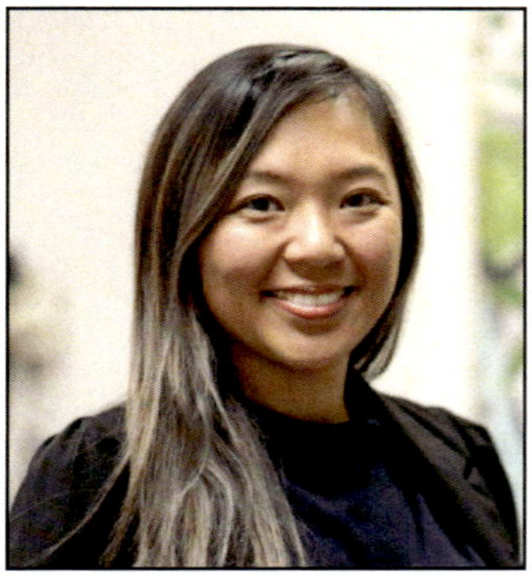

Janny Lee is a dedicated Registered Nurse with a multifaceted background spanning intensive care, community, and emergency care. Currently, Janny is a Clinical Nurse Specialist in Geriatrics in Toronto, Canada, where she is involved in age-friendly initiatives and improving care for older adults. In addition, Janny is an Adjunct lecturer and health tech consultant, offering strategic advisory and clinical transformation. Janny's academic journey is a testament to her commitment to lifelong learning. She earned her Bachelor's in Nursing from the University of New Brunswick, a Master's in Nursing from Athabasca University, and a Master's in Business Administration from the Frankfurt School of Finance and Management. Her dedication to staying abreast of the latest advancements in geriatrics is evident in her active engagement in continuing education. Janny's unwavering dedication to patient care and his diverse experiences and academic achievements exemplify her commitment to excellence in healthcare delivery. She is driven by a profound sense of compassion and empathy, striving to positively impact the lives of those she serves.

Word Roots, Prefixes, and Suffixes by Chapter

Chapter 1 Introduction to Gerontology

geront/o: old age

senesc/o: to grow old

presby/o: old age

somat/o: body

chron/o: time

bio-: life, living

poly-: many

anti-: against, opposite

pre-: before

-logy: the study of

-itis: inflammation

-pathy: disease

-osis: condition, usually abnormal

-genic: causing, producing

Chapter 2 Evolutionary Biology of Aging

Sen- (from Latin senex, meaning old)

Ger- (from Greek geras, meaning old age)

Chrono- (from Greek chronos, meaning time)

Aging (from Old English agen): central concept referring to the process of getting older.

Cyt- (from Greek kytos, meaning cell):

Hist- (from Greek histos, meaning tissue)

Gen- (from Greek genos, meaning origin or race)

Osteo- (from Greek osteon, meaning bone)

Chapter 3 Principles and Theories of Aging

Anti-: Against, opposite

Bio-: Life, living matter

Pro-: Before, forward

Senso-: Sensation, perception

Hyper-: Excessive, above normal

-logy: Study

-genic: Producing, forming

-plasia: Formation, growth

-genesis: Formation, origin

-opathy: Disease, disorder

Chapter 4 Toxicology and the Aging Process: A Critical Examination

Toxi-: Pertaining to poison or toxicity.

Cyto-: Relating to cells, often used in the context of cellular toxicity.

Hepato-: Relating to the liver, where toxins are processed and detoxified.

Neuro-: Referring to nerves or the nervous system, relevant in neurotoxicology.

Eco-: Relating to ecology or the environment, relevant in ecotoxicology.

-ology: Denotes the study or science of a particular subject

-toxic: Indicates toxicity or the capacity to cause harm

-emia: Refers to presence in the blood

-pathy: Denotes a disease or disorder

Chapter 5 The Biology of Aging

Anti-: Against

Bi-: Two, double

Meta-: Change, beyond

Poly-: Many, much

Pro-: Before, forward

Aging: The process of growing old

Bio-: Life

Chrono-: Time

Gen-: Origin, race, kind

Phago-: To eat

-logy: Study of

-lysis: Breakdown, dissolution

-osis: Condition, process

-stasis: Stopping, controlling

Chapter 6 The Impact of the Environment on Age-Related Diseases and Organ Function Changes

Aging-: Relating to the process of aging.

Geronto-: Referring to old age or the elderly.

Sen-: Pertaining to old age.

Ger-/Gero-: Root meaning old age.

Chrono-: Root meaning time, often used in the context of age-related changes.

Sarc-: Root meaning flesh, often used in medical terms related to muscle changes with age.

-pathy: Suffix indicating disease or disorder.

-genesis: Suffix indicating origin or development.

-plasia: Suffix indicating formation or growth.

Chapter 7 The Science of Dietary and Nutritional Interventions in Aging

Bio- (relating to life or living organisms)

Nutri- (related to nutrition)

Geronto- (related to aging)

Meta- (beyond, change)

Poly- (many, much)

Micro- (small, microscopic)

Nutri- (nutrition)

Vent- (to come, to go)

Suffixes:

-ology (study of)

-ical (related to)

-ation (action or process)

-al (relating to, pertaining to)

Chapter 8 Physiological Changes Across the Lifespan

Hypo-: Below, deficient

Hyper-: Above, excessive

Dys-: Abnormal, difficult

Physio-: Relating to nature or function of the body

-Logy: Study or science of

-Gen: Producing, forming

-ic: Pertaining to

-ism: Condition or state of

-osis: Condition, often abnormal condition

Chapter 9 Age-Related Cognitive Decline

Co- (together): e.g., co-cognition (shared cognition)

Meta- (beyond, transcending): e.g., metacognition (thinking about thinking)

Peri- (around, near): e.g., pericognition (cognition around a specific topic)

Cogni- (related to knowledge or thinking): e.g., cognition (the process of acquiring knowledge)

Gnos- (to know): e.g., agnosia (loss of ability to recognize familiar objects)

-tion (act or process of): e.g., cognition (process of acquiring knowledge)

-itive (relating to): e.g., cognitive (relating to cognition)

-sis (process): e.g., diagnosis (process of identifying a disease)

Table of Contents

LIST OF FIGURES

LIST OF TABLES

PREFACE

Aging is a natural process that every individual undergoes at their own unique pace and timing. It encompasses all the transformations that occur throughout a person's life, starting from birth, through growth, development, and eventual maturity. While aging may be perceived as an exciting journey in youth, it gradually presents more visible changes as one enters middle age, such as graying hair, wrinkled skin, and a noticeable decline in physical abilities. These changes are inevitable, affecting even the healthiest and most aesthetically fit individuals.

As people age further, they often experience a gradual decline in physical function and an increase in dependency. This can lead to functional disabilities and a greater need for assistance in daily activities during old age. According to the World Health Organization, aging is an intrinsic biological reality that begins at conception and concludes with death. It is a natural process beyond human control, characterized by its own set of dynamics.

However, societal perceptions and constructions of old age also play a significant role in shaping the experience of aging. In many developed countries, for instance, the age of 60 is commonly regarded as the retirement age and marks the beginning of old age. These societal constructs influence how individuals perceive and navigate the aging process.

In this book, readers will understand the aging processes and associated physiological changes. By exploring these topics, readers can gain a deeper understanding of aging and its impact on individuals and society as a whole. This book is an up-to-date and realistic view on physiopathological mechanisms of aging and age-related diseases.

The book "Gerontology" presents a comprehensive and interdisciplinary overview of the field of gerontology, focusing on the biological, psychological, and social aspects of aging. It aims to address the complex challenges and opportunities associated with the aging process, offering insights into how individuals, families, communities, and societies can promote healthy aging and enhance the quality of life for older adults.

It also examines the biological processes of aging, including cellular and molecular changes that occur with age. Covering topics of genetics, cellular senescence, and age-related diseases, the book seeks to deepen the reader's understanding of the aging process at a fundamental level.

It explores the psychological aspects of aging, including cognitive function, mental health, and psychosocial well-being including topics such as memory and cognition, personality development, and coping mechanisms, the book aims to provide insights into the unique psychological challenges faced by older adults and how these challenges can be addressed.

The book also aims to highlight the social dimensions of aging, including the impact of social relationships, cultural factors, and societal attitudes on the aging experience.

This book is designed to cater to a wide range of readers interested in the field of aging and the study of older adults. It is particularly relevant for students, researchers, and professionals in various disciplines, including geriatrics, psychology, sociology, nursing, and social work.

For students, especially those pursuing degrees in gerontology or related fields, the book offers a comprehensive introduction to the multidimensional aspects of aging. It provides foundational knowledge that can be applied to future research or clinical practice.

Researchers will find the book valuable for its in-depth exploration of current theories, research findings, and methodologies in gerontology. It can serve as a reference for designing and conducting studies on aging-related topics.

Professionals working with older adults, such as healthcare providers, social workers, and policymakers, can benefit from the book's insights into the challenges and opportunities associated with aging. It offers practical strategies for promoting healthy aging and improving the quality of life for older individuals.

Additionally, caregivers and family members of older adults may find the book informative in understanding the aging process and providing better care and support for their loved ones. Therefore, the book aims to be accessible and informative for anyone interested in learning more about aging and its implications for society.

Chapter 1

INTRODUCTION TO GERONTOLOGY

Contents

Introduction

With an understanding of gerontology, individuals can make informed decisions about their health, finances, and living arrangements as they age. They can anticipate potential challenges and plan for them accordingly, ensuring a higher quality of life in their later years. For example, knowing the risk factors for age-related diseases can prompt individuals to adopt healthier lifestyles, potentially delaying or preventing the onset of such conditions.

Communities and legislators can also benefit from an understanding of gerontology. By recognizing the unique needs of older adults, they can implement policies and programs that promote healthy aging and support older adults' well-being. This might include improving access to healthcare, creating age-friendly environments, and implementing social programs that combat isolation and loneliness.

As we continue to lead longer and healthier lives, the collective wisdom and experience of older adults become increasingly valuable. Their insights can inform decision-making at all levels, from individual choices to public policy. However, to fully realize the benefits of an aging population, we must address the challenges that come with it. This includes ensuring access to affordable healthcare, affordable housing, and opportunities for social engagement.

Orientation and Directional Terms:

Term	Definition	Illustration
Gerontology	The study of aging and the challenges encountered as individuals grow older. This field examines the biological, psychological, and sociological aspects of aging.	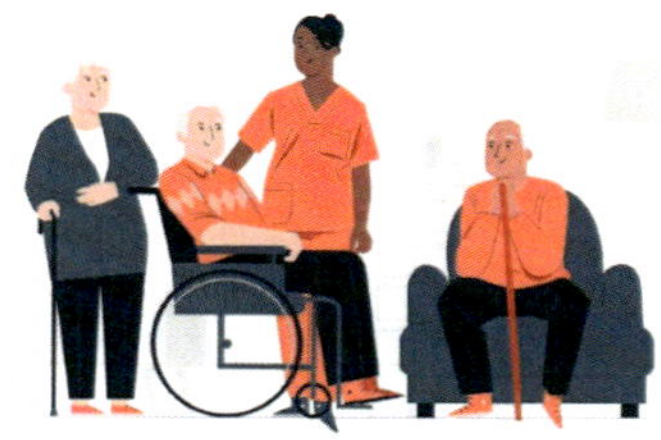
Senescence	The gradual deterioration of functional characteristics in organisms that leads to aging. This includes cellular aging, where cells lose the ability to divide and function, leading to age-related diseases.	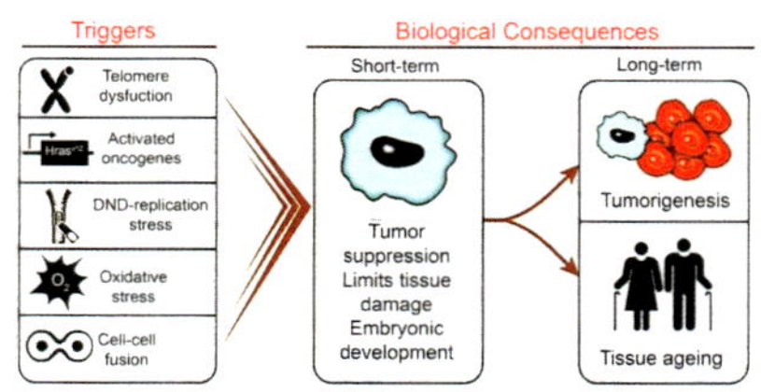
Life Expectancy	The average period a person is expected to live based on statistical averages. Life expectancy varies by region, gender, and other demographic factors and is influenced by healthcare, lifestyle, and genetics.	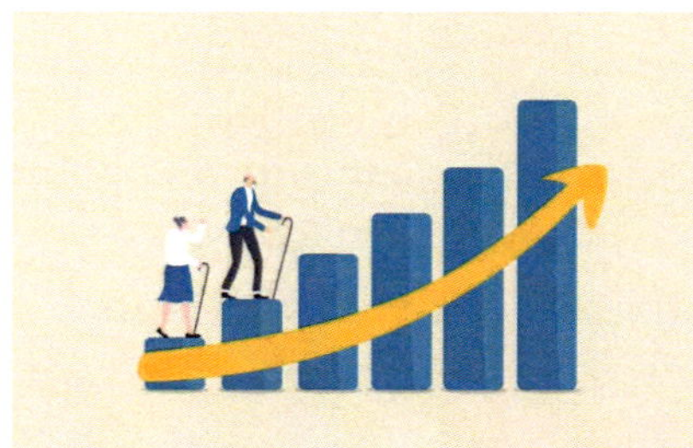
Ageism	Discrimination and prejudice against individuals based on their age. This often involves stereotypes, myths, and misconceptions about older adults, impacting their social status and access to services.	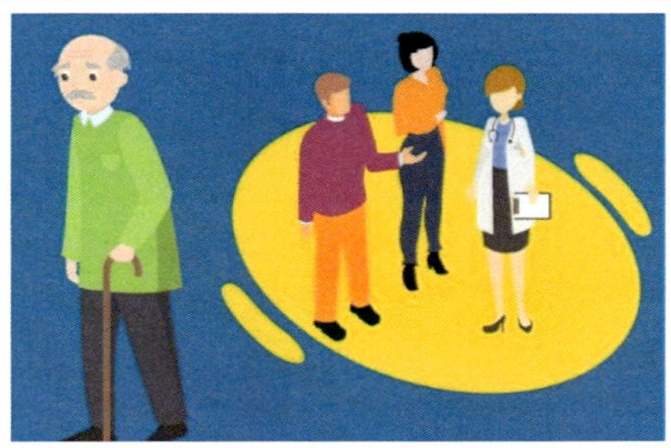
Geriatrics	A branch of medicine focused on the health care of elderly people. It aims to promote health by preventing and treating diseases and disabilities in older adults.	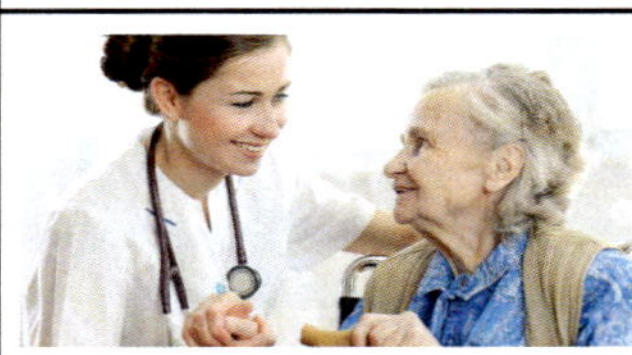

1.1. Definition of Gerontology

Gerontology is the study of aging and older adults. The science of gerontology has evolved as longevity has improved. Researchers in this field are diverse and are trained in areas such as physiology, social science, psychology, public health, and policy. A more complete definition of gerontology includes all of the following:

- Scientific studies of processes associated with the bodily changes from middle age through later life;
- Multidisciplinary investigation of societal changes resulting from an aging population and ranging from the humanities (e.g., history, philosophy, literature) to economics; and
- Applications of this knowledge to policies and programs.

Gerontology is the study of aging. It comes from the Greek words geron, meaning "old man," and -ology, a suffix meaning "the study of." Gerontology is a multidisciplinary field. It involves the scientific study of physical, mental, and social changes that occur in older people, the investigation of societal changes from an economic, historical, and philosophical standpoint, and the carrying out of policies and procedures to aid older people with information from gerontology in mind. Gerontologists in the field of biology study the biological changes that occur in older individuals. Gerontology is not to be confused with geriatrics, which specifically refers to the medical care and treatment of older people.

1.2. History of Gerontology

People have been fascinated with aging since ancient times. Of course, many ancient cultures, much like today's society, were highly interested in slowing the aging process or reversing it. The earliest known recipe for an anti-aging ointment is from an Egyptian papyrus dating back to 2800–2700 B.C. called "The Book for Transforming an Old Man into a Youth of Twenty." It claimed to beautify the skin and remove any disfiguring signs of age. Another ancient papyrus from 1550 B.C. describes some of the biological changes that can occur with aging, such as heart pain, deafness, blindness, and what would later be known as cancer.

Gerontology research, and other forms of scientific research, really took off during the 19th Century, when the use of the compound microscope became widespread. Many scientists at first began to study bacteria under the microscope to study senescence or aging, but this proved difficult because bacteria reproduce by dividing themselves into two cells and do not become senescent in the way that the cells of multicellular organisms do. Multicellular animal models had to be used instead, and this is one reason why the use of mice became so ubiquitous in research. With the use of the microscope, scientific knowledge advanced a great deal. For the first time, researchers could examine the processes of aging at the cellular level, and really begin to understand the specific changes that take place in the cells of older people. People began to develop theories about why aging occurs; August Weissman, a German embryologist, proposed that lifespan was related to an evolutionary selective advantage, and that species with different body sizes, intelligence, and ecology had different lifespans. The term gerontology was coined in 1903 by Élie Metchnikoff, a Russian zoologist who did immunology research and won the Nobel Prize in Physiology or Medicine for his work.

In the mid-20th century when the structure of DNA was uncovered, another paradigm shift occurred in gerontology research. Scientists could now study genetics relating to aging; for example, they looked at unique mutations in abnormally long-lived or short-lived fruit flies. Other ways of extending an organism's lifespan were also found, like putting mice on calorie-restricted diets or putting fruit flies in very small cages so that they couldn't fly as much. Further progress was made when age-related decline in certain hormones, like growth hormone, thyroid hormone, and estrogen, was discovered. More recently, genome sequencing has been used to identify genes associated with aging.

1.3. A New Concept: Aging is Not an Event But a Process

For the development theorists and practitioners aging is one of the most neglected issues mainly because aged people are considered as disempowered and non-resourceful persons. They are not considered as a class category or status group either by economists or sociologists. Though aging is universal, till a decade back aging is considered a natural and evolutionary process and hence it is not taken seriously. Till the 1980s, the problems of the old were not known to the state in developing countries and therefore they were not attended. There are many ways to reduce the child population but the old population cannot be stopped as developing countries like Asian countries methodically ignore the structure of the population. Aging can generally be described as the process of growing old and is an intricate part of the life cycle, it is a multi-dimensional process and affects almost every aspect of human life. Introduction to the study of human aging have typically emphasized changes in demography focusing on the aging of population'- a trend, which has characterized industrial societies throughout the twentieth century but in recent decades, has become a worldwide phenomenon.

Population aging is the most significant result of the process known as the demographic transition. Two dimensions of demographic transition are:

a. Reduction of fertility that leads to a decline in the proportion of the young in the population.

b. Reduction of mortality which means a longer life span for individuals.

Jean Bourgeois Pichat (1979) has called attention to two process in aging which reflect the two dimensions of demographic transition.

a. Aging at the base

b. Aging at the apex. Aging at the base occurs when fertility falls, thus decreasing the proportion of children and aging at the apex occurs when the proportion of aged persons increases presumably due to declining mortality at older ages.

Population aging involves a shift from high mortality / high fertility to low mortality / low fertility and consequently, an increased proportion of older people in the total population (Prakash,1999).

1.4. Dimensions and Definition of Aging

Aging has been defined in various ways by different scholars and it is measured in many ways according to the academic background of the person who studies them. Some have regarded aging as a period of physiological deterioration, others regard it as simply the advancement of years and still others have emphasized that aging involves a restriction on cultural roles. According to Bhatia (1983) the term aging' is a broad one and can be studied under three types - Biological, Psychological, and Socio-cultural.

In the broadest sense, Charles S Becker (1959) defines aging as those changes occurring in an individual, which are the result of the passage of time.' These may be, according to him, anatomical, physiological, psychological and even social and economic. He further adds: Aging consists of two simultaneous components – anabolic building up and catabolic breaking down. In the middle years, there is an essential balance between expansion and decay, while growth predominates in youth; degenerative changes that start occurring very clearly in life pre-dominate in the late life span. Edward J. Stieglitz (1960) defines aging as the element of time in living.' According to him, aging is a part of living. Aging begins with conception and terminates with death. It cannot be arrested unless we arrest life.

According to Tibbitts (1960), aging may be best defined as the survival of a growing number of people who have completed the traditional roles of making a living and child rearing and years following the completion of these tasks represent an extension of life. He also says, aging is an inevitable and irreversible biological process.

According to Hooyman and Kiyak (1994), the gerontologists view aging in terms of the following four distinct process or dimensions:

Four dimensions of aging are commonly identified: chronological, biological, psychological and social aging.

- Chronological Aging: Refers to the number of years since someone was born Chronological age also provides individuals with a means of distinguishing roles and relationships in terms of the behavior and expectations that are linked to different chronological groupings. However, it is generally not recognized as an adequate measure of the extent of aging because, as a process, it is thought to vary between individuals.
- Biological Aging: Often known as senescence (declines of a cell or organism due to aging) and sometimes functional aging, refers to biological events occurring across time that progressively impair the physiological system so that the organism becomes less able to withstand disease, ultimately increasing its susceptibility to death. From this perspective, the aging process stems from several physiological factors, and is modified throughout the life course by environmental factors (such as nutrition), experiences of disease, genetic factors and life stage. This is usually associated with the decline in the regulation and proper functioning of the vital organs of the body. However, not all people experience decreased organ function in the same proportion. Some individuals have healthier hearts at age 80 than others do at age 60.
- Psychological Aging: Focuses upon changes that occur during adulthood to an individual's personality, mental functioning (e.g., memory, learning and intelligence) and sensory and perceptual processes. Jegede (2003) stated that the indices of psychological aging include feelings, motivation, memory, emotions, and experience and self-identify. For instance, people who had the intention of traveling abroad may decide to drop the idea and contribute to the growth of their own economy. Psychological aging is heterogeneous and continuous as an individual passes through life.
- Social Aging: Refers to the changing

experiences that individuals will encounter in their roles and relationships with other people and as members of broader social structures (such as a religious group) as they pass through different phases of their life course. In sociological aging, personal or attitude and interaction within the community are used to assess a person's maturation and aging. As a person ages socially, he/she calculates his/her utterances, limits the use of vulgar language, prunes relationships with mature friends, changes his/her mode of dressing, and reduces nocturnal clubs. As a person ages socially, he/she tends to be guided by the norms of the society to which the person belongs. As an individual experience, social aging affects perceptions of who we are, but can also be shaped or 'constructed' by social and cultural contexts that dictate the normative expectations about the roles, positions and behavior of older people in society.

While all three dimensions of biological, social and psychological aging generally interact, the pace at which each dimension is experienced may be different for the same individual. This is usually how a person relates with others in the society.

Strehler (1962) has proposed four criteria for aging, reported in Tyagi (1999). They are: Aging is universal, which means it occurs in all members of a population.

- Aging is progressive, a continuous process.
- Aging is intrinsic to the organism
- Aging is degenerative

Thus, aging is an inevitable, ubiquitous and universal phenomenon of human life because it is a natural process. Finally, population aging, sometimes referred to as societal aging, is a process whereby a group (such as a country or an ethnic group) experiences the progressive increase in the actual numbers and proportion of older people within its total population. This change, brought about largely by socio-economic improvements in health and living standards, progressively reduces mortality and fertility, resulting in increased life expectancy and fewer births, and ultimately, an increase in the older population in relation to younger age groups. Population aging has long-term implications for governments in terms of, for example, of the cost of health and social care for an increasingly important number ofolder people.

Cavanaught (1993) in Osunde and Obiunu (2005) divided aging into three types, the primary aging, the secondary aging and the tertiary aging.

- Primary Aging: Primary aging is considered as the normal process which has nothing to do with illness. It simply involves changes in the biological, social and psychological domains. These occur due to the wear and tear of vital organs of the body.
- Secondary Aging: This process is associated with different kinds of terminal illnesses that prevent the normal functioning of the individual.
- Tertiary Aging: This occurs when there are loses brought about by death or disasters like war(s) on a family member or close friends that could lead to a gradual decline in the proper functioning of the individual.
- Demographic Dividend: The growing

global economic support ratio could have beneficial effects on the macroeconomy, through the so-called demographic dividend. The demographic dividend is defined as the increase in per capita consumption brought about by a growing economic support ratio. Demographic dividend, as defined by the United Nations Population Fund (UNFPA) means, —the economic growth potential that can result from shifts in a population's age structure, mainly when the share of the working-age population (15 to 64) is larger than the non-working-age share of the population (14 and younger, and 65 and older). In other words it is —a boost in economic productivity that occurs when there are growing numbers of people in the workforce relative to the number of dependents. UNFPA stated that "A country with both increasing numbers of young people and declining fertility has the potential to reap a demographic dividend."

1.5. Demographic Profile of the Older Population

Aging is taking place in the global adult population and within the older population itself. The proportion of persons aged 80 years or over within the older population increased from 7 percent in 1950 to 14% in 2013.

According to the projection, this proportion of —oldest-old within older persons is expected to reach 19% in 2050 and 28% in 2100.

If this projection is realized, there will be 830 million persons aged 80 years or over by the end of the century, seven times as many as in 2013.

The rise in the population aged 80 years or over is occurring at a faster pace in the less developed regions than in the more developed regions.

In 1950, there were 6 million people aged 80 years or over in the less developed regions and 8 million in the more developed regions, but by 2013, people aged 80 years or over are already slightly more numerous in the less developed regions than in the more developed regions

The present number of persons aged 80 years or over is the result of

- The birth rates of many decades ago, which determined the initial size of these cohorts
- The survival rates, which have been improving dramatically since these cohorts were born. The number and proportion of centenarians (people aged 100 years or more) is growing even faster. The number of centenarians in the world is projected to increase rapidly from approximately 441,000 in 2013 to 3.4 million in 2050 and 20.1 million in 2100.

Aging is a global phenomenon. Aging plays a vital role in the global demographic transition. According to projections by the UN Population Division, there will be two old age persons for every child in the world by 2050. This implies that the aged 60 and above, which currently constitute less than 20% of the population will account for 32% of the population by 2050. The world old age population (aged 60+) in 1980 accounted for 8.6% of the total population and is fast growing and would reach 12.9% in the year 2020. The old age population is growing twice as fast in developing countries. The old age people in India accounted for 5.7% in 1990 and it is estimated to reach 12.6% in the year 2020 AD. Other predictions indicate that India will have the second-largest population of elderly in the world in 2025 with 13% of the total population. The projected increase in both the absolute and relative size of the old age population in many third-world countries is a subject of concern. Thus the aged population is becoming an important segment of the population pyramid for public policy making. In India, the population of the old age is growing rapidly and is emerging as a serious area of concern for the government and the policy planners. According to data on the age of India's population, as per the Census 2001, there are a little over 76.6 million people above 60 years, constituting 7.2 percent of the population. The number of people over 60 years in 1991 was 6.8 percent of the country's population. Recently, with 90 million persons over 60 years of age, India has the second largest population of older people in the world. Furthermore, between now and 2050 the Indian population over 60 years of age will almost quadruple. The low level of benefits and their limited coverage push large numbers of older people, particularly older women, to continue working in the informal economy. The combination of old-age, lack of access to decent work, poverty and exclusion is therefore of great concern .

According to Irudaya Rajan in 2008, globally, life expectancy at birth increased from 47 years in the 1950s to 67 in 2008, an increase of 20 years in the space of half a century. In India, the increase has been 21 years. On average, an older person is expected to live 18–20 years upon reaching 60. Some consequences of aging population are declining participation in the economy by the old age people, financial strains on account of retirement trends and increasing demand for health care and other welfare measures. In India the process of industrialization and urbanization has weakened the joint family system. Migration of youth to other cities and developed regions had brought problems to old age people, which were unheard of in the past. Hence research on aging in India has gained importance and is very vital for the allocation of resources, effective planning and utilization of human resources and to design of welfare packages. According to Easwaramoorthy 1995, the concept of quality of life has gained significance in Gerontology due to the need for an integrated approach towards understanding the aged and the requirement for an outcome measure for health care and welfare policies. Moreover, aging is a multidimensional phenomenon and this is in fact empirically well-established. There are economic, physical, psychological and social dimensions acting on an aging individual, variables related to these dimensions are interactive and interdependent and can be best understood in the light of a multidimensional approach. Many governments in the world, including the Government of India, have their support systems in place for old age persons such as social security welfare measures and free or discounted medical care. For example, however, most of these systems were built on the premise that there will always be significantly fewer older persons than younger or middle- aged individuals living at one time. Because of declining death rates, these systems are beginning to feel a strain that will only increase over time. Additionally, the older-person support ratio is falling in both more and less-developed regions, which could further lessen the ability of societies and governments to care for their aging populations. These demographic trends create unique challenges for all people, particularly for the governments of nation-states around the globe.

There is also a prevalent belief among many that old age persons are worthless in today's fast-paced, globalized and increasingly industrialized world. Obviously, with the number of old age population is rising rapidly, there is an increased urgency to address the rights and roles of old age persons in our world. The family provides the ambiance for affection and social bonding throughout the life-cycle. It is not only supportive by nature but also contributes to the social integration of old age people. It is within the domain of the family that the old age people seek care and for emotional, social, economic and health support in old age. Caring for old age people constitutes a major concern for most families, especially in rural sector and remains a problem, despite changes such as accelerated aging, urbanization, industrialization and modernization taking place in society. These are likely to have consequences on family structure and individual lifestyles. These, in turn, will have a bearing on the well-being of the old age people. The life expectancy has also gone beyond 70 years today. Better medical facilities, care and liberal family planning policies made the old age persons the fastest within four-walls, that's why only a few cases of violation of human rights of old age people come out. Ever-increasing numbers of distress calls from older persons clearly indicate disturbing conditions of the Human Rights of Old age Persons in India. According to the Universal Declaration of Human Rights Definition as per Article 25, "Everyone has the right to a standard of living adequate for the health and well-being of himself and of his family, including food, clothing, housing and medical care and necessary social services, and the right to security in the event of unemployment, sickness, disability, widowhood, old age or other lack of livelihood in circumstances beyond his control."

1.6. Health of the Older Population

The health profile of populations has changed in parallel with the demographic transition. The importance of communicable or infectious diseases has declined and that of non- communicable or chronic diseases has increased. This phenomenon is referred to as the epidemiological transition. Its implications, particularly for the delivery of health and long-term care services to older persons, need to be examined.

While episodes of communicable disease can have disabling consequences, non- communicable diseases, such as cardiovascular disease and cancer, often bring about a long period of poor health and diminished functioning. In addition, some non-fatal (but often chronic) conditions can have an important impact on the quality of life and healthcare costs for older individuals. Examples of such conditions include hearing and vision loss, musculoskeletal conditions such as osteoarthritis, and cognitive impairments including Alzheimer's disease and other dementias.

Increasing life expectancy raises the question of whether longer life spans result in more years of life in good health, or whether it is associated with increased morbidity and more years spent in prolonged disability and dependency.

The major causes of disability and health problems in old age are non-communicable diseases including the —four giants of geriatrics, namely:

1. Memory loss
2. Urinary incontinence
3. Depression and falls or immobility
4. Communicable diseases and injuries

As population aging takes place, health

expenditures tend to grow rapidly since older persons usually require more health care in general and more specialized services to deal with their more complex pathologies. The number of deaths also increases sharply due to the exponential increase in mortality with age. Furthermore, older women generally experience higher rates of morbidity and disability than older men, in large part because of their longer life expectancy (WHO, 2007).

The global crude death rate is defined as the ratio of annual total deaths to the total population. This is increasing because population aging shifts the age distribution towards the older ages, which are subject to a higher risk of mortality. Because of this, population aging causes two seemingly contrasting situations:

a. An increase in the crude death rates despite the increasingly longer life expectancy and
b. Highest crude death rates observed in regions with the lowest overall levels of mortality.

The annual number of deaths in the world was rather stable, even slightly declining from 1960 to 1970, a decade in which the lowest level—51 million—of deaths per annum was recorded.

- From then on, the annual number of deaths has been rising; in 2010, it reached 64 million.
- The global crude death rate is expected to reach its lowest point in 2015 with about 8.0 deaths per 1,000 population per year, and to gradually increase thereafter, reaching 9.8 deaths per 1,000 population by 2050.
- In 1950–1955, 45% of deaths were of children under the age of 15, while deaths of persons aged 65 years or older represented only 22% of the total.
- As countries have made progress in their demographic transitions, the distribution of deaths has shifted towards older ages.
- In 2005–2010, over half (53 percent) of all deaths in the world were concentrated in the population aged 65 years or over, while the proportion of deaths among children (aged 0–14) had declined to 15 percent.

As more people are living longer almost everywhere in the world, the causes of death and disability are changing from infectious to non-communicable diseases, and in some countries, to injuries. The disability-adjusted life years (DALY) measure the burden of disease, injury and death in a given population. The main causes of DALY for the older population are almost everywhere non-communicable diseases such as heart disease, cancer and diabetes, in all development groups.

The distribution of DALYs by age group varies greatly across development regions and it is closely associated with the level of development.

In the more developed regions, 33% of persons aged 60 years or above in 2004 had Disability Adjusted life years.

By contrast, in the less developed regions, only around 12% were affected with DALY, and in the least developed countries, the proportion was even lower, of only 6 percent. At the world level, 85% of persons aged 60 years or above died from non-communicable diseases in 2008.

The percentage by region of persons aged 60 years or above who died from non-communicable diseases are

- More developed regions –92%;
- Less developed regions --83%; and
- Least developed countries–74%.

Furthermore, the increasing levels of exposure to risk factors such as tobacco use, unhealthy diet, physical inactivity, sedentary lifestyle and the harmful use of alcohol enhances the chances of non-communicable diseases (Palloni, 2013).

Communicable diseases are also responsible for death among the elderly but they vary according to region. In 2008, the proportions of old-age deaths due to communicable diseases were more:

Developed regions –5%, Less developed regions –13%, and Least developed countries–21%.

Deaths caused by communicable diseases are commonly associated with low income, poor diets and limited sanitary, health care infrastructure, low awareness, and less government intervention found in developing regions (WHO and U.S. NIA, 2011). Per capita health expenditure, both public and private, tends to increase with population aging. Population aging is associated with higher health expenditure due to the increase in the proportion of older persons, which have a higher prevalence of morbidity and demand for health care than younger adults. Again, because of scientific developments life expectancy has increased which leads to survival of all old age groups (60 and above) and this lengthens the period between the onset of significant morbidity or disability and death.

In the more developed regions with comprehensive social security systems, the majority of the health expenditure is covered by social insurance schemes. In the less developed regions with low levels of health care coverage, health expenditure is mainly financed with private spending by individuals.

Most people are not comfortable hearing that they are aging or growing old. This is simply because it tends to suggest advances in age, a decline of organ function, and loss of flexibility, hearing and vision decline, lessening of muscular strength, the flexibility of the skin and blood vessels, the appearance of wrinkles on the skin, etc. But it is a known fact that the process of maturation and aging in living organisms (human beings) are inevitable because the life cycle continues and is not reversible until death comes. Aging, should be conceived as a natural stage of development that comes when it should come. Aging comes about as a result of the cessation of cell division that takes place in human beings. Today, aging and anti-aging have become a global phenomenon and the endless struggle against becoming old, the refusal to accept changes in the body and the millions of money spent on cosmetic and plastic surgery all point to the fact that nobody wants to get old. However, aging just like death, is inevitable. No matter how you try to conceal it, it will definitely manifest with time. Osunde and Obiunu (2005) stated that aging goes beyond biological change. It includes physical, mental, social, and intellectual decline. All these negative indicators which show a decline in the functions of body organs due to aging make the adult person feel uncomfortable being associated with aging. This feeling affects the adult person emotionally, and psychologically. The aging population (the retired and the retrenched adult person) needs relevant adult education programs to enable them to cope and adjust to changing and challenging conditions of their lives and to enable them to feel they are still relevant in human society. Such adult education programs should be able to motivate the retired adult and make him feel that he can still learn new tricks to continue to exist comfortably in a human environment or society. Osunde and Obiunu (2005) stated that for elderly adults to say they are too old to learn makes them shun their responsibilities as active members of society.

The aging process can be viewed from three major perspectives; namely, biological aging, sociological aging and psychological aging.

Biological Aging: This is usually associated with decline in the regulation and proper functioning of the vital organs of the body. However, not all people experience decreased organ function in the same proportion. Some individuals have healthier hearts at age 80 than others do at age 60.

Sociological Aging: This is usually how a person relates with others in the society. In sociological aging, personal or attitude and interaction within the community are used to assess a person's maturation and aging.

As a person ages socially, he/she calculates his/her utterances, limits the use of vulgar language, prunes relationship to mature friends, changes his/her mode of dressing, and reduces nocturnal clubs. As a person ages socially, he/she tends to be guided by the norms of the society to which the person belongs. Psychological Aging: Jegede (2003) stated that the indices of psychological aging include feelings, motivation, memory, emotions, and experience and self-identify. For instance, people who had the intention of traveling abroad may decide to jettison the idea and contribute to the growth of their own economy. Psychological aging is heterogeneous and continuous as an individual passes through life. Cavanaught (1993) in Osunde and Obiunu (2005) divided aging into three viz, the primary aging, the secondary aging and the tertiary aging.

1.7. Gerontology

Gerontology is derived from two Greek words "geron" which means "old man" and "logos" which means "discourse" or "study." Gerontology is the study of the phenomenon of old age. It is the study of the social psychological and biological aspects of aging in an adult person. Gerontology is distinguished from geriatrics which is the branch of medicine that studies the diseases and care of the elderly person. The elderly adult deserves intensive medical at tension as he continues to grow old. The Oxford Mini reference Dictionary defines gerontology as the study of aging. The new Webster's Dictionary of English Language (1994) edition, defines gerontology as a study of the phenomenon of old age. Also, the encyclopedia on aging (volume 2, 297–298) defined gerontology as the scientific study of aging and older population. As the adult advances in age, the need for gerontology becomes necessary. Contemporary gerontology concerns itself with the aging population. Considering the above definitions and explanations, gerontology encompasses the following:

i. Studying the physical, mental and social changes in people (adults) as they age.
ii. Investigating the aging process itself (biogerontology).
iii. Investigating the interface of normal aging and age-related diseases (geroscience).
iv. Investigating the effects of our aging population on our society; including the fiscal effects of pensions, entitlements, life and health insurance and retirement planning.
v. Applying knowledge to policies and programs; including a macroscopic perspective i.e., (running a nursing home). These five scopes of gerontology can simply be referred to

as multidisciplinary. This is so because there are a number of sub-fields in it, as well as psychology and sociology. The field of gerontology is relatively a late developed field of study. This simply means it is a recent field of study. This made it possible for it to lack the structural and institutional support required. However, the huge increase in the elderly population in the postindustrial Western nations made gerontology become the most rapidly growing field of study. Currently, gerontology is a well-paid field for many all over the world.

1.8. The Myths and Stereotypes of Aging

Ageist stereotypes about seniors are unfortunately pervasive in our culture. In films, on television and even in the jokes we hear, misconceptions about aging and seniors are ever-present.

- Some of the Top Myths and Stereotypes of Aging Include

1. Myth: Aging Dulls Wits: While aging can create cognitive changes, older people may perform better in certain areas of intelligence and poorer in others. While seniors may have slower reaction times, "mental capabilities that depend most heavily on accumulated experience and knowledge, like settling disputes and enlarging one's vocabulary, clearly get better over time," writes Patricia Cohen in the New York Times.
2. Myth: Aging Erases Your Libido: Discussing the love and sex lives of seniors is largely taboo and has led to the stereotype that the elderly are sexless. This stereotype is harmful because it can cause seniors to have conflicted feelings or unnecessary guilt about their sexuality, while simultaneously causing younger people to hold misconceptions about aging and the elderly. As a State of Oregon document notes: "Research has found that sexual activity and enjoyment do not decrease with age. People with physical health, a sense of well-being and a willing partner are more likely to continue sexual relations. People who are bored with their partner, mentally or physically tired, afraid of failure or overindulge in food or drink are unlikely to engage in sexual activity. These reasons do not differ a great deal when considering whether or not a person will engage in sex at any age."
3. Myth: Aging Is Depressing: Contrary to the myth that aging is depressing, many studies find that seniors are among the happiest age groups. Happiness levels by age follow a U-shaped curve, with self-reported levels of happiness at their lowest at age 40, but then growing thereafter.
4. Myth: Aging Leads to Loneliness: Though social isolation can be a problem for seniors, especially for those who have limited mobility, most seniors are able to stay socially engaged. Activities with family and friends and visits at places such as the local senior center or a place of worship, also help seniors stay active and happy.
5. Myth: Aging Makes You Less Creative: Countless examples dispel the myth that aging makes you less creative. In fact, many artists actually find their calling or achieve mastery in their later years. A great example is the American artist "Grandma Moses," who held her first one-woman art show in 1940 when she was 80 and continued to

paint until she was 101.

6. Myth: Aging Makes You More Religious: Seniors certainly have a higher rate of religious attendance, but this is a generational phenomenon rather than an aging phenomenon. If you regularly attended church growing up, you're likely to continue to do so as you age. Today's seniors haven't become more religious with time. Instead, they grew up in a time when more people went to church, which is why seniors are the most religious age group.
7. Myth: Aging Makes You Unable to Adapt to New Situations: Older people are not only able to adapt to new situations, they are actually experts at adapting. By the time one has become a senior, they have had to adapt to innumerable changes and transitions in life. Seniors may be slower to change their opinions, but one of humanity's greatest traits, adaptability, is generally retained as we grow old.
8. Myth: Aging Makes You Unproductive: Though retired people may have left the workforce, they are hardly unproductive. They contribute countless hours to activities like helping with child-rearing and volunteering, which makes an enormous impact on society. In fact, a report by the Bureau of Labor Statistics indicates that 24% of senior citizens report engaging in volunteer work after retirement.

A Closer Look

Aging

Aging is a complex and multifaceted process that affects every individual differently. It involves a combination of biological, psychological, and social changes. Biologically, aging is marked by the gradual decline in the functionality of cells and organs. This decline is influenced by genetic factors, lifestyle choices, and environmental conditions. Common biological signs of aging include decreased bone density, reduced muscle mass, and the accumulation of cellular damage. This cellular damage, often caused by oxidative stress and the shortening of telomeres, contributes to the aging process and the onset of age-related diseases such as Alzheimer's, cardiovascular diseases, and arthritis.

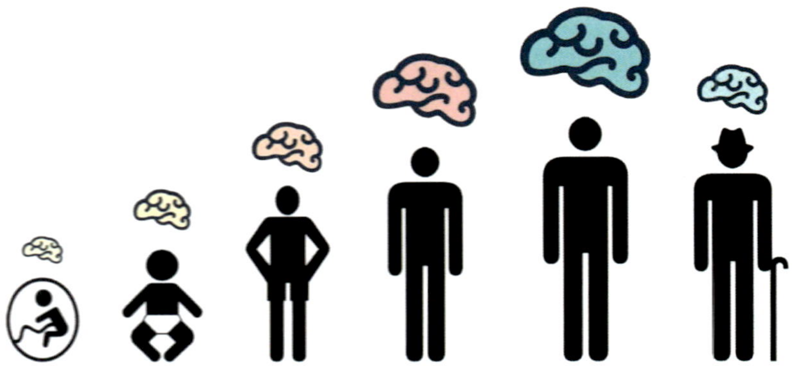

Psychologically, aging can impact cognitive functions, emotional well-being, and mental health. While some cognitive decline is a normal part of aging, significant impairments such as those seen in dementia are not. Emotional well-being in older adults can be influenced by factors such as social support, physical health, and a sense of purpose. Mental health issues, including depression and anxiety, are also prevalent among the elderly, often exacerbated by isolation and loss of loved ones.

Socially, aging affects individuals' roles and interactions within their communities and families. Retirement, changes in family dynamics, and shifts in social networks can all impact an older adult's sense of identity and belonging. Ageism, or discrimination based on age, can further marginalize elderly individuals, affecting their self-esteem and access to resources.

Advances in gerontology and geriatrics aim to improve the quality of life for older adults. These fields focus on understanding the aging process and developing interventions to mitigate its negative effects. Promoting healthy aging involves encouraging physical activity, balanced nutrition, mental stimulation, and social engagement. With an aging global population, fostering supportive environments and policies that address the unique needs of older adults is increasingly important.

Understanding and addressing the diverse aspects of aging, we can enhance the well-being and dignity of older adults, ensuring that they can lead fulfilling and productive lives in their later years.

Summary

- This chapter provides a comprehensive overview of the study of aging, exploring its biological, psychological, and sociological aspects. The field of gerontology has become increasingly important as the global population ages, presenting both challenges and opportunities for individuals and society as a whole.
- One of the key themes in gerontology is the concept of aging as a multidimensional process. It is not just about the physical changes that occur as we age, but also about the psychological and social changes that accompany the aging process. Understanding these dimensions of aging is crucial for developing effective strategies to promote healthy aging and enhance the quality of life for older adults.
- Another important topic in gerontology is the study of age-related changes in health and functioning. Gerontologists examine the factors that contribute to these changes, such as genetics, lifestyle choices, and environmental factors. They also study the impact of these changes on individuals' well-being and independence, and develop interventions to help older adults maintain their health and independence for as long as possible.
- Gerontology also explores the social aspects of aging, including the role of social relationships, support networks, and societal attitudes toward aging. It examines how these factors influence the experiences of older adults and how they can be improved to enhance the quality of life for older adults.

References

1. Altman, J. (1962). Are new neurons formed in the brains of adult mammals? *Science, 135*(3509), 1127–1128. https://doi.org/10.1126/science.135.3509.1127.
2. Arenaza-Urquijo, E. M., & Vemuri, P. (2018). Resistance vs resilience to Alzheimer disease: Clarifying terminology for preclinical studies. *Neurology, 90*(15), 695–703. https://doi.org/10.1212/WNL.0000000000005303.
3. Bäckman, L., Lindenberger, U., Li, S. -C., & Nyberg, L. (2010). Linking cognitive aging to alterations in dopamine neurotransmitter functioning: Recent data and future avenues. *Neuroscience & Biobehavioral Reviews, 34*(5), 670–677. https://doi.org/10.1016/j.neubiorev.2009.12.008.
4. Bigio, E. H., Hynan, L. S., Sontag, E., Satumtira, S., & White, C. L. (2002). Synapse loss is greater in presenile than senile onset Alzheimer disease: Implications for the cognitive reserve hypothesis. *Neuropathology and Applied Neurobiology, 28*(3), 218–227. https://doi.org/10.1046/j.1365-2990.2002.00378.x.
5. Blennow, K., Hampel, H., Weiner, M., & Zetterberg, H. (2010). Cerebrospinal fluid and plasma biomarkers in Alzheimer disease. *Nature Reviews Neurology, 6*(3), 131–144. https://doi.org/10.1038/nrneurol.2010.4.
6. Blennow, K., Vanmechelen, E., & Hampel, H. (2001). CSF total tau, Aβ42 and phosphorylated tauprotein as biomarkers for Alzheimer's disease. *Molecular Neurobiology, 24*(1–3), 87–97. https://doi.org/10.1385/MN:24:1-3:087.

7. Braak, H., & Braak, E. (1995). Staging of Alzheimer's disease-related neurofibrillary changes. *Neurobiology of Aging, 16*(3), 271–278. https://doi.org/10.1016/0197-4580(95)00021-6.

8. Braak, H., & Braak, E. (1996). Evolution of the neuropathology of Alzheimer's disease. *Acta Neurologica Scandinavica, 94*(165), 3–12. https://doi.org/10.1111/j.1600-0404.1996.tb05866.x.

9. Brayne, C., Ince, P. G., Keage, H. A., McKeith, L. G., Matthews, F. E., Polvikoski, T., & Sulkava, R. (2010). Education, the brain and dementia: Neuroprotection or compensation? *Brain, 133*(8), 2210–2226. https://doi.org/10.1093/brain/awq185.

10. Bruandet, A., Richard, F., Bombois, S., Maurage, C. A., Masse, I., Amouyel, P., & Pasquier, F. (2008). Cognitive decline and survival in Alzheimer's disease according to education level. *Dementia and Geriatric Cognitive Disorders, 25*(1), 74–80. https://doi.org/10.1159/000111128.

11. Buerger, K., Ewers, M., Pirttila, T., Zinkowski, R., Alafuzoff, I., Teipel, S. J., & Hampel, H. (2006). CSF phosphorylated tau protein correlates with neocortical neurofibrillary pathology in Alzheimer's disease. *Brain, 129*(11), 3035–3041. https://doi.org/10.1093/brain/awl269.

12. Cabeza, R. (2002). Hemispheric asymmetry reduction in older adults: The HAROLD model. *Psychology and Aging, 17*(1), 85–100. https://doi.org/10.1037/0882-7974.17.1.85.

13. Cabeza, R., Albert, M., Belleville, S., Craik, F., Duarte, A., Grady, C., & Rugg, M. D. (2018). Cognitive neuroscience of healthy aging: Maintenance, reserve, and compensation. *Nature Reviews Neuroscience, 19*(11), 701–710. https://doi.org/10.1038/s41583-018-0068-2.

14. Cabeza, R., Anderson, N. D., Locantore, J. K., & McIntosh, A. R. (2002). Aging gracefully: Compensatory brain activity in high-performing older adults. *Neuroimage, 17*(3), 1394–1402. https://doi.org/10.1006/nimg.2002.1280.

15. Cappa, S. F. (2017). Cognitive reserve and successful aging. *Journal of Gerontology and Geriatrics, 65*(6), 296–298. https://doi.org/10.11138/jger.2017.65.6.296.

16. Carapelle, E., Serra, L., Modoni, S., Falcone, M., Caltagirone, C., Bozzali, M., & Avolio, C. (2017). How the cognitive reserve interacts with β-amyloid deposition in mitigating FDG metabolism: An observational study. *Medicine, 96*(9), e5876. https://doi.org/10.1097/MD.0000000000005876.

17. Clifford Jr., R. J. (2014). PART and SNAP. *Acta Neuropathologica, 128*(6), 773–776. https://doi.org/10.1007/s00401-014-1322-3.

18. Clifford, R. J., Jr., Bennett, D. A., Blennow, K., Carrillo, M. C., Dunn, B., Haeberlein, S. B., & Phelps, C. H. (2018). NIA-AA research framework: Toward a biological definition of Alzheimer's disease. *Alzheimer's & Dementia, 14*(4), 535–562. https://doi.org/10.1016/j.jalz.2018.02.018.

19. Cobb, J. L., Wolf, P. A., Au, R., White, R., & D'Agostino, R. B. (1995). The effect of education on the incidence of dementia and Alzheimer's disease in the Framingham Study. *Neurology, 45*(9), 1707–1712. https://doi.org/10.1212/WNL.45.9.1707.

20. Crystal, H., Dickson, D., Fuld, P., Masur, D., Scott, R., Mehler, M., & Wolfson, L. (1988). Clinico-pathologic studies in dementia: Nondemented subjects with pathologically confirmed Alzheimer's disease. *Neurology, 38*(11), 1682. https://doi.org/10.1212/WNL.38.11.1682.

21. Davies, C. A., Mann, D. M. A., Sumpter, P. Q., & Yates, P. O. (1987). A quantitative morphometric analysis of the neuronal and synaptic content of the frontal and temporal cortex in patients

with Alzheimer's disease. *Journal of Neurological Sciences, 78*(2), 151–164. https://doi.org/10.1016/0022-510X(87)90057-4.

22. Davis, D. G., Schmitt, F. A., Wekstein, D. R., & Markesbery, W. R. (1999). Alzheimer neuropathologic alterations in aged cognitively normal subjects. *Journal of Neuropathology & Experimental Neurology, 58*(4), 376–388. https://doi.org/10.1097/00005072-199904000-00009.

23. DeKosky, S. T., & Scheff, S. W. (1990). Synapse loss in frontal cortex biopsies in Alzheimer's disease: Correlation with cognitive severity. *Annals of Neurology, 27*(5), 457–464. https://doi.org/10.1002/ana.410270502.

24. Dowling, N. M., Johnson, S. C., Gleason, C. E., & Jagust, W. J. (2015). Alzheimer's Disease Neuroimaging Initiative. The mediational effects of FDG hypometabolism on the association between cerebrospinal fluid biomarkers and neurocognitive function. *NeuroImage, 105*, 357–368. https://doi.org/10.1016/j.neuroimage.2014.10.042.

25. Dubois, B., Feldman, H. H., Jacova, C., Cummings, J. L., Dekosky, S. T., Barberger-Gateau, P., & Scheltens, P. (2010). Revising the definition of Alzheimer's disease: A new lexicon. *Lancet Neurology, 9*(11), 1118–1127. https://doi.org/10.1016/S1474-4422(10)70223-4.

26. Edison, P., Archer, H. A., Hinz, R., Hammers, A., Pavese, N., Tai, Y. F., Hotton, G., Cutler, D., Fox, N. C., Kennedy, A., & et al. (2007). Amyloid, hypometabolism, and cognition in Alzheimer disease: An [11C]PIB and [18F]FDG PET study. *Neurology, 68*(7), 501–508. https://doi.org/10.1212/01.wnl.0000244749.20056.7e.

27. Evert, J., Lawler, E., Bogan, H., & Perls, T. T. (2003). Morbidity profiles of centenarians: Survivors, delayers, and escapers. *Psychological Science, 58A*(3), 232–237. https://doi.org/10.1093/geront/58.3.232.

28. Ewers, M., Insel, P. S., Stern, Y., & Weiner, M. W. (2013). Cognitive reserve associated with FDG-PET in preclinical Alzheimer disease. *Neurology, 80*(12), 1194–1201. https://doi.org/10.1212/WNL.0b013e31828970c8.

29. Fagan, A. M., Roe, C. M., Xiong, C., Mintun, M. A., Morris, J. C., & Holtzman, D. M. (2007). Cerebrospinal fluid tau/beta-amyloid(42) ratio as a prediction of cognitive decline in nondemented older adults. *Archives of Neurology, 64*(3), 343–349. https://doi.org/10.1001/archneur.64.3.343.

30. Fotenos, A. F., Mintun, M. A., Snyder, A. Z., Morris, J. C., & Buckner, R. L. (2008). Brain volume decline in aging: Evidence for a relation between socioeconomic status, preclinical Alzheimer disease, and reserve. *Archives of Neurology, 65*(1), 113–120. https://doi.org/10.1001/archneurol.2007.27.

31. Fratiglioni, L., Grut, M., Forsell, Y., Viitanen, M., Grafström, M., Holmén, K., Ericsson, K., Bäckman, L., Ahlbom, A., & Winblad, B. (1991). Prevalence of Alzheimer's disease and other dementias in an elderly urban population: Relationship with age, sex, and education. *Neurology, 41*(12), 1886–1892. https://doi.org/10.1212/WNL.41.12.1886.

32. Grady, C. L., Springer, M. V., Hongwanishkul, D., McIntosh, A. R., & Winocur, G. (2006). Age-related changes in brain activity across the adult lifespan. *Journal of Cognitive Neuroscience, 18*(2), 227–241. https://doi.org/10.1162/089892906775783705.

33. Grady, C., McIntosh, A. R., Horwitz, B., Maisog, J., Ungerleider, L. G., Mentis, M. J., Pietrini, P., Schapiro, M. B., & Haxby, J. V. (1995). Age-related reductions in human recognition memory due to impaired encoding. *Science, 269*(5221), 218–221. https://doi.org/10.1126/science.7618082.

34. Hampel, H., Vassar, R., De Strooper, B., Hardy, J., Willem, M., Singh, N., & Nisticò, R. (2020). The β-secretase BACE1 in Alzheimer's disease. *Biological Psychiatry, 89*(9), 745–756. https://doi.org/10.1016/j.biopsych.2020.01.002.

35. Hansson, O., Zetterberg, H., Buchhave, P., Londos, E., Blennow, K., & Minthon, L. (2006). Association between CSF biomarkers and incipient Alzheimer's disease in patients with mild cognitive impairment: A follow-up study. *Lancet Neurology, 5*(3), 228–234. https://doi.org/10.1016/S1474-4422(06)70355-6.

36. Herholz, K. (2003). PET studies in dementia. *Annals of Nuclear Medicine, 17*(2), 79–89. https://doi.org/10.1007/BF02988425.

37. Herholz, K., Salmon, E., Perani, D., Baron, J. C., Holthoff, V., Frölich, L., Schönknecht, P., Ito, K., Mielke, R., Kalbe, E., & et al. (2002). Discrimination between Alzheimer dementia and controls by automated analysis of multicenter FDG PET. *NeuroImage, 17*(1), 302–316. https://doi.org/10.1006/nimg.2002.1162.

38. Herholz, S. C., Herholz, R. S., & Herholz, K. (2013). Non-pharmacological interventions and neuroplasticity in early stage Alzheimer's disease. *Expert Review of Neurotherapeutics, 13*(11), 1235–1245. https://doi.org/10.1586/14737175.2013.845086.

39. Ingber, A. P., Hassenstab, J., Fagan, A. M., Benzinger, T. L., Grant, E. A., Holtzman, D. M., Morris, J. C., & Roe, C. M. (2016). Cerebrospinal fluid biomarkers and reserve variables as predictors of future "non-cognitive" outcomes of Alzheimer's disease. *Journal of Alzheimer's Disease, 52*(4), 1055–1064. https://doi.org/10.3233/JAD-160011.

40. Insua, D., Suarez, M. L., Santamarina, G., Sarasa, M., & Pesini, P. (2010). Dogs with canine counterpart of Alzheimer's disease lose noradrenergic neurons. *Neurobiology of Aging, 31*(4), 625–635. https://doi.org/10.1016/j.neurobiolaging.2008.05.018.

41. Jack, C. R., Knopman, D. S., Jagust, W. J., Shaw, L. M., Aisen, P. S., Weiner, M. W., Petersen, R. C., & Trojanowski, J. Q. (2010). Hypothetical model of dynamic biomarkers of the Alzheimer's pathological cascade. *Lancet Neurology, 9*(1), 119–128. https://doi.org/10.1016/S1474-4422(09)70299-6.

42. Johnson, K. A., Minoshima, S., Bohnen, N. I., Donohoe, K. J., Foster, N. L., Herscovitch, P., Karlawish, J. H., Rowe, C. C., Hedrick, S., Pappas, V., & et al. (2013). Update on appropriate use criteria for amyloid PET imaging: Dementia experts, mild cognitive impairment, and education. *Journal of Nuclear Medicine, 54*(7), 1011–1013. https://doi.org/10.2967/jnumed.112.112998.

43. Katzman, R., Terry, R., DeTeresa, R., Brown, T., Davies, P., Fuld, P., & Peck, A. (1988). Clinical, pathological, and neurochemical changes in dementia: A subgroup with preserved mental status and numerous neocortical plaques. *Annals of Neurology, 23*(2), 138–144. https://doi.org/10.1002/ana.410230206.

44. Kesler, S. R., Adams, H. F., Blasey, C. M., & Bigler, E. D. (2003). Premorbid intellectual functioning, education, and brain size in traumatic brain injury: An investigation of the cognitive reserve hypothesis. *Applied Neuropsychology, 10*(3), 153–162. https://doi.org/10.1207/S15324826AN1003_03.

45. Knopman, D. S., Parisi, J. E., Salviati, A., Floriach-Robert, M., Boeve, B. F., Ivnik, R. J., & McDonald, W. C. (2003). Neuropathology of cognitively normal elderly. *Journal of Neuropathology & Experimental Neurology, 62*(11), 1087–1095. https://doi.org/10.1093/jnen/62.11.1087.

46. Koberskaya, N. N., & Tabeeva, G. R. (2019). The modern concept of cognitive reserve. *Neurology, Neuropsychiatry, Psychosomatics, 11*(4), 96–102. https://doi.org/10.14412/2074-2711-2019-4-96-102.

47. Lazarov, O., & Marr, R. (2013). Of mice and men: Neurogenesis, cognition and Alzheimer's disease. *Frontiers in Aging Neuroscience, 5*, 43. https://doi.org/10.3389/fnagi.2013.00043.

48. Lyness, S. A., Zarow, C., & Chui, H. C. (2003). Neuron loss in key cholinergic and aminergic nuclei in Alzheimer disease: A meta-analysis. *Neurobiology of Aging, 24*(1), 1–23. https://doi.org/10.1016/s0197-4580(02)00057-x.

49. Meng, X., & D'arcy, C. (2012). Education and dementia in the context of the cognitive reserve hypothesis: A systematic review with meta-analyses and qualitative analyses. *PloS ONE, 7*(6), e38268. https://doi.org/10.1371/journal.pone.0038268.

50. Mortimer, J. A., Borenstein, A. R., Gosche, K. M., & Snowdon, D. A. (2005). Very early detection of Alzheimer neuropathology and the role of brain reserve in modifying its clinical expression. *Journal of Geriatric Psychiatry and Neurology, 18*(4), 218–223. https://doi.org/10.1177/0891988705281860.

51. Mortimer, J. A., Snowdon, D. A., & Markesbery, W. R. (2003). Head circumference, education and risk of dementia: Findings from the Nun Study. Journal of Clinical and Experimental Neuropsychology, 25(5), 671–679. https://doi.org/10.1076/jcen.25.5.671.14584.

52. Nelson, P. T., Head, E., Schmitt, F. A., Davis, P. R., Neltner, J. H., Jicha, G. A., Abner, E. L., Smith, C. D., Van Eldik, L. J., Kryscio, R. J., & et al. (2011). Alzheimer's disease is not "brain aging": Neuropathological, genetic, and epidemiological human studies. Acta Neuropathologica, 121(5), 571–587. https://doi.org/10.1007/s00401-011-0826-y.

53. Nelson, P. T., Schmitt, F. A., Lin, Y., Abner, E. L., Jicha, G. A., Patel, E., & Sonnen, J. A. (2011). Hippocampal sclerosis in advanced age: Clinical and pathological features. Brain, 134(5), 1506–1518. https://doi.org/10.1093/brain/awr053.

54. Ott, A., Van Rossum, C. T., Van Harskamp, F., Van De Mheen, H., Hofman, A., & Breteler, M. M. B. (1999). Education and the incidence of dementia in a large population-based study: The Rotterdam Study. Neurology, 52(3), 663–666. https://doi.org/10.1212/wnl.52.3.663.

55. Otto, M., Wiltfang, J., Tumani, H., Zerr, I., Lantsch, M., Kornhuber, J., & Poser, S. (1997). Elevated levels of tau-protein in cerebrospinal fluid of patients with Creutzfeldt–Jakob disease. Neuroscience Letters, 225(3), 210–212. https://doi.org/10.1016/s0304-3940(97)00197-9.

56. Pascual-Leone, A., Freitas, C., Oberman, L., Horvath, J. C., Halko, M., Eldaief, M., & Vahabzadeh-Hagh, A. M. (2011). Characterizing brain cortical plasticity and network dynamics across the age-span in health and disease with TMS-EEG and TMS-fMRI. Brain Topography, 24(3), 302–315. https://doi.org/10.1007/s10548-011-0196-8.

57. Perls, T. T. (2006). The different paths to 100. American Journal of Clinical Nutrition, 83(2), 484S–487S. https://doi.org/10.1093/ajcn/83.2.484S.

58. Petrie, E. C., Cross, D. J., Galasko, D., Schellenberg, G. D., Raskind, M. A., Peskind, E. R., & Minoshima, S. (2009). Preclinical evidence of Alzheimer changes: Convergent cerebrospinal

fluid biomarker and fluorodeoxyglucose positron emission tomography findings. Archives of Neurology, 66(5), 632–637. https://doi.org/10.1001/archneurol.2009.46.

59. Raz, N., Lindenberger, U., Rodrigue, K. M., Kennedy, K. M., Head, D., Williamson, A., & Acker, J. D. (2015). Regional brain changes in aging healthy adults: General trends, individual differences and modifiers. Cerebral Cortex, 15(11), 1676–1689. https://doi.org/10.1093/cercor/bhi044.

60. Rodrigue, K. M., Kennedy, K. M., Devous, M. D., Sr., Rieck, J. R., Hebrank, A. C., Diaz-Arrastia, R., & Park, D. C. (2012). β-Amyloid burden in healthy aging: Regional distribution and cognitive consequences. Neurology, 78(6), 387–395. https://doi.org/10.1212/WNL.0b013e318245d295.

61. Satz, P. (1993). Brain reserve capacity on symptom onset after brain injury: A formulation and review of evidence for threshold theory. Neuropsychology, 7(3), 273–295. https://doi.org/10.1037/h0083588.

62. Schmand, B., Smit, J. H., Geerlings, M. I., & Lindeboom, J. (1997). The effects of intelligence and education on the development of dementia. A test of the brain reserve hypothesis. Psychological Medicine, 27(6), 1337–1344. https://doi.org/10.1017/S0033291797005461.

63. Schoonenboom, N. S. M., Pijnenburg, Y. A. L., Mulder, C., Rosso, S. M., Van Elk, E. J., Van Kamp, G. J., & Scheltens, P. (2004). Amyloid β (1–42) and phosphorylated tau in CSF as markers for early-onset Alzheimer disease. Neurology, 62(10), 1580–1584. https://doi.org/10.1212/01.WNL.0000123230.32136.9A.

64. Serra, L., Cercignani, M., Petrosini, L., Basile, B., Perri, R., Fadda, L., Spano, B., Marra, C., Giubilei, F., Carlesimo, G. A., & et al. (2011). Neuroanatomical correlates of cognitive reserve in Alzheimer disease. Rejuvenation Research, 14(2), 143–151. https://doi.org/10.1089/rej.2010.1093.

65. Serrano-Pozo, A., Qian, J., Monsell, S. E., Blacker, D., Gómez-Isla, T., Betensky, R. A., Growdon, J. H., Johnson, K. A., Frosch, M. P., Sperling, R. A., & et al. (2014). Mild to moderate Alzheimer dementia with insufficient neuropathological changes. Annals of Neurology, 75(4), 597–601. https://doi.org/10.1002/ana.24125.

66. Soldan, A., Pettigrew, C., & Albert, M. (2018). Evaluating cognitive reserve through the prism of preclinical Alzheimer disease. Psychiatric Clinics, 41(1), 65–77. https://doi.org/10.1016/j.psc.2017.10.011.

67. Soldan, A., Pettigrew, C., & Albert, M. (2020). Cognitive reserve from the perspective of preclinical Alzheimer disease: 2020 update. Clinics in Geriatric Medicine, 36(2), 247–263. https://doi.org/10.1016/j.cger.2020.01.009.

68. Stern, Y. (2002). What is cognitive reserve? Theory and research application of the reserve concept. Journal of the International Neuropsychological Society, 8(3), 448–460. https://doi.org/10.1017/S1355617702813248.

69. Stern, Y. (2006). Cognitive reserve and Alzheimer disease. Alzheimer Disease & Associated Disorders, 20(2), S69–S74. https://doi.org/10.1097/01.wad.0000213815.20177.19.

70. Stern, Y. (2009). Cognitive reserve. Neuropsychologia, 47(10), 2015–2028. https://doi.org/10.1016/j.neuropsychologia.2009.03.004.

71. Stern, Y. (2012). Cognitive reserve in ageing and Alzheimer's disease. The Lancet Neurology, 11(11), 1006–1012. https://doi.org/10.1016/S1474-4422(12)70191-6.

72. Stern, Y., Alexander, G. E., Prohovnik, I., & Mayeux, R. (1992). Inverse relationship between education and parietotemporal perfusion deficit in Alzheimer's disease. Annals of Neurology, 32(3), 371–375. https://doi.org/10.1002/ana.410320308.

73. Terry, R. D., Masliah, E., Salmon, D. P., Butters, N., DeTeresa, R., Hill, R., & Katzman, R. (1991). Physical basis of cognitive alterations in Alzheimer's disease: Synapse loss is the major correlate of cognitive impairment. *Annals of Neurology, 30*(4), 572–580.

74. Tripathi, M., Tripathi, M., Damle, N., Kushwaha, S., Jaimini, A., D'Souza, M. M., Sharma, R., Saw, S., & Mondal, A. (2014). Differential diagnosis of neurodegenerative dementias using metabolic phenotypes on F-18 FDG PET/CT. *Neuroradiology Journal, 27*(1), 13–21.

75. Tripathi, R. K., & Tiwari, S. C. (2013). Cognitive functioning of community dwelling urban older adults with reference to socio-demographic variables. *Indian Journal of Clinical Psychology, 40*(1), 92–102.

76. van Harten, A. C., Kester, M. I., Visser, P. J., Blankenstein, M. A., Pijnenburg, Y. A., van der Flier, W. M., & Scheltens, P. (2011). Tau and P-tau as CSF biomarkers in dementia: A meta-analysis. *Clinical Chemistry and Laboratory Medicine, 49*(3), 353–366.

77. Visser, P. J., Verhey, F., Knol, D. L., Scheltens, P., Wahlund, L. O., Freund-Levi, Y., & Bürger, K. (2009). Prevalence and prognostic value of CSF markers of Alzheimer's disease pathology in patients with subjective cognitive impairment or mild cognitive impairment in the DESCRIPA study: A prospective cohort study. *The Lancet Neurology, 8*(7), 619–627.

78. Xu, W., Yu, J. T., Tan, M. S., & Tan, L. (2015). Cognitive reserve and Alzheimer's disease. *Molecular Neurobiology, 51*(1), 187–208.

Chapter 2

EVOLUTIONARY BIOLOGY OF AGING

Contents

Introduction

Significant progress has been made in evolutionary research on senescence over the last two decades. The field has evolved from early numerical genetic studies to the integration of advanced molecular techniques, leading to a more comprehensive understanding of aging processes.

Early studies by Edney & Gill (1968), Luckinbill et al. (1984), and Rose & Charlesworth (1980) laid the foundation for investigating senescence concepts. Evolutionary scientists now use advanced molecular techniques to study aging, integrating natural molecular methodologies to gain a cohesive understanding of the process. Molecular science senescence recognizes biological evolution as a significant factor in understanding senescence, more so than other fields of natural ecology.

Debates among scholars have centered on the hypothesis of antagonistic pleiotropy by George Williams (Williams, 1957) and Tom Kirkwood's theory of recyclable soma (Kirkwood, 1977). The study of antagonistic pleiotropy has been furthered by researchers like Campisi (2003).

Efforts have been dedicated to examining traditional evolutionary hypotheses about senescence, such as those proposed by Hughes & Charlesworth (1994), Promislow et al. (1996), and Rose & Charlesworth (1980). The field is transitioning beyond testing pre-existing hypotheses, but its future trajectory remains uncertain.

Evolutionary research on aging is distinguished from other fields by its focus on ultimate questions, such as the evolutionary reasons for aging and the selective pressures driving the evolution of genes influencing lifespan. In contrast, non-evolutionary scientists tend to focus on proximate questions, such as the mechanisms and genetic factors underlying age-related processes.

Recent years have seen a convergence between evolutionary and non-evolutionary biology, with evolutionary theory inspiring molecular geneticists to investigate individual genes involved in aging (Walker et al., 2000; Campisi, 2003). Evolutionary scientists have also adopted methodologies based on contemporary molecular biology (Tatar et al., 2001; Pletcher et al., 2002), further bridging the gap between these disciplines.

Orientation and Directional Terms:

Term	Definition	Illustration
Evolutionary Biology	The study of the evolutionary processes that have shaped life on Earth, including aging.	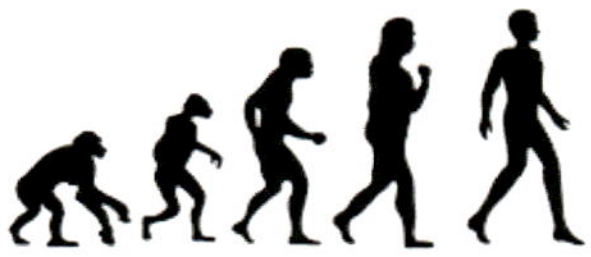
Aging	The process of becoming older, characterized by a progressive decline in physiological function.	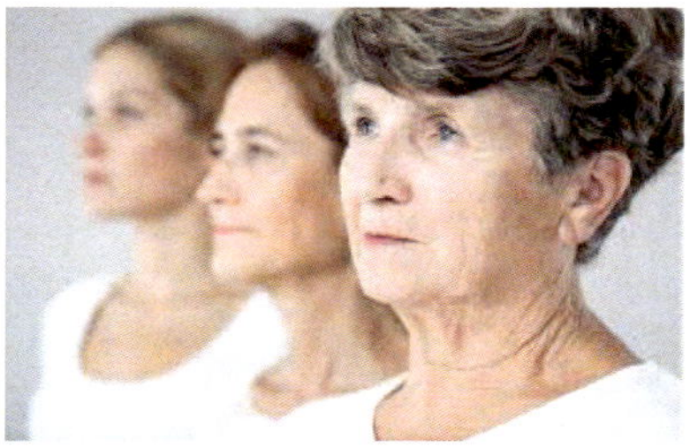
Genetics of Aging	Study of how genetic factors contribute to the aging process and longevity.	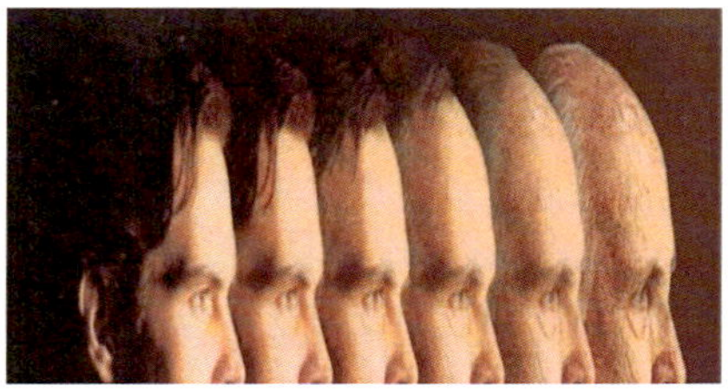
Gene-environment	Interaction between genetic predispositions and environmental factors.	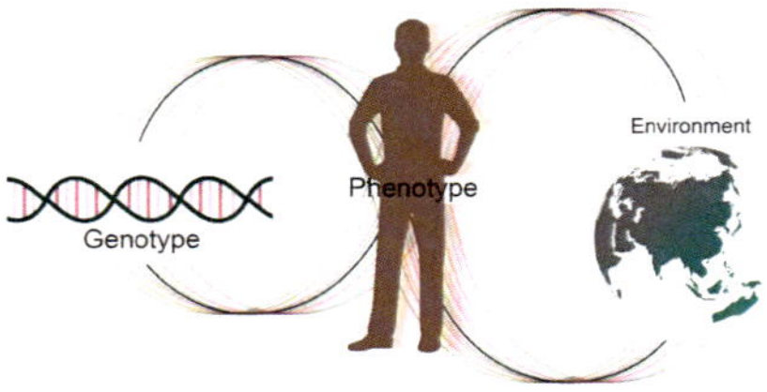
Molecular geneticists	Scientists who study the genetic basis of biological processes at the molecular level.	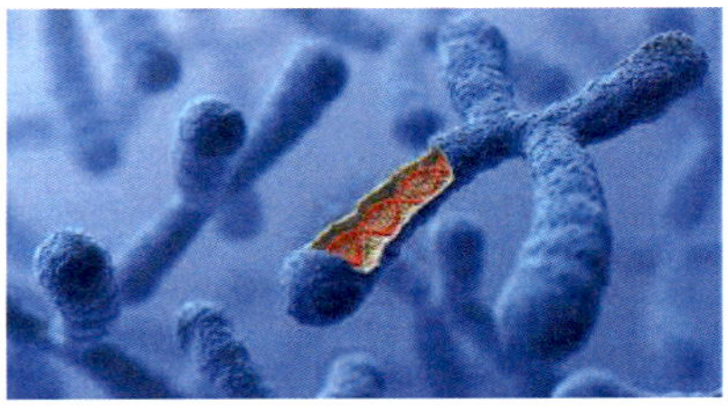

2.1. History

Evolutionary biologists at the present time make use of contemporary research methodologies. On the other hand, the most significant evolutionary advancements in the field of research on aging can be traced back to approximately fifty years ago. The idea that the benefits of getting older lay in the fact that it contributed to the continuation and expansion of the species was the prevalent one up until the middle of the 1900s. It was Weismann in 1891. Since the 1940s, there has been a shift away from the argument that was presented earlier, which is now regarded as being fallacious. Building on the earlier works of Fisher (1930) or Haldane (1941), Medawar (1946) proposed that aging is an unavoidable consequence of a decline in the capacity for selection with increasing age. This idea was based on the fact that this decline occurs with increasing age. Let us consider a hypothetical situation in which there is an unusual change in the germ line that results in a shorter lifespan at a particular age. There is a consistent decrease in the likelihood of an organism surviving to reproduce at any given age if it experiences a decrease in survival occurring prior to reaching maturity. It is possible that a mutation that causes deleterious effects would be subjected to significant negative selection, and it would eventually be eradicated from the population.

On the other hand, a gene mutation that reduces the likelihood of survival at a later stage of life, when the majority of individuals within the population have already passed away, would be subject to weak selective pressure and could potentially proliferate through stochastic genetic drift. There is a consistent elimination of early-acting harmful mutations throughout the course of evolution by the selective process, while late-acting mutations gradually accumulate. According to the hypothesis that Medawar has developed concerning the accumulation of change, it is impossible to avoid the fact that every individual carries a significant burden of harmful mutations that become apparent later in life and have been handed down to our group from our ancestors. As people get older, they are more likely to experience the effects of genetic mutations, which can lead to a decrease in their ability to survive physically and to reproduce.

After ten years had passed, George Williams put forward a theory that came to be known as antagonistic pleiotropy. According to Williams (1957), this theory proposes that senescence may take place if late-acting harmful mutations are favored by choosing due to the early-acting beneficial impacts that they have. It is believed that the phenomenon of senescence is the result of a tradeoff between the benefits that the individual experiences early in life and the drawbacks that they experience later in life. The subsequent theory of recyclable soma that Tom Kirkwood developed (Kirkwood, 1977) was an expansion of this concept that he had previously developed. It has been fifty years since the works of Medawar and Williams, and biologists who study evolution are still working hard to determine which of the two theories presented above provides the best explanation for senescence (Charlesworth & Hughes, 1996; Charlesworth, 2001; Hughes et al., 2002; Partridge & Gems, 2002a; Snoke & Promislow, 2003). In recent times, molecular historians have demonstrated a growing inclination towards these concepts, specifically focusing on identifying mutations that exhibit antagonistic pleiotropy (Campisi, 2003; Walker et al., 2000).

The contemporary emphasis in the field of biological evolution on aging includes three primary domains:

1. The mission of the ongoing research endeavors is to outline the hereditary framework of the aging process; the

inquiry pertains to determining an explanation for the genetic variability that is associated with senescence. Additionally, it seeks to determine whether or not allelic variations in "growing older genes" that have been discovered to extend lifespan in laboratory settings correlate with longevity in naturally occurring isolates. In addition, the purpose of the investigation is to determine the influence that aging has on the genes, gender, and the external environment in which they take place. (Nuzhdin et al., 1997; Fry et al.,1998, Leips and Mackay in 2000).

2. An additional body of research has concentrated on the configuration of mortality patterns, intending to elucidate the factors that contribute to the exponential increase in mortality rates that occurred with increasing age. According to Abrams and Ludwig (1995) and Charlesworth (2001), there is a topic of interest that pertains to the phenomenon of mortality rates decreasing in later life situations in certain instances. (For additional information, see Finch and Pike (1996), Mueller and Rose (1996), and Vaupel et al. (1998). Service (2000), Linnen et al. (2001), and Mueller et al. (2003).
3. Recently, evolutionary scientists have demonstrated a growing interest in investigating the potential significance of the hormonal system in the process of shaping a person's "life the past strategy." This approach takes into account a wide range of characteristics, including the ages at which maturation occurs, the rate of growth, the dimensions of the body, fertility, and the length of life. (Tatar et al., 2003).
4. A number of different sources contained information regarding the progression of aging, more specifically with regard to the three subjects in question. Subsequently, rather than reiterating topics that have been extensively researched, the subsequent chapter will investigate five domains that have received relatively less attention although they have the potential to advance natural investigations on aging. Indeed, they include.

i. One of the most important areas of research concern in the field of biology is the investigation of molecular evolution and gene networks.
ii. the point of intersection between physiology and population;
iii. the relationship between parasites and immunity is an important area of investigation in the field of medicine;
iv. the topics of interest are sexual disputes and gender selection.
v. inherited variation in human populations is the fifth factor.

2.2. Genetics of Senescence

Over the course of nearly twenty years, researchers in the fields of biological evolution and molecular biology who were investigating the biology of aging appeared to be concentrating on different issues, with very little interaction between the two groups of researchers involved. This communication gap may be analogous to the divide that exists between researchers who study cell death and those who investigate aging in animal models. Recently, evolutionary biologists have shifted their attitudes toward adopting contemporary molecular methods, while geneticists have begun to explore and evaluate evolutionary hypotheses. Both of these developments have occurred in recent years. The first-ever comprehensive microarray analysis of gene expression patterns associated with senescence across the entire genome of a fly was the result of a collaborative effort between researchers in the fields of natural and molecular biology. According to Pletcher et al. (2002) through the sequencing of complete genomes, it has become much simpler to identify genes that are associated with the aging process in a wide variety of taxonomically distinct organisms. Because of this, it has become possible to identify mechanisms of aging that have profound evolutionary roots. To determine whether the genetic factors associated with aging were species-specific, that is, governed by "private" processes, or whether they remained constant throughout the course of evolutionary history, George Martin proposed a hypothesis. referred to as "public" mechanisms (Martin, 1997). Sirtuins and insulin signaling are two gene pathways that have been identified as potential mechanisms linked to getting older. These pathways are believed to be widely recognized (Tissenbaum & Guarente, 2001; Partridge & Gems, 2002). Both of these gene pathways have been identified as potential mechanisms.

The current research on the molecular biology of aging is primarily focused on elucidating the roles that genes play in the process. There has been prior identification of these gene pathways, as well as the discovery of new genes. Events of significant importance are taking place at this particular location. The inquiry is concerned with the position of evolutionary biology within the framework of this molecular endeavor. Within the context of the discourse, the introductory section focused on the variation in the intensity of selection as a function of age. Identifying how selection intensity operates not only on demographic characteristics but also on the particular genes that influence those demographic characteristics is a significant challenge that needs to be overcome. If one can accomplish this, then the development of an evolutionary genetic framework for aging that makes it easier to predict genes that are associated with aging might be possible. Using either of two different methods, it is possible to improve the selection evaluation process at each gene and genome level. A framework for life span assessments is incorporated into the first approach, which involves the integration of molecular evolutionary investigations of DNA sequences or genomes. The second method involves analyzing the networks of gene-protein interactions as well as between proteins.

2.2.1. Molecular Evolution and Aging

The field of molecular biology is a scientific discipline that investigates the mechanisms of evolution by analyzing variations in the sequences of amino acids and genetic material both within and between different species. There have been a great number of researchers working within this field who have focused their attention on investigating the historical and currently occurring patterns of genetic selection. Whether it was primarily due to choosing or the random movement of neutral and almost-neutral mutations, this field of study was initiated with the discourse surrounding the predominant cause of variation in genetics (Kimura, 1968). This discourse was the beginning of this field of study. There are some similarities between the history of the neutralist–selectionist debate in molecular evolution and the history of the mutation accumulation–antagonistic pleiotropy debate in senescence. In the wake of a protracted debate between neutralists and selectionists, the majority of evolutionary biologists have concluded that certain genes have evolved in a neutral environment. Other species, on the other hand, have developed primarily as a result of selective forces.

Nevertheless, Kimura's debate served as the impetus for decades of research that was both exciting and fruitful. There is a striking similarity between the historical trajectory of the neutralist-selections discourse in molecular evolution and the course of the mutational accumulation-antagonistic plurality discourse in senescence. The view that certain genes have undergone evolution under neutral circumstances is the one that has gained the majority of support among evolutionary scientists after a lengthy debate between supporters of the neutralist and selectionist schools of thought. On the other hand, the majority of the others have taken on the form of selective pressures. Kimura's discourse, on the other hand, was the impetus for several years of investigation that was both stimulating and fruitful. To a similar extent, in the field of developing aging, some have undergone an evolution as a consequence of the accumulation of mutations, while others have done so as a result of opposing pleiotropy. On the other hand, the debate that surrounds which hypothesis offers a more compelling explanation has resulted in significant advancements in research.

The significant academic value of the correlation between the evolution of molecules and research on aging is not limited to its historical significance; rather, it holds significant value in the academic world. The study of the evolution of DNA has led to significant advancements in our understanding of the biological aspects of organisms. These kinds of advancements have the potential to offer insightful suggestions for research projects that will be carried out in the field of gerontology in the future.

Significant portions of the genomes of a variety of organisms have been found to be composed of elements that are capable of being transposed (TEs), according to research that has been conducted on the genetic makeup of these organisms. According to McDonald (1993), mobile genetic elements, also known as "jumping genes," have the potential to function as parasitic entities within the genetic material of the organisms that serve as hosts. This ability can result in significant increases in the frequencies of mutations that are occurring beneath the surface. Assuming that age-related elevations have an effect on the aging process in somatic mutation rates, TEs have the potential to have a significant impact on the aging process. Remarkably, only a small number of studies have been conducted to investigate the relationship between transposable elements (TEs) and the aging process (Woodruff & Nikitin, 1995; Nikitin & Shmookler Reis, 1997). There is a particular study that introduces a noteworthy observation that is worthy of attention. The research highlights the fact that putting out a gene by inserting a P-element, which is a transposable element found in flies, may have a cautionary implication when it comes to identifying genes that are linked to longevity in Drosophila. This is because the simple insertion of the P-element has the potential to influence the lifespan of the living thing, regardless of the impact it has on the gene that is being targeted. (Kaiser et al. 1997). Investigating the role that transposable elements (TEs) play in this phenomenon would be a worthwhile endeavor. Quantifying the extent to which the aging process is attributed to the accumulation of somatic mutations associated with aging would be a valuable pursuit.

Throughout evolutionary history, certain genes have been subjected to significant periods of intense selection, while other genes have been subjected to significant influences from drift. This is according to the findings of molecular research. (Li, 1997). Not only could the observed variation in choosing potentially result in differences between genes, but it could also potentially result in differences between tissues. Krumbiegel (1929) researched on the fat body for aging Drosophila is a good example of the initial research endeavors that investigated the deterioration of specific tissues in parallel with the progression of age. Recent studies have shown that the rate of decline that is associated with aging varies not only between different types of tissues but also between ages. The aging process of muscle cells in nematodes appears to occur at a significantly accelerated rate in comparison to the aging process of nerve cells, (Herndon et al., 2002) Furthermore, the influence of gene expression on lifespan is frequently exclusive to particular cells (Libina et al., 2003; Hwangbo et al., 2004). A challenge that appears to be present is determining whether or not there are differences in the rate of aging that occur between different tissues as a result of different selection mechanisms that are at work on each tissue. There is a possibility that the potential fitness outcomes that result from the failure of a cell to generate a hair follicle will be significantly different from those that result from the failure of a pancreatic cell to produce insulin. This is because there is a variation in the rate of getting older that is specific to different tissues. Another name for this phenomenon is "senescent heterochrony," which can be thought of as the opposite of the "one hoss shay" impact. Given the profound evolutionary roots of this phenomenon, it would be worthwhile to investigate the possibility of shared genetic and epigenetic modification etiologies that are the basis for this trend.

Comparing the complete genomes of various species allows for the identification of physiological mechanisms based on the patterns of genetic variation. For example, Eisen and Hanawalt (1999) assessed the distribution of various DNA repair genes in over 20 different species of microorganisms. By employing the technique known as "phylogenomics," the researchers were able to ascertain the prevalence of a number of different fix or gene routes and make predictions regarding the repair characteristics of various microorganisms based on their genotypes. The findings of the study demonstrated that certain repair mechanisms, such as those associated with the recA gene, display remarkable conservation across a wide range of species, whereas other mechanisms have undergone relatively recent changes throughout evolution. When it comes to repair, different species have different genetic foundations, and in some instances, specific repair systems have developed in a way that is converging across different taxonomic communities. Scientists who study biogerontology ought to take note of these findings as a cautionary tale. While it is possible that certain genes associated with aging, such as those involved in the glucose signaling network, have deep historical roots, it is also possible that our attention to these widespread pathways may cause us to miss numerous other genes that develop rapidly and exhibit significant species-specific variation. Within the next few years, we are confident that "phylogenomic" techniques will result in the production of a fundamental understanding of the evolution and development of genetic pathways that are responsible for the process of aging.

2.2.2. Gene Networks

Over the course of human history, conventional research on aging has traditionally relied on either forward or changing genetic methodologies to isolate particular genes that are responsible for extending the lifespan. It is a simplified perspective to consider the possibility of attributing one gene to a single characteristic (Wright, 1932; Lewontin and White, 1960). In recent years, there has been a growing recognition of the complex interaction that occurs between protein genes, which has an effect on the development of the ultimate phenotype from an evolutionary perspective (Wolf et al.2000; Gibson and Honeycutt, 2002). Previous research has shown that there have been significant discoveries made within the population of worms and flies (Shook & Johnson, 1999; Leips & Mackay, 2000; Jackson et al., 2002). These discoveries have shown that the influence of a specific allele on the lifespan of an organism can vary depending on the presence of other alleles at other genetic locations. (Spencer et al., 2003).

On the other hand, the shift from focusing on individual genes to investigating epistatic interactions between pairs of loci needs to be much more complicated. It is of the utmost importance to begin contemplating the changes that occur in entire networks of interdependent components as a result of advancing age. Recent studies have shown that the interaction of genes and proteins within a complex structure can confer resilience to the network in a manner that would not be possible if its components were to interact with one another. It is believed that the structural organization of a network is responsible for this resilience (Albert et al., 2000 Wagner, 2000; Siegal & Bergman, 2002; Maslov et al., 2004; Flatt, 2005).

According to Albert and Barabási (2002), the term "degree" or "connectivity" refers to the number of edges that a node possesses. This includes the distribution of frequencies of connectivity among all of the nodes in a network, which is collectively and collectively referred to as the network's degrees distribution. The majority of nodes exhibit a low degree, typically having only one or two borders, and the level of distribution of biological systems frequently displays a power law distribution (Albert & Barabási, 2002). Nevertheless, some entities might have a large number of edges, anywhere from tens to hundreds.

According to the findings of research on network durability, the network context in which a particular gene functions has a significant impact on the degree of selection that acts upon that gene. It is possible, for instance, to propose that alleles or proteins that have higher levels of connectivity are subject to more intense selection. The fact that more densely connected proteins develop (Fraser et al., 2002,) lends support to this theory. These proteins are more likely to result in a lethal phenotype (Jeong et al., 2001). According to Krylov et al. (2003), so there is a lower probability that these genes will vanish as a result of evolution.

Based on these discoveries, we have come to the conclusion that the composition of gene or protein communication networks may affect the genes that are associated with senescent decline. (Sozou and Kirkwood, 2001). During his investigation into a yeast protein-protein interactions system, Promislow (2004) discovered that proteins that displayed a higher level of connectivity were more likely to be associated with replicative aging in comparison to proteins that had lower levels of interaction. In addition, it was discovered that genes that are associated with the process of aging displayed a higher degree of operational pleiotropy than what would be expected under the assumption of random chance. According to the observations that Promislow (2004) made, the antagonistic pluralism theory of aging appears to be the most plausible explanation. Nevertheless, the reasons that lie beneath these patterns continue to be a subject of investigation that is still progressing.

Investigations at the molecular level have shed light on the senescence process, specifically the insulin-like/insulin growing factor signaling pathway in *C. elegans* cells and *D. melanogaster* cancer cells. These studies have shed light on the complex pathways that have an effect on the aging process. According to Van Swinderen and Greenspan (2005), one is present with the exciting task of employing traditional genetics methodologies at present. It has been possible to shed light on the complex gene networks that may affect the aging process through the utilization of microarray analyzes. At the same time, it is of the utmost importance to have theoretical models that are capable of predicting the utilization of the network of node locations that a single gene communicates with in order to make predictions.

2.3. From Physiology to Demography

According to the publication that Michael Rose wrote about the evolutionary process of aging, senescence is defined as a gradual decline in the age-specific fitness attributes of a living thing as a result of an internal physical decline (Rose, 1991, page 20). The reduction of age-specific fitness components, specifically mortality and fertility, is the primary area of concentration for geneticists who study senescence. Physiologists have directed their attention toward age-related alterations in various physiological systems (Masoro, 1995); more emphasis should be placed on examining the proposition that population senescence is a result of internal physiological decay, as Williams (1999) proposed. In addition, there has been a limited amount of research conducted on the possibility that physiological equilibrium could be used to mitigate the decline in survival or fecundity that is associated with senescence (Kowald & Kirkwood, 1996).

To determine the likelihood of a gene being passed down to subsequent generations, the conventional evolutionary models make use of a metric that is solely comprised of age-specific survival and fecundity. Researchers in the field of evolutionary biology have a strong interest in the changes that occur in the number of genes over time. It is therefore a reasonable method for determining the age of an organism by observing the declines in survival and fecundity that are associated with increasing age. When it comes to explaining age-related changes in the survival or fecundity, evolutionary historians have traditionally considered physiological factors to be of less significance. On the other hand, this viewpoint has been called into question in very recent times. Although there is no evidence of biological deterioration, there are many models that suggest that age-related senescence could still occur. Rather than a decline in the physiological conditions that are associated with aging, the research that was carried out by Houston and McNamara (1999) demonstrated that death rates might increase with increasing age due to individuals' optimization of reproductive effort. There have been instances in which evolutionary scientists have investigated demographic and physiological variables, and the results have occasionally been unexpected. Further, Reznick et al., (2004) discovered that the study discovered that guppies that originated from high-predation circumstances exhibited a greater decline in motor function than those that did not originate from such circumstances. On the other hand, they showed a longer lifespan and fewer signs of sexually active getting older than guppies in conditions where there was low predation. Because of this, there may be no direct correlation between the physiological process of aging and the decline in population percentage.

However, establishing these associations is of the utmost importance. Determining the correlation between genetic makeup, physiological, and demographics aging is a challenging endeavor; however, finding these associations is essential. There will be a significant increase in the social or medical expenses that are associated with the physiological deterioration that is observed in individuals who are getting older over the course of the next few decades. To maximize the potential benefits, it may be beneficial to shift the focus of evolutionary aging studies from demographic measures of quality of life to physiological measures of quality of life. A more consolidated methodology that combines demography and physiology can result in a more all-encompassing comprehension of the biological science of the aging process.

There are three primary domains in which this can manifest itself. Specifically, it is imperative that we (1) It is recommended to advance further the development of theoretical representations of senescence that are grounded in physiological principles; (2) Traditional quantitative genetic methodologies can be employed to ascertain whether the genetic factors that regulate the pace of physiological deterioration are identical to those that govern the pace of the demographic state of decline(3) It is possible to use conventional quantitative genetic methods to determine whether or not the genetic factors that govern the rate of physiological deterioration are the same as those that govern the rate of the overall demographic state of decline. The subsequent section makes use of the term "physiology" in its broadest sense, referring to the entirety of an organism's functioning, which is the essence of the field. This encompasses a wide range of aspects, including the efficiency of organs, the functionality of systems (including immunity), the shape of cells, the behavior of organisms, and other factors related to these aspects. Considering the fact that non-demographic characteristics have the potential to involve intricate overlap and interaction, which will ultimately determine the fitness criteria for specific age growth, fecundity, and survival, it is necessary to have a comprehensive definition of these characteristics.

2.3.1. Physiological Models of Senescence

Some investigations have not ignored the physiological factors that are involved in the theory of aging. Within the framework of life-history models, Mangel (2001) incorporated the energy level of a living thing as well as the overall damage to the metabolism as a state of health. All of the models that have been presented thus far are intended to make predictions regarding the influence that calorie restriction and development have on the morphology of the mortality curve. According to the physiologically organized model that Mangel and Bonsall (2004) developed, the shape of the death curve may be affected by physiological mechanisms such as the levels of development and repair. It is possible to develop models that depict the relationship between physiological retirement and demographic retirement, and these models are becoming increasingly accurate as research on the genetic regulation of deteriorating organ functioning continues to emerge (Wessells et al., 2004) (Figure 2.1).

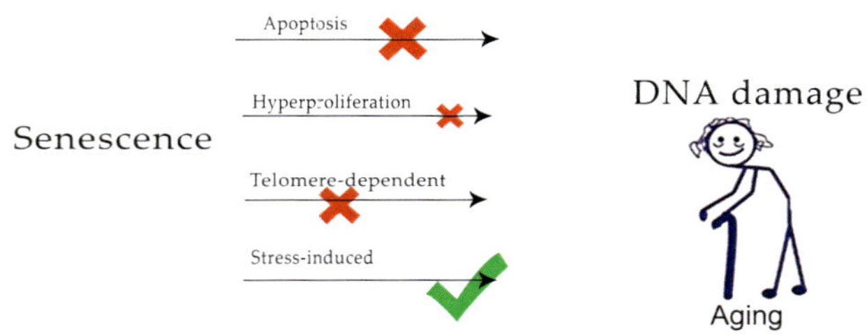

Figure 2.1. *Physiological and pathological consequences of senescence.*

Source: https://en.wikipedia.org/wiki/File:Graphical_Abstract_for_Cellular_Senescence.jpg.

2.3.2. Quantitative Genetic Analyzes of Physiology and Demography

Earlier on the importance of developing a framework that is more complex and nuanced regarding the genetic makeup of the aging process was outlined. Therefore, the incorporation of physiological factors is required to achieve a comprehensive understanding of the genetic aspects of demographic aging. On the other hand, the genetic correlation between biological and demographic aging may present a scenario that is more complicated than expected. Physiological aging has the potential to act as the functional mediator that connects the "longevity genes" and demographics of retirement. There is a possibility that the same genes, albeit one that operates independently, are responsible for the regulation of senescence interest rates in both demographics and biological processes. As a result, it is possible that the decline in population is not solely attributable to the biological processes already mentioned. In conclusion, the two processes are capable of functioning independently from one another, both in terms of their genetic makeup and their operational characteristics. Wessells et al., (2004) investigated the changes in the rate of heart failure that occur in Drosophila as a result of aging.

According to the findings of the study, insulin-signaling mutations that were associated with longer lifespans exhibited significantly lower rates of coronary artery disease. The current study demonstrates the correlation between a particular gene that affects mortality rates and a biological parameter. On the other hand, the nature of the causal connection between heart failure and how fruit fly larvae age and die is still not fully understood.

Quantitative genetic studies have demonstrated that there is a significant relationship between the rate of aging-specific survival reduction and the rate of survival respectively, fecundity (Charlesworth 1994; Promislow et al., 1996; Tatar et al., 1996) and Hughes and In a wide variety of taxa, ranging from cows and goats to Drosophila, there is a substantial body of evidence that suggests the presence of gene variation for physiological characteristics (Kiddy, 1979; Zera & Harshman, 2001). This evidence is quite convincing. Numerous studies, such as Djawdan et al. (1998) and Gibbs et al. (1997), have demonstrated that there is a correlation between the genetic variations in durability and the physiological variations that are responsible for those variations.

On the other hand, there is a paucity of information concerning gene variation and the rate of loss of bodily functions that is associated with aging (Wessells et al., 2004). We still have a limited understanding of the genetic correlation that exists between death parameters and longevity and death parameters.

It is necessary to address a specific set of questions to establish a connection between the genotype or physiological factors and the demographic retirement: Does there appear to be a connection between genotypes that display a rapid decline in physiological characteristics and an accelerated increase in the inherent mortality rate with increasing age? If a strategy extends life by decreasing the rate of death that is specific to age, is it also possible for it to reduce the rate of physiological decline? Let's say that a certain intervention reduces the initial mortality rate, which means that it increases the lifespan.

If this is the case, it is important to inquire about whether the rate of physiological decline stays the same, as Gavrilov Gavrilova explains in Chapter 1 of his book. Williams (1957) proposed that there is a regulatory system that governs the rate of degradation of all physiological characteristics. Does this system exist, and does it share characteristics with other physiological characteristics? Alternatively, is the genetic foundation for the pace of decline of one trait distinct from the genetic foundation for the pace of decline of a different trait?

2.3.3. Molecular Genetic Analyzes of Physiology and Demography

Researchers working in the field of molecular biology have, similar to natural geneticists, focused their attention primarily on demographic characteristics when studying the aging process. One of the most important motivating factors behind this endeavor has been the search for genes that confer longevity on organisms, regardless of the physiological condition of the organisms.

According to Arantes-Oliveira et al. (2003), the majority of biogerontologists have the goal of discovering methodologies that can improve the longevity and well-being of individuals during their later stages of life. To be successful in accomplishing this objective, it is essential to put into action a strategy for conducting research that takes into account a comprehensive approach that takes into account both biological and demographic points of view.

There is, thankfully, evidence that there has been a shift in emphasis toward the perspective that is more elevated. In their study on *C. elegans* mutations, Huang et al. (2004) found that there was a positive correlation between the age-related decrease in oral pumping and body movement and the life span of the subjects.

This proposition suggests that a decrease in physiological processes may result in a decrease in the likelihood of survival, or that a common mechanism governs the deterioration of physiology and survival. Both of these hypotheses are plausible. In subsequent research endeavors, the focus should be on explicitly testing the two hypotheses, as was mentioned earlier, while also incorporating demographic variables that go beyond longevity.

According to the findings of Huang et al. (2004), the decrease in oral transport or movement of the body that occurs as a result of aging does not correlate with a self-fertile reproductive span. According to the authors' hypothesis, there might be a connection between the deterioration of physiological function and other indicators of the advancing years of reproductive age. It is possible for genes that influence the aging process to have pleiotropic effects on the movement and survival of an organism at the same time that they do not have an effect on the reproductive capacity of the organism. There is an expectation that the field of cell biology will undergo significant advancements. For the purpose of examining the aging process in C. elegans, Herndon et al. (2002) utilized a histological approach. In their research, they found that age-1 mutants that lived for longer periods of time had a slower rate of degradation in the ultrastructure of their cells. Particularly noteworthy is the fact that the decreased rates were only observed in particular cellular categories (Figure 2.2).

As Huang et al. (2004) demonstrated, the findings of the two studies that were conducted on *C. elegans* in conjunction with one another indicate that there is a correlation between physiology and certain demographic characteristics. In addition, Herndon et al. (2002) found that there was a correlation between certain physiological characteristics and demographic characteristics. To establish a comprehensive research program that encompasses genetics, biology, and demographics, the current task requires the collaboration of conceptual, quantitative, and molecular genetic experts. This will result in the development of a more cohesive approach to the study of biogerontology.

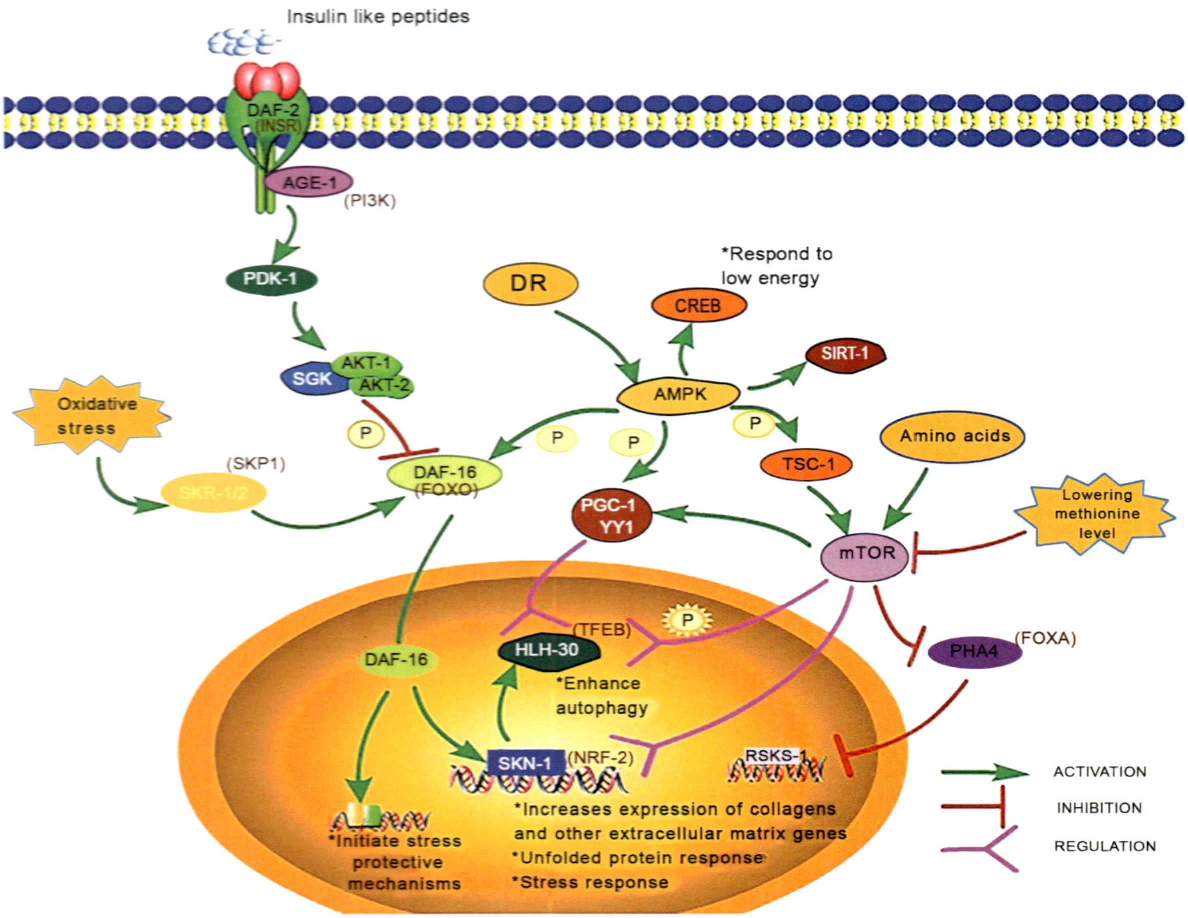

Figure 2.2. *Major longevity pathways and longevity-associated transcription factors in C. elegans. The IIS pathway is one of the most studied longevity pathways. DAF-2, AGE-1, and DAF-16 are its three key genes. Mutations in DAF-2 and AGE-1 and low IIS activity prolong lifespan via DAF-16 and downstream gene expression. AMPK is another crucial metabolic energy sensor that links nutrient availability to lifespan by binding and phosphorylating a set of transcriptional (co)activators. The mTOR pathway is another critical pathway that links nutrient availability and metabolism to longevity; however, its mechanism remains to be fully elucidated.*

Source: Zhang S, Li F, Zhou T, Wang G and Li Z (2020) Caenorhabditis elegans as a useful model for studying aging mutations. Front. Endocrinol. 11:554994. doi: 10.3389/fendo.2020.554994 C. elegans. (Source: Wikipedia).

2.4. Parasites and Immune Function

Within the preceding section, it was argued that evolutionary gerontologists are confronted with a significant challenge when it comes to bringing together the disparity between biology and demography in their investigations of the aging process. Several specific approaches were proposed as possible solutions to address this issue of concern. The presence of parasites is a potentially pervasive factor that has the potential to link the physiological and demographic aspects of aging. Personal experiences and numerous studies on model organisms that demonstrate the impact that parasites have on reducing lifespan are evidence that indicates that parasites are known to have negative effects on individuals. In a similar vein, it has been observed that an individual's lifespan is lengthened when they do not have their typical bacterial flora (Croll et al., 1977; Min & Benzer, 1997; Garigan et al., 2002; Houthoofd et al., 2002; Larsen & Clarke, 2002). Recent research has led to the discovery of molecules that have overlapping effects on both immune function and survival. The release of juvenile hormone (JH) from the body is considered to be an essential component in some important reproductive pathways within insects, including the production of spermatophores (Wigglesworth, 1965). However, previous studies have shown that increased levels of juvenile hormone titers can harm the immune system's functionality in the Tenebrio Molitor beetle and other insects (Rolff and Siva-Jothy, 2002; Rantala et al., 2003. In their study from 2001, Herman and Tatar found that the monarch butterfly had a shorter lifespan than it had previously been. The physiological conflict that exists between reproduction, immunity, and survival may have a significant impact on the aging process of insects.

In spite of the fact that the immediate effects of parasites on lifespan may be easily discernible and uncomplicated, there are connections between hosts and their parasites that are more nuanced and intriguing, and these connections may continue to emerge throughout the course of evolution. It is believed that parasites have a significant impact on the development of a variety of biological characteristics, including the beginning of sexual reproduction. Hamilton (1980) describes the phenomenon of avian species exhibiting a coloration that is both striking and distinct (Hamilton and Zuk, 1982). This refers to the ability of living things to establish themselves in new environments (Wolfe, 2002; Torchin et al., 2003). The relationship between parasitic organisms and life-history strategies has been the subject of recent research endeavors. According to Rolff and Siva-Jothy (2003) and Williams and Day (2001), parasites, according to the author's hypothesis, have the potential to influence the mechanisms that natural selection uses to shape senescence trends.

2.4.1. From Immunosenescence to Demographic Senescence

Immunosenescence, also known as decreased immunocompetence, is a physiological phenomenon that is commonly associated with aging (Walford, 1969). This phenomenon is a significant physiological aspect that deserves attention. There is a significant amount of knowledge regarding the immediate factors that contribute to immunosenescence in the human population. In the course of its existence, for instance, the region of the thymus that is responsible for the development of T cells has suffered a decline. It is because of this that thymic tissue loses its capacity to control essential immunological processes, such as the regeneration of T cells in the lymphatic system (Hirokawa and Makinodan, 1975). In addition, the origins of B lymphocytes, which are capable of precisely matching a protein that is present in an invading virus, diminish over time (Leslie, 2004). It is possible that this loss, in conjunction with an aging T-cell population, will result in a diminished antibody reaction to the majority of antigens (Weksler and Schwab, 1992). These immune system modifications that are specific to aging are indicative of a severe physiological decline that occurs in later life and may have a significant impact on demographic patterns associated with aging (Figure 2.3).

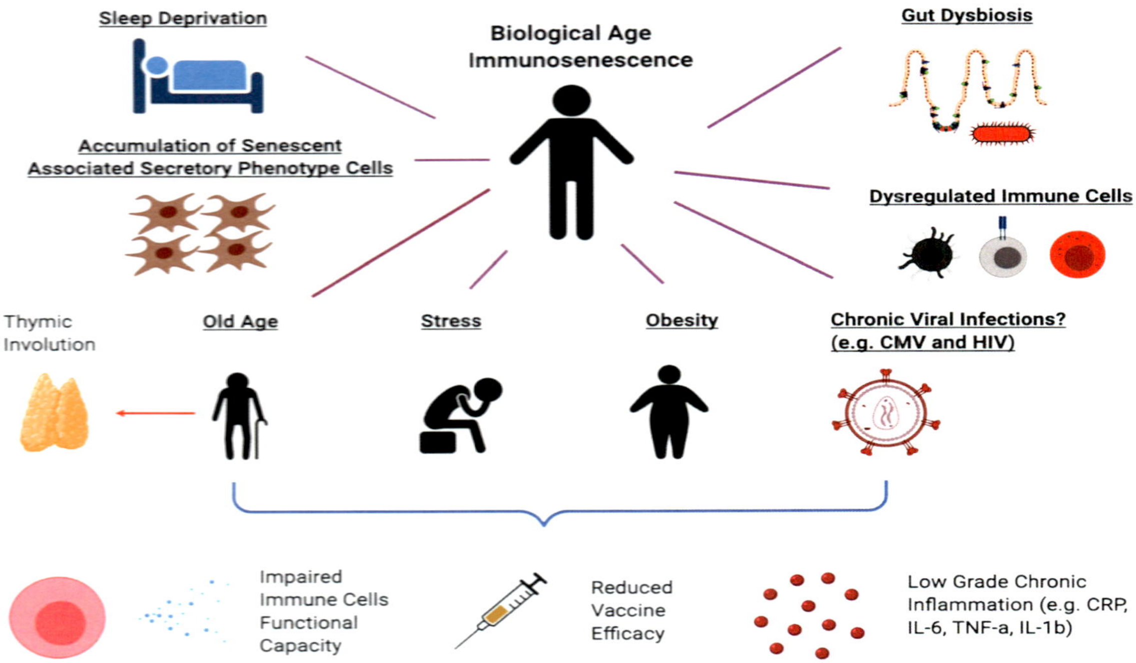

Figure 2.3. *Immunosenescence and Aging.*

Source: Xu, W., Wong, G., Hwang, Y.Y. et al. The untwining of immunosenescence and aging. Semin Immunopathol 42, 559–572 (2020). https://doi.org/10.1007/s00281-020-00824-x.

According to Torroba and Zapata (2003), this immune senescence overall pattern is observed in an astonishingly wide variety of taxa, including fish, birds, and amphibians. This is although the specifics of the immune system vary from cell to cell. There is a discernible age-related shift that occurs in several immune system components of insect species, such as bumble honeybees, crickets, and overall dragonflies. This shift frequently leads to higher parasitism rates and mortality rates (Adamo et al. (2001); Rolff, 2001; Doums et al., 2002). Laws et al. (2004) examined the relationship between increasing age and an increased susceptibility to infections brought on by bacteria in the nematode species *C. elegans*. They found that there was a correlation between the two. The current state of knowledge regarding the existence of a causal connection between immune senescence and the age-related decline in fitness is still uncertain. This is according to the current state of knowledge. The process of immune aging may be a contributor to the general decline in the various functions of the body. Because the immune system is subject to aging, it may require additional resources in order to maintain its current state. As a consequence of this, there may be a reduction in the amount of funding available for other costly systems within the body. In the case of the caught flycatcher, also known as *Ficedula albicollis*, it has been observed that the aging process in females leads to a decrease in both the humoral immunity and the size of the children (Cichon et al., 2003). In order to determine whether or not the reduction in offspring dimensions can be attributed to the increased energy requirements of an immune system that is maturing, additional research is required. On the other hand, the alterations in the immune system observed in elderly individuals may serve as a surface-level indicator of other fundamental mechanisms contributing to the aging process. If this is the case, immune senescence has the potential to be an important biomarker for determining physiological age in upcoming research endeavors.

2.4.2. Immunocompetence Tradeoffs

By taking into account only the survival and fecundity rates that are unique to each age group, Hamilton's research demonstrated that it is possible to anticipate a reduction in the intensity of selection with age. According to de Jong and van Noordwijk (1992), previous theoretical frameworks have proposed that there is an inverse relationship between these two characteristics. This is because there is a limited amount of resources available for investment. In Kirkwood's recyclable soma theory, which explains the evolutionary process of senescence (Kirkwood, 1977), the concept of tradeoff is an essential component. Having said that, this framework may be missing some components. There is a recommendation that, in addition to allocating resources to reproductive and survival functions, it may be beneficial to incorporate other physiological factors that act as intermediaries as separate elements of the model. These parts may include neurons, circulatory, and immune system functioning if there is an immediate connection between the expenditure of immune function as well as both age-specific development and specific to age surviving, such as when the physiological expenses of immunity impact fecundity along with survival concurrently, it is plausible that immune operation may be responsible for the correlation among fecundity and surviving. The phenomenon will, as was mentioned earlier, result in a decrease in choosing strength with increasing age (Figure 2.4).

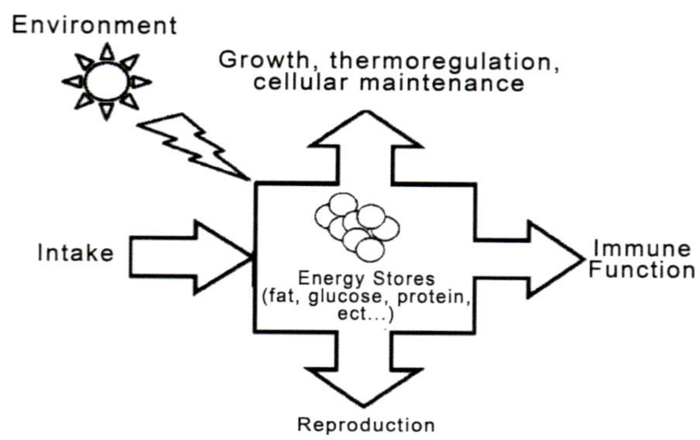

Figure 2.4. *Physiological tradeoffs.*

Source: Researchgate.net. Ecological immunology: The organism in context. 2009; 49(3):246-53. DOI:10.1093/icb/icp032.

Prospective hosts employ a wide variety of defensive mechanisms, such as preventative measures and post-infection responses, to stay away from the parasite and avoid becoming infected. The implementation of these defensive measures, on the other hand, might result in sizeable financial costs. There is an example of this phenomenon that can be seen in situations where there is an increase in the allocation of resources towards enhancing immunity, which is frequently accompanied by a decrease in reproductive output (Zuk & Stoehr, 2002). A decrease in the survival rate is observed, on the other hand, in the case of individuals who increase the proportion of the resources that they devote to reproduction (Partridge & Harvey, 1985). Additionally, it is important to bear in mind that immunocompetence is also an essential component to take into consideration (for example, Fedorka et al., 2004). The majority of the instances of immune expenses that are incurred during reproduction are derived from the study of insects. In a study that was carried out by Helle et al. (2004) on women from Finland during the 18th and 19th centuries, it was discovered that those women who gave birth to identical twins at any point during their reproductive life expectancy had a higher likelihood of contracting an infectious illness after menopause in comparison to those women who only gave birth to singletons. Even after taking into account the total number of offspring that each female had produced, this finding remained unchanged.

It is necessary to carry out this to gain an understanding of the mechanisms that are responsible for the conversion of the costs associated with a parasitic relationship with the immune system into the metric of demographic aging. The evaluation of how the physiological costs associated with the initiation of an immune system reaction and the fatality costs linked to parasitism vary across different age groups is an important area of concern. There is a possibility that the alterations will result in complex and counterintuitive variations in mortality rates. According to the conventional models for host-parasite cooperation or senescence, there is an increase in the number of deaths in the population, and there is a corresponding increase in the rates of infectiousness and getting older. They conducted two theoretical investigations, which indicate that the interaction between external sources of death and the physical condition of the organism in question in a nonadditive manner can decrease infectiousness as the background rate of death rises (Williams and Day, 2001); Day, 2003). A theoretical framework that incorporates the models of parasitism and senescence that Williams and Day have proposed is currently required because of the current need for such a framework. In addition, it is of the utmost importance to carry out empirical investigations to assess the validity of the existing theoretical constructs. It is anticipated that these models will be of assistance in determining how the patterns of age-specific expenditure on immunity and age-specific survival, as well as the potential interaction between the two, should be influenced by choosing.

2.4.3. Parasites and the Genetics of Aging

Research that investigates the relationship between aging and immunity has the potential to improve our understanding of the genetic framework that underlies the process of senescence. Many studies have shown that a close connection exists between immune defense mechanisms and a large number of genes that influence lifespan (Lagaay et al., 1991; Ivanova et al., 1998; Caruso et al., 2001; Garsin et al., 2003; Laws et al., 2004). Immunity may be the immediate mechanism that is responsible for the development of genes that exhibit antagonistic pleiotropy in certain situations. Studies conducted on older human adults have shown that there is a significant correlation between the length of one's lifespan and the Major Histocompatibility Complexity (MHC) haplotypes (Lagaay et al., 1991; Ivanova et al., 1998; Caruso et al., 2001). Caruso et al. (2000) published a study in which they hypothesized that the 8.1 AH leukocyte antigen haplotype might confer a distinct advantage during the early stages of infancy because it might offer a potential defense against infectious diseases. In spite of this, this haplotype has been associated with susceptibility to many autoimmune conditions that become apparent during reproductive maturity. These conditions include sarcoidosis and chronic lupus erythematosus (Lio et al., 1997; Price et al., 1999). It is important to note that this particular haplotype confers a sex-specific advantage for male carriers in their later years, whereas female carriers continue to experience premature mortality and morbidity in their later years (Caruso et al., 2000).

Genes that are associated with the immune system may frequently involve compromises of this kind, which is a plausible hypothesis. C28Y is the name of the MHC mutation that is responsible for the generation of an additional instance. It has been observed that the mutation described above improves the intestinal absorption process of iron, which is an essential component in several immune systems (Salter-Cid et al., 2000). According to Waheed et al. (1997), the variant that is believed to be associated with the condition in homozygotes is a medical condition that is characterized by a decrease in lifespan due to an excessive buildup of iron within the organs and a simultaneous decrease in immunity. A number of researchers have proposed the existence of possible connections between tuberculosis and Tay-Sachs syndrome (Spyropoulos, 1988), as well as between cholera and cystic fibrosis (CF) (Gabriel et al., 1994). Biologists have recently shifted their focus to investigate the implications of tradeoffs associated with immunity for the course of evolution (DeVeale et al., 2004). There is, however, a lack of a comprehensive connection between this research field and the process of aging. It is necessary to conduct additional research to investigate the prevalence of such tradeoffs and their potential manifestation of age-specificity concerning the opposing pluralism hypothesis concerning senescence. A compelling challenge awaits individuals who are interested in establishing an evolutionary perspective on immunosenescence, and that challenge is the identification of these genes.

When it comes to the biology of aging, parasites have the potential to exert a more widespread influence (Brummel et al., 2004) New research has shown that the presence of bacterial flora is one of the factors that determine whether or not certain genes have the ability to increase longevity. An example of this would be the fact that the administration of antibiotics rendered the benefits of longevity that DJ817 mutant-carrying flies had become obsolete. According to the research that was presented earlier, it was found that male *Drosophila melanogaster*, when they were not exposed to their typical bacterial complement during the early stages of their adulthood, experienced a significant reduction in their lifespan. Taking into consideration the intriguing findings, it is of the utmost importance to investigate the extent to which the expression of genes related to longevity is dependent upon the presence of microbes and to identify the specific bacterial species that serve as early-age symbiotics in *Drosophila*.

2.4.4. Parasites and Sex Differences in Longevity

It is possible that research on parasites, the immune system, and senescence could shed light on the factors that contribute to the distinct aging patterns that are observed in males and their female counterparts. (Lagaay et al., 1991; Lio et al., 2002) Research on immunosenescence has shown that several MHC haplotypes that are associated with a longer lifespan exhibit patterns that are specific to only one gender. Among the three MHC alleles that are associated with human durability, research found that two of them exhibited a sex-specific impact (Ivanova et al., 1998). In their study on variations in a promoter region of the IL-10 gene, Lio et al. (2002) found that there was a statistically significant male bias among centenarians. There is a prevailing consensus that interleukin-10 (IL-10) acts as an inhibitor of the pro-inflammatory immune system reaction, which is a process that is responsible for the elevated mortality rates that are observed in elderly individuals. There is a plausible explanation for the observed patterns, and that explanation is the prevalence of gender disparities in immunity. Reduced immunity is a common occurrence in males and mammals (Klein and Nelson, 1997). Parasitic infections are more common in males than they are in females (Radhika et al., 1998; Kurtz et al., 2000; Adamo et al., 2001; Kurtz and Sauer, 2001; Rolff, 2001; Moore and Wilson, 2002). All found that males of invertebrate species exhibited a similar pattern throughout their lives. There is a complex structure of life-history compromises that can make it difficult to predict sexual dimorphism in the immune system (Moret & Schmid-Hempel, 2000; Doums et al., 2002; Zuk & Stoehr, 2002; Zuk et al., 2004). This can make it difficult to predict sexual dimorphism in the immune system. With regard to the selective forces that affect immunity and lifespan, the observed patterns that are specific to each sex indicate that males and females are subject to different selective forces.

There is a hypothesis that suggests that differences in immunity between the sexes could be a factor in the observed differences in lifespan between males and females. As we move on to the following section, we will shift our attention away from resistance and delve more deeply into the fundamental factors that contribute to gender-based differences in lifespan.

2.5. Sex, Sexual Selection, and Sexual Conflict

Lifespan differences between men and women are extremely common. One of the most frequently observed phenomena is that female creatures tend to have a longer lifespan in comparison to their male counterparts. Males have been observed to have a longer lifespan than females, with the possible exception of certain cases, such as between anthropoid primates that exhibit extended fatherly care (Allman et al., 1998). This has been observed, with the possible exception of certain cases, such as between anthropoid primates. On the other hand, avian species display a pattern that is in contrast to that of nematodes (McCulloch & Gems, 2003) and nematodes (Promislow et al., 1992). It has been observed that the male gender tends to outlive the female gender. A wide variety of hypotheses are being put forward in order to explain these patterns. These hypotheses range from variations in hormonal profiles (for example, increased levels of male hormones in males) to variations in susceptibility to predation (for example, the increased susceptibility of nesting females) (Figure 2.5).

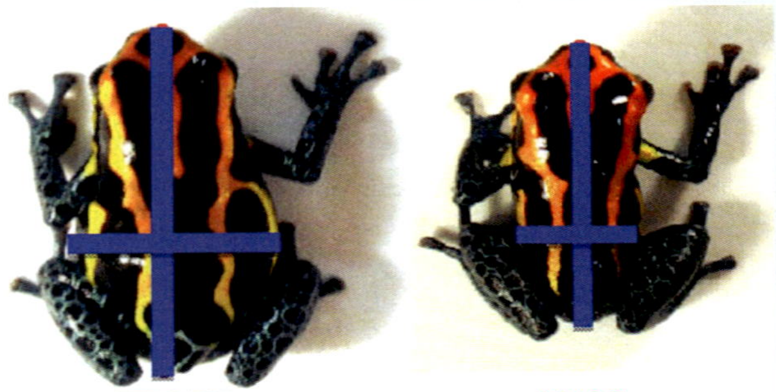

Figure 2.5. *Sexual size dimorphism.*

Source: M., C. (2013). The evolution of sexual dimorphism: Understanding mechanisms of sexual shape differences. InTech. doi: 10.5772/55154.

In order to account for some of these variations, there is likely a fundamental difference in the methods of reproduction. There may be significant differences between the optimal reproduction strategy of a male and that of a female population. Rice (1996) made this statement. The differences that exist between the sexes can lead to age-specific selection stresses that are distinct from one another and have a different impact on each of them. To this day, we are still trying to get a full understanding of the implications that these differences have. In the following section, we will outline three distinct domains that have the potential to improve our understanding of aging patterns that are specific to each gender. These domains include the costs that are associated with reproduction, the immediate and evolutionary outcomes of female selection, and the discord that exists between the sexes themselves.

2.5.1. Cost of Reproduction

A number of different organisms can experience an increase in their mortality rate as a consequence of development (Sgrò & Partridge, 1999; Fedorka et al., 2004). Nevertheless, there may be substantial differences in these costs between males and females in a variety of organisms (Michener & Locklear, 1990; Rocheleau & Houle, 2001; Lyons & Dunne, 2003). Males and females may allocate their resources differently when it comes to the production of gametes, providing support for parents, and cooperating with one another in the workplace. Different levels of reproductive expenditure can lead to different levels of susceptibility to predation or infections that are transmitted through sexual activity, as well as different levels of assets that are devoted to somatic maintenance. As a result of the development of sexually multifaceted characteristics, which can be attributed to either female preference or male rivalry, the manifestation of sex-specific costs can be observed. Boys frequently exhibit amplified secondary sexual characteristics, such as vivid feather patterns or hues, prominent vocalizations, or substantial antlers, to increase their reproductive success due to either the attraction of a mate or the competition with other males. On the other hand, these characteristics may also act as a magnet for potential predators or make it more difficult for the male to escape from unsafe situations. Furthermore, the aforementioned characteristics incur a substantial physiological cost, which may lead to a reduction in the resources intended for immune defense and other characteristics, which ultimately leads to a reduction in the percentage of individuals who survive (Andersson, 1994). The changes in longevity may, in the future, lead to gender-specific variations in the weakening of selection pressure with increasing age. To facilitate the identification of how differences in mortality risk between the sexes could result in variations in aging rates, it is necessary to provide examples that are specific to each gender separately.

2.5.2. Choice of a Female Partner

Numerous studies conducted on a wide range of species have uncovered substantial evidence suggesting that females frequently choose to engage in sexual reproduction with males under their genetic makeup. According to Andersson (1994). As a result of engaging in this behavior, selective females have the potential to influence the process of aging and its evolution. According to the findings of the research conducted by Hamilton and Zuk in 1982, female avian species have been observed to utilize the conspicuous coloration of their male counterparts in order to evaluate their inherent capacity to combat parasitic infections. If the selection of females increases the population's overall immunity, there is a possibility that the average survival interest rates additionally rise. Consequently, there is a possibility that the selective pressures that bring about senescence will change.

Female preference has the potential to immediately influence the process of senescence within a particular population. This is because females prefer to mate with males who belong to a particular age cohort (Hansen and Price, 1995; Kokko, 1998; Beck and Powell, 2000). They have proposed that females may have a preference for mating with older males because older males have been in existence for a longer period of time. The computer models revealed that in situations where females were given the freedom to select males based on age, they generally preferred older males (Beck et al., 2002). It has been observed that older males, in comparison to their younger counterparts, have a higher frequency of alleles that are associated with a longer lifespan. This is the case in a population that is characterized by genetic heterogeneity. There is a correlation between the preference of females for older males and a decrease in the mortality rate of the offspring of the selective female. In addition, this phenomenon contributes to an increase in the average lifespan of the evolution of every collective.

It has been demonstrated through empirical research carried out on Drosophila that the theoretical conclusions that selectivity can result in an increased lifespan are consistent with observations. In the research carried out by Promislow et al. in 1998, a comparison was made between the mortality rates of strains that were subjected to enforced polygamy for multiple generations and those that allowed female choice in addition to male-male rivalry. According to the findings of the study, strains that exhibited higher levels of reproductive selection experienced a decrease in death rates. This occurred over the course of time. According to the findings of a study conducted by Promislow et al., in 1992, female survival rates are generally higher in avian species that are subjected to intense sexual selection. It is necessary to conduct additional empirical research to determine whether or not the tendency of females to gravitate toward older men can alter the structures of senescence that are present in the natural world.

2.5.3. Sexual Conflict

Several researchers have suggested that the impact of sexual disagreement is a significant factor in the development of aging. When there is a disparity between males and females in terms of the reproductive strategy that is most advantageous, sexual disagreement can arise. By engaging in multiple copulations with a variety of males, she has been able to improve her physical condition in certain instances. This behavior, on the other hand, may be detrimental to the health of all of her partners because it has the potential to lower the quality of their sperm due to the presence of sperm from males who are competing with them. There is a possibility that these conflicts will result in a situation in which males eventually develop the ability to maximize their reproductive success (Promislow, 2003; Svensson & Sheldon, 1998).

It has been known for a considerable amount of time that male behavior can appear to be female. In 1980, Parker and Thompson observed the dung fly, also known as *Scatophaga stercoraria*. They discovered that male dung flies, in their quest to find potential mates, would frequently drown them, resulting in their death. Because of this behavior, there is a clear opposition between the interests of the male and those of the female. As a result of male Cimex lectularius bedbugs engaging in forced copulation, which involves penetrating the abdominal cavity of females through their needle-like genitals, there is a significant mortality rate among the female population (Stutt & Siva-Jothy, 2001). There is the potential for conflict to materialize on the level of the molecular. The transfer of the gland amino acids (ACPS) from male Drosophila species to females occurred during the process of copulation. It has been discovered that these ACPS have the potential to decrease the sexual receptivity of the female, render sperm that was previously provided inactive, prevent subsequent years of sperm eviction, and increase the rate of oviposition. (Chapman et al., 1995; Heifetz et al., 2000). Moreover, it has been observed that ACPS have a dose-dependent effect on reducing the average lifespan of females (Chapman et al., 1995; Lung et al., 2002). This is something that has been observed repeatedly. In 1996, Moshitzky et al., have shown that there is a direct connection between ACPS and longevity. To be more specific, they discovered that an amino acid found in the ejaculate of the male, which is classified as one of the sex peptides, can stimulate the production of the young hormone, which is closely associated with an increased lifespan.

To determine the potential impact of sexual conflicts on the rate of aging and the differences in senescence structures that are observed between the sexes, additional research is required. Does there appear to be a connection between higher rates of aging and increased levels of sexual conflict among species? Could there be a connection between the degree of sexual dimorphism in getting older rates and the level of competition that exists within a species or between the two? Could there be a connection between genes that are associated with conflicts, such as ACPS in Drosophila, and differences in the length of life spans of individuals of both sexes?

2.6. Genetic Variation in Natural Populations

According to the findings of several studies (Sgrò & Partridge, 2000; Linnen et al., 2001), the introduction of living organisms into laboratory environments can inadvertently expose them to unprecedented selection challenges and length of life. As a result, the information attained in laboratory settings concerning the genetic factors that contribute to the aging process might not necessarily apply to natural environments. It had been believed that senescence did not occur very often in natural environments (Comfort, 1979). This was because it was more likely for organisms to die from accidental causes before they reached the stage of senescence. Previous studies have shown that senescence is not a fictitious phenomenon that occurs as a result of optimal conditions in laboratories; rather, it is a phenomenon that is common among native populations of animals (Promislow, 1991) and birds (Ricklefs, 1998—2000). It is possible to observe senescence in natural communities of insects. By observing the phenomenon of aging in male antlers that were operating with a very short lifespan in their natural habitat, Bonduriansky and Brassil (2002) made the observation. In mayflies, which are notorious for having an extremely short lifespan, Carey (2002) also reported finding evidence of getting older. Recent studies on the aging process in short-lived species of animals have shown that there is the potential for the creation of independent model organisms that can be used to investigate the genetic mechanisms that are responsible for the aging process.

Several studies have provided evidence that a genetic component of the variability in aging prices found in natural populations is responsible for the observed variation. Investigations conducted in laboratories have provided the majority of the information that we have regarding the genetic mechanisms that are responsible for the aging process. When drawing conclusions about whether or not the information learned in a laboratory setting can be directly applied to situations that occur in the real world, it is essential to exercise appropriate caution. Some people believe that an allele that confers an extended lifespan under laboratory incubation conditions would also confer an extended lifespan in a natural environment. This is a fairly common hypothesis. We regret to inform you that the introduction of naturally occurring groups into laboratory settings has the potential to significantly alter demographic data due to the influence of environmental selection pressures (Tatar et al., 1997; Bronikowski et al., 2002; Reznick et al., 2004).

There is a tendency for organisms that have adapted to laboratory conditions to display accelerated maturation, increased fecundity during the early stages of life, and a significantly reduced lifespan. Clark (1987), Promislow and Tatar (1998), Sgrò and Partridge (2000), Miller et al. (2002), and Houle and Rowe (2003), are some of the studies that have studied this topic. According to Linnen et al. (2001), one could argue that the life-prolonging effects of new mutations or artificial selection merely reinstate the lifespan of laboratory strains that have a shorter lifespan in comparison to their natural counterparts.

There are two distinct factors that need to be taken into consideration before making assumptions about the applicability of laboratory findings to natural populations. These factors were discovered through recent research focused on insects and flies. The influence of a mutation can differs depending on the environment in which the organism is located. This is because of the interaction that occurs between genes and the external environment, which is commonly known as gene-environment (G × E) interplay. Furthermore, several research studies have suggested that it may be possible to extend one's life without incurring any additional costs. In controlled laboratory settings, the daf-2 change that was observed in *C. elegans* has the potential to significantly increase lifespan, while at the same time exhibiting no discernible decline in fertility or physical activity (Kenyon et al., 1993). The persistent mutant, on the other hand, continues to be greater than the normal strain when both the normal strain and a daf-2 mutation that has a long lifespan are present in the same cultures (Jenkins et al., 2004). When transferred to a natural setting, genes that increase longevity in the laboratory may have implications that are unexpectedly detrimental to fitness.

The question of whether or not alleles that are associated with longevity in laboratory settings exhibit functionalities that are comparable in populations that occur naturally has been the subject of a great deal of research interest. There is a variation in the abundance of methuselah, a gene that is found in Drosophila and has the potential to significantly increase longevity across different geographic regions (Lin et al., 1998). This observation was made by Schmidt et al. in the year 2000. Within the methuselah of a gene, the researchers discovered that there was no significant correlation between clinal variation in durability and clinal variation within a single nucleotide polymorphism. The results of previous studies have shown that the translation of laboratory-derived findings to real-world groups yields more favorable outcomes. Using wild-derived inbred cultivars of Drosophila, Geiger-Thornsberry and Mackay (2004) carried out a laboratory study to investigate the genetic variability of genes that are associated with the aging process.

After conducting quantitative enhancement tests, it was discovered that there was a variation in genes at these loci within natural populations. This was discovered through the application of these tests. In addition to this, it was discovered that this genetic variation displayed a correlation in the varying levels of longevity that were observed between different strains. The current task entails determining whether the observations made by Geiger-Thornsberry and Mackay regarding the INR or adh DNA are anomalous or representative, as well as determining how natural selection has influenced the characteristics of these genetic loci throughout the course of development.

There is a significant amount of importance in determining whether or not genes that have been discovered in people Flies that have been raised in a laboratory are effective in extending the life span of naturally occurring populations. There is, however, a more significant challenge that has presented itself. Is it possible to extrapolate results obtained in a laboratory to populations found in nature across a wide range of taxonomic categories? To what extent is it possible to extrapolate the genetic findings obtained from laboratory experiments conducted on flies or worms to groups of vertebrates that exist in the real world? Studies conducted in academic institutions have suggested that certain species of fish, such as killifish (Herrera & Jagadeeswaran, 2004), guppies (Gerhard, 2003; Gerhard & Cheng, 2002), and zebrafish (Reznick, 1997), could be suitable candidates to conduct research. To facilitate the connection between invertebrate taxa and mammalian taxa within the context of research on aging, the utilization of ideal models can serve as a valuable tool. Reznick examined the hypothesis that groups with increased extrinsic death rates exhibit increased senescence prices by conducting an empirical study using an actual population of guppies (Reznick et al., 2004). Despite widespread agreement, the data did not provide support for the theory. As mentioned earlier in this chapter, this demonstrates the importance of having simulations that are physiologically plausible to gain a better understanding of the development of retirement.

Studies have suggested that avian species (Holmes et al. 2001), chiropterans (Wilkinson and South, 2002), and other organisms with a tendency to age more slowly (Austad, 2001) could be useful model systems for the study of senescence. These hypotheses have been supported by a number of researchers. It may be possible to determine the extent to which the processes that occur during the aging process are conserved across different taxa if the scope of taxa that are used in the investigation of aging is expanded. The study of long-lived organisms in their natural habitat or in laboratory settings has the potential to introduce a novel perspective to the field of aging studies. This is although there are obvious benefits associated with the study of short-lived species (Holmes and Ottinger, 2003).

A Closer Look

Sexual Disagreement

Sexual conflict in aging arises from the differing evolutionary strategies between males and females, leading to potential trade-offs in reproductive success and survival as individuals age. In many species, males often exhibit reproductive behaviors that prioritize mating opportunities and fertilization success, while females typically invest more in parental care and longevity. These divergent strategies can create conflicts over resource allocation and lifespan trade-offs between the sexes.

One aspect of sexual conflict in aging involves the physiological costs associated with reproductive effort. In species where males compete intensely for mates, such as through aggressive behaviors or elaborate courtship displays, the energy and resources allocated to these activities can accelerate physiological aging and reduce lifespan. Conversely, females may face trade-offs between investing in current offspring versus maintaining their own health and longevity.

Sexual conflict can manifest in genetic and molecular mechanisms that influence aging. Evolutionary pressures may favor genes that enhance reproductive success early in life but contribute to age-related decline later on. This can result in physiological pathways that promote rapid aging in males or impose constraints on female longevity.

Understanding sexual conflict in aging is crucial for comprehending the evolutionary forces shaping lifespan and reproductive strategies across species. It underscores the complexity of biological aging, where the interplay between sexual selection, reproductive investment, and longevity has profound implications for individual fitness and population dynamics. By studying these dynamics, researchers can gain insights into how natural selection acts differently on males and females throughout their lifespans, shaping patterns of aging and reproductive success in diverse ecological contexts.

Summary

- The initial conceptual frameworks that were developed by Medawar (1946; 1952) and Williams (1957) served as the foundation for the primary theoretical advancements that were made in the process of comprehending the progression of senescence. In the past half-century, there has been a substantial advancement in the understanding of evolutionary processes and patterns, ranging from the process of adapting to altruism and evolution to the study of gender ratios. This advancement is a direct result of the ground-breaking collaboration between Medawar and Williams. For the most part, the significant conceptual advancements in this field have occurred independently of evolutionary investigations of the aging process. However, there are a few exceptions to this rule.
- Through the course of this chapter, we have investigated five different areas that have the potential to significantly advance our understanding of the progression of aging. The aforementioned topics include the genetic composition of senescence, the correlation between physiological and demographic deterioration, the significance of parasites and immunity, gender differences in behavior or aging, and investigations of aging in natural habitats. All of these topics are discussed in greater detail below. Researchers in the field of evolutionary biology who work in areas other than the study of aging have made significant advancements in several different fields. The overarching question of which factors will influence the reduction in the strength for being chosen that occurs with advancing age is the factor that connects all of these phenomena together.
- The inquiries that are currently being presented in this context will serve as a catalyst for an increased number of evolutionary biologists to address the problem of aging evolution. Molecular investigations, which reveal an exceptional discovery rate regarding novel genes and gene routes that impact aging, are the primary focus of the majority of biogerontological scholarly investigations. In light of the rapid advancements in genome sequencing and microarray technology, it is permissible to question whether or not an evolutionary perspective is still applicable. An individual thinks that a fully integrated study poses an exciting challenge for all those who are directly involved. For this program, researchers in the field of molecular evolutionary biology would work together. Molecular biologists would pose questions about evolution, and evolutionary biologists would carry out research using sophisticated molecular techniques. The resolution of previous challenges will, as a consequence of this integration, give rise to novel and intriguing inquiries at an accelerated pace. This will ensure that the investigation of aging continues to be a field that is both stimulating and illuminating.

References

1. Armanios, M.; Alder, J.K.; Parry, E.M.; Karim, B.; Strong, M.A.; Greider, C.W. Short telomeres are sufficient to cause the degenerative defects associated with aging. Am. J. Hum. Genet. 2009, 85, 823–832.
2. Blackburn, E.H.; Greider, C.W.; Szostak, J.W. Telomeres and telomerase: The path from maize, Tetrahymena and yeast to human cancer and aging. Nat. Med. 2006, 12, 1133–1138.

3. Calderwood, S.K.; Murshid, A.; Prince, T. The shock of aging: Molecular chaperones and the heat shock response in longevity and aging—A mini-review. Gerontology 2009, 55, 550–558.
4. Corral-Debrinski, M.; Horton, T.; Lott, M.T.; Shoffner, J.M.; McKee, A.C.; Beal, M.F.; Graham, B.H.; Wallace, D.C. Marked changes in mitochondrial DNA deletion levels in Alzheimer brains. Genomics 1994, 23, 471–476.
5. Corral-Debrinski, M.; Shoffner, J.; Lott, M.; Wallace, D. Association of mitochondrial DNA damage with aging and coronary atherosclerotic heart disease. Mutat. Res. 1992, 275, 169–180.
6. De Sandre-Giovannoli, A.; Bernard, R.; Cau, P.; Navarro, C.; Amiel, J.; Boccaccio, I.; Lyonnet, S.; Stewart, C.L.; Munnich, A.; Le Merrer, M. Lamin a truncation in Hutchinson-Gilford progeria. Science 2003, 300, 2055.
7. Fontana, L.; Partridge, L.; Longo, V.D. Extending healthy life span—From yeast to humans. Science 2010, 328, 321–326.
8. Freije, J.M.; López-Otín, C. Reprogramming aging and progeria. Curr. Opin. Cell Biol. 2012, 24, 757–764.
9. Glickman, M.H.; Ciechanover, A. The ubiquitin-proteasome proteolytic pathway: Destruction for the sake of construction. Physiol. Rev. 2002, 82, 373–428.
10. Harrison, D.E.; Strong, R.; Sharp, Z.D.; Nelson, J.F.; Astle, C.M.; Flurkey, K.; Nadon, N.L.; Wilkinson, J.E.; Frenkel, K.; Carter, C.S. Rapamycin fed late in life extends lifespan in genetically heterogeneous mice. Nature 2009, 460, 392–395.
11. Hartl, F.U.; Bracher, A.; Hayer-Hartl, M. Molecular chaperones in protein folding and proteostasis. Nature 2011, 475, 324–332.
12. Herrera, E.; Samper, E.; Martin-Caballero, J.; Flores, J.M.; Lee, H.W.; Blasco, M.A. Disease states associated with telomerase deficiency appear earlier in mice with short telomeres. EMBO J. 1999, 18, 2950–2960.
13. Hoenicke, L.; Zender, L. Immune surveillance of senescent cells—Biological significance in cancer-and non-cancer pathologies. Carcinogenesis 2012, 33, 1123–1126.
14. Hsu, A.-L.; Murphy, C.T.; Kenyon, C. Regulation of aging and age-related disease by DAF-16 and heat-shock factor. Science 2003, 300, 1142–1145.
15. Kanfi, Y.; Naiman, S.; Amir, G.; Peshti, V.; Zinman, G.; Nahum, L.; Bar-Joseph, Z.; Cohen, H.Y. The sirtuin SIRT6 regulates lifespan in male mice. Nature 2012, 483, 218–221.
16. Kirkwood, T.B. Understanding the odd science of aging. Cell 2005, 120, 437–447.
17. Leak, R.K. Heat shock proteins in neurodegenerative disorders and aging. J. Cell Commun. Signal. 2014, 8, 293–310.
18. Lee, H.W.; Blasco, M.A.; Gottlieb, G.J.; Horner, J.W., II; Greider, C.W.; DePinho, R.A. Essential role of mouse telomerase in highly proliferative organs. Nature 1998, 392, 569–574.
19. Levine, B.; Klionsky, D.J. Development by self-digestion: Molecular mechanisms and biological functions of autophagy. Dev. Cell 2004, 6, 463–477.
20. Liu, G.; Rogers, J.; Murphy, C.T.; Rongo, C. EGF signalling activates the ubiquitin proteasome system to modulate C. elegans lifespan. EMBO J. 2011, 30, 2990–3003.

21. Longo, V.D.; Antebi, A.; Bartke, A.; Barzilai, N.; Brown-Borg, H.M.; Caruso, C.; Curiel, T.J.; De Cabo, R.; Franceschi, C.; Gems, D. Interventions to slow aging in humans: Are we ready? Aging Cell 2015, 14, 497–510.

22. López-Otín, C.; Blasco, M.A.; Partridge, L.; Serrano, M.; Kroemer, G. The hallmarks of aging. Cell 2013, 153, 1194–1217.

23. Lord, C.J.; Ashworth, A. The DNA damage response and cancer therapy. Nature 2012, 481, 287–294.

24. Masoro, E.J. Overview of caloric restriction and ageing. Mech. Ageing Dev. 2005, 126, 913–922.

25. Olovnikov, A.M. Telomeres, telomerase, and aging: Origin of the theory. Exp. Gerontol. 1996, 31, 443–448.

26. Peleg, S.; Sananbenesi, F.; Zovoilis, A.; Burkhardt, S.; Bahari-Javan, S.; Agis-Balboa, R.C.; Cota, P.; Wittnam, J.L.; Gogol-Doering, A.; Opitz, L.; et al. Altered Histone Acetylation Is Associated with Age-Dependent Memory Impairment in Mice. Science 2010, 328, 753–756.

27. Powers, E.T.; Morimoto, R.I.; Dillin, A.; Kelly, J.W.; Balch, W.E. Biological and chemical approaches to diseases of proteostasis deficiency. Annu. Rev. Biochem. 2009, 78, 959–991.

28. Rogina, B.; Helfand, S.L. Sir2 mediates longevity in the fly through a pathway related to calorie restriction. Proc. Natl. Acad. Sci. USA 2004, 101, 15998–16003.

29. Rubinsztein, D.C.; Mariño, G.; Kroemer, G. Autophagy and aging. Cell 2011, 146, 682–695.

30. Rudolph, K.L.; Chang, S.; Lee, H.W.; Blasco, M.; Gottlieb, G.J.; Greider, C.; DePinho, R.A. Longevity, stress response, and cancer in aging telomerase-deficient mice. Cell 1999, 96, 701–712.

31. Tissenbaum, H.A.; Guarente, L. Increased dosage of a sir-2 gene extends lifespan in Caenorhabditis elegans. Nature 2001, 410, 227–230.

32. Tomaru, U.; Takahashi, S.; Ishizu, A.; Miyatake, Y.; Gohda, A.; Suzuki, S.; Ono, A.; Ohara, J.; Baba, T.; Murata, S. Decreased proteasomal activity causes age-related phenotypes and promotes the development of metabolic abnormalities. Am. J. Pathol. 2012, 180, 963–972.

33. Tomás-Loba, A.; Flores, I.; Fernández-Marcos, P.J.; Cayuela, M.L.; Maraver, A.; Tejera, A.; Borrás, C.; Matheu, A.; Klatt, P.; Flores, J.M. Telomerase reverse transcriptase delays aging in cancer-resistant mice. Cell 2008, 135, 609–622.

34. Wallace, D.C. A mitochondrial paradigm of metabolic and degenerative diseases, aging, and cancer: A dawn for evolutionary medicine. Annu. Rev. Genet. 2005, 39, 359–407.

35. Westerheide, S.D.; Anckar, J.; Stevens, S.M.; Sistonen, L.; Morimoto, R.I. Stress-inducible regulation of heat shock factor 1 by the deacetylase SIRT1. Science 2009, 323, 1063–1066.

Chapter 3

PRINCIPLES AND THEORIES OF AGING

Contents

Introduction

Gerontology is the scientific study of the processes and problems of aging from all aspects — biological, clinical, psychological, sociological, legal, economic and political. Geriatrics is the branch of medicine concerned with the diagnosis, management and prevention of medical problems associated with senility and aging.

Although the terms "aging" and "senescence" are sometimes used interchangeably, they are often distinguished by biologists. For example, Leopold (1978), a plant biologist, said that aging consists of "the processes associated with the increase in maturity over time, while senescence can be defined as the deteriorative processes that are natural causes of death." This means that aging begins at birth.

However, most gerontologists are primarily concerned with the age-related changes in structure and function that occur after maturation. Maturation is usually defined as the attainment of sexual maturity and the adult stage of morphology and physiology.

Furthermore, most gerontologists would not consider phenomena that are strictly linked to chronological time as fundamental, intrinsic aging processes. For example, changes (racemization) of amino acids in the lens of the eye indicate how old an animal is, but do not distinguish between the aging rate of a short-lived mammal, such as a mouse, and that of a long-lived mammal, such as a human.

No one disputes that the developmental events before maturation are of enormous importance in setting the stage for the patterns of postmaturational aging.

Thus, it is conceivable that disruption of some aspect of development (e.g., alteration of some stem cell pools due to environmental influences) would have drastic effects on some aging processes decades later. For example, depletion of the progenitors of substantia nigra neurons could increase the likelihood of early onset of Parkinson's disease. A change in the apparent thresholds for many other pathophysiologic phenomena associated with aging could be in part such a cause.

However, the elderly population is the focus of gerontology and this report because they may be particularly susceptible to many environmental factors due to normal age-related changes in cellular structure and function, a general reduction in the ability to maintain physiologic homeostasis, and acquired changes due to environmental exposures. It is conceivable that environmental agents act at every stage of the life cycle.

Exactly how they affect aging processes is not known, as this topic has not yet been sufficiently researched and the aging processes themselves have not been adequately described.

Variations in environmental exposure and genetic constitution make it very difficult to establish general indices of aging, and a satisfactory analysis of aging processes must deal with the complexity of the relationships between gene expression and environment. In humans in particular, genetic heterogeneity and environmental heterogeneity are so great that no two individuals are likely to manifest aging in exactly the same way — not even identical twins.

The genetic concepts of genotype and phenotype need to be defined. Johannsen (1909) originally defined the genotype, now commonly referred to as the genome, as the sum of the genetic information contained in the chromosomes of an organism. Today we know that non-chromosomal inheritance exists (e.g., via mitochondrial DNA), and the term "genotype" is used to encompass all possible forms of genetic information that define a cell or organism, and to refer to the particular form (allele) of a single gene or small group of genes. Until the advent of recombinant DNA technology, the genotype of an organism was largely derived from mating experiments. Now a specific DNA segment can be directly isolated, clonally amplified and analyzed.

Johannsen (1909) defined the phenotype as the sum of the observable characteristics (structural, biochemical and physiological) of an organism or cell. The phenotype of senescence (or the phenotype of aging) can be described as the totality of properties that are generally assumed to characterize senescence (or aging). Gerontologists disagree on the extent to which age-related diseases should be considered integral features of this phenotype. One view is that every age-related degenerative or proliferative disease has a pathogenesis that does not necessarily involve an underlying component of intrinsic aging.

Another view is that many common age-related human diseases are ultimately an expression of an underlying, slowly progressive and insidious aging process — for example, various forms of arteriosclerosis, including atherosclerosis and medial calcinosis; microvascular disease; glomerulosclerosis, osteoarthritis, osteoporosis, adult-onset diabetes, chronic obstructive pulmonary disease, presenile dementia, Parkinson's disease, cataracts, macular degeneration and a variety of atrophies, hyperplasias and neoplasms.

Phenotypic expression is the result of the interaction between inherited genetic potential and the mosaic of environmental experiences.

Due to differences in inheritance and environmental experiences, patterns of phenotype, including disease, vary. However, lifespan is a constitutional trait of a species, and although environmental influences can easily modulate the lifespan of populations, in most cases lifespan is not affected. Since lifespan appears to be under polygenetic control, encompassing multiple aging processes, one would not expect a single environmental intervention to have global effects on lifespan.

Advances in experimental genetics may make it possible to critically examine the structural and regulatory role of allelic variation and mutation at specific genetic loci. The mouse *Mus musculus domesticus*, the worm *Caenorhabditis elegans* and the fruit fly *Drosophila melanogaster* are the preferred organisms for such studies. The maximum lifespan of *C. elegans*, for example, is directly genetically controlled (Johnson, 1987). In rodents, considerable progress is being made in dietary restriction as a means of extending lifespan in experimental cohorts.

These two approaches, genetic and dietary, may help to identify the fundamental features of aging and thus set the stage for more rational research into the environmental factors that promote aging.

Any number of toxic environmental influences can shorten life. One task of the gerontologist is to determine which of them can influence intrinsic aging processes. A substance that accelerates the onset or progression of a particular process or processes could be labeled "gerontogenic."

Such environmental exposures can be expected to cause the premature onset or accelerated progression of functional decline and age-related disease, thereby affecting quality of life in later decades. However, much more research into the basic mechanisms of aging is needed before we can definitively assess possible environmental factors that influence the aging process.

Both longitudinal studies on the environmental influences on aging in individuals and large-scale cross-sectional studies on population groups will be important to find out how aging and the environment are related. In longitudinal studies, observations are linked to different points in time.

In cross-sectional studies, measurements of cause and effect are linked to one point in time. Cross-sectional studies are prone to interpretation difficulties, particularly cohort and selection effects over time.

Figure 3.1 illustrates the differences between comparable data collected in cross-sectional and longitudinal studies (in this case, data on cognitive function).

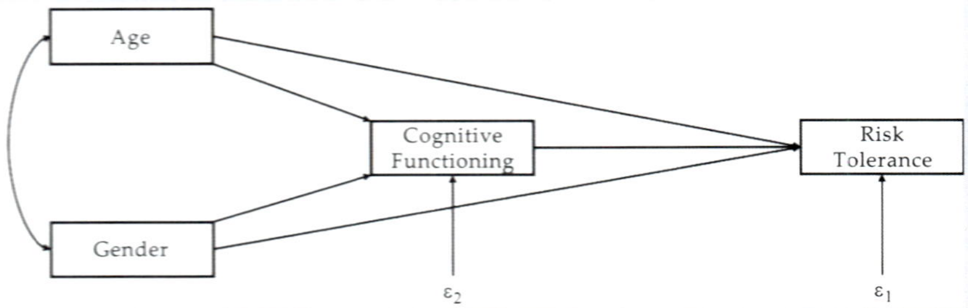

Figure 3.1. Cross-sectional and longitudinal differences with age in performance on a test of cognitive function.

Source: *Sharma M, Chatterjee S. Cognitive functioning: An underlying mechanism of age and gender differences in self-assessed risk tolerance among an aging population. Sustainability. 2021; 13(4):2361. https://doi.org/10.3390/su13042361.*

The development of changes with age has fascinated evolutionary biologists for at least 40 years. Normally, aging is not beneficial to either the individual or the species, but it seems likely that the changes are inevitable consequences of the action of selective forces (Charlesworth, 1980). They may be due to the accumulation of late-acting deleterious genes (Medawar, 1952) or to the action of genes that are beneficial early in life but deleterious later (Williams, 1957). Various theories of the evolution of aging have been put forward, but the "throwaway soma" theory of Kirkwood (1985), which states that "fitness is maximized at a level of repair lower than would be required for indefinite somatic survival," seems to encompass most of the alternatives .

Orientation and Directional Terms:

Term	Definition	Illustration
Theories of aging	Various hypotheses explaining the biological processes that lead to aging, including genetic, cellular, and environmental factors.	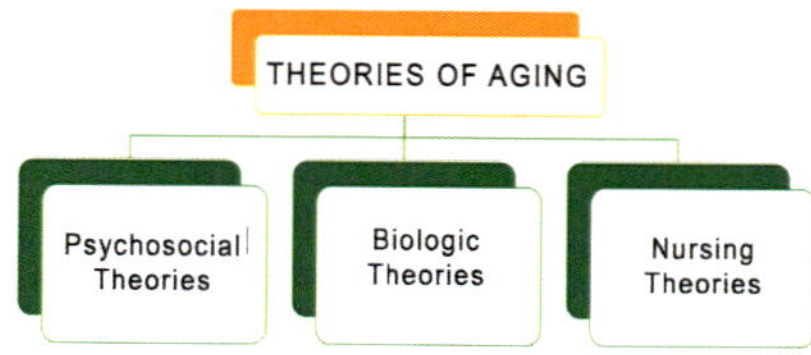
Osteoporosis	A medical condition characterized by weakened bones, increasing the risk of fractures, often due to loss of bone density as a result of aging, hormonal changes, or deficiencies.	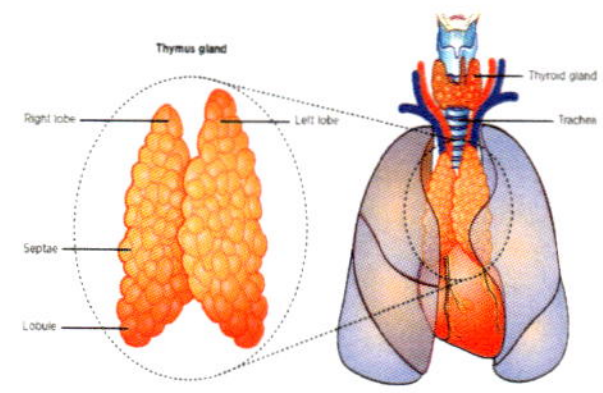
Thymic hormones	Hormones produced by the thymus gland involved in the regulation of the immune system, particularly in the development and function of T lymphocytes.	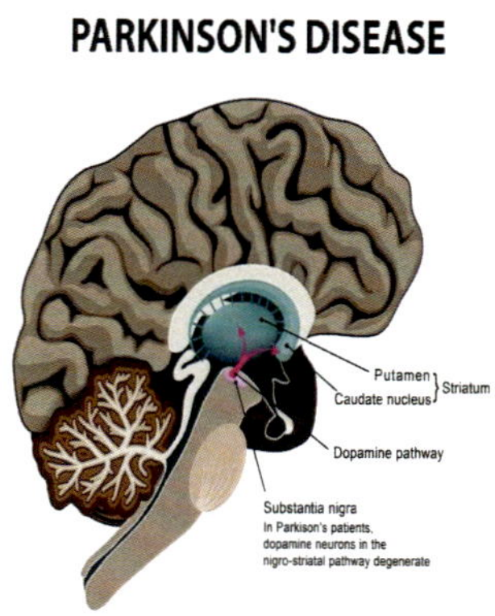
Parkinson's disease	A neurodegenerative disorder affecting movement, characterized by tremors, rigidity, bradykinesia (slowness of movement), and postural instability.	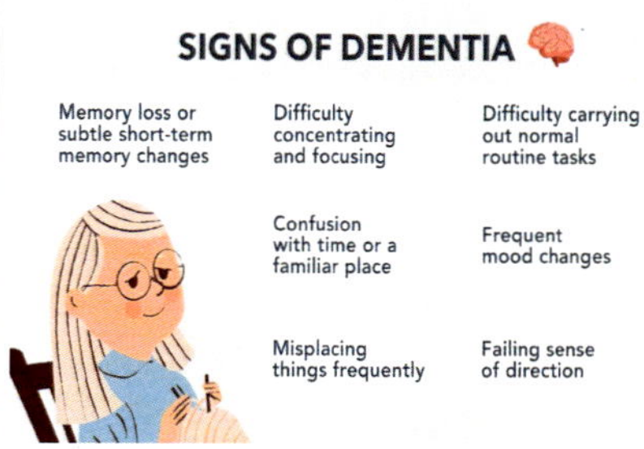
Dementia	A group of symptoms affecting memory, thinking, and social abilities severely enough to interfere with daily functioning, often caused by neurodegenerative diseases.	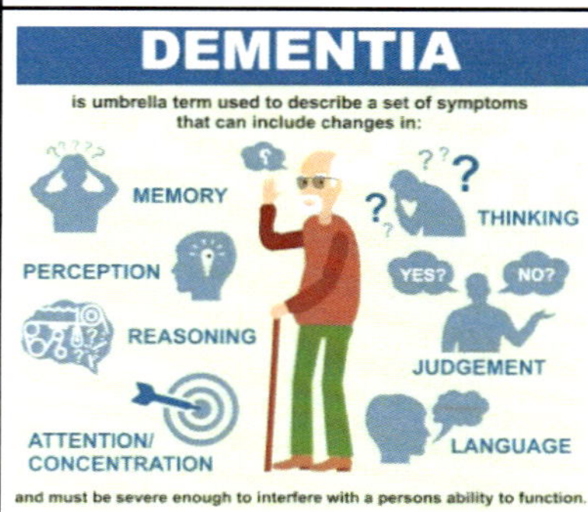

3.1. Theories of Aging

Theories of aging generally fall into two broad categories: those that invoke deterministic or 'program' changes in gene expression or structure, and those that invoke a variety of stochastic or 'random' changes in the structure and function of macromolecules, cells and organ systems.

However, this distinction has its limitations, as stochastic changes in individual cells can lead to predictable phenomena in a large population of cells. An example of the blurring of deterministic and stochastic categorization is the use of terminal differentiation to explain the limited replicative lifespan of somatic cells — that is, cell populations cease to divide because they have differentiated into more specialized cells. For each individual cell, this differentiation is a random event. At the level of a population of many cells, however, the process appears deterministic (Martin et al., 1974; Bell et al., 1978).

Although the idea of terminal differentiation has been applied primarily to the cell culture model of cell senescence (Hayflick and Moorhead, 1961), it could also be applied to cohorts of stem cells in vivo (Martin, 1979). If this idea is correct, any environmental agent, such as retinoic acid, that depletes subsets of cells or alters the state of differentiation could be an important modulator of senescence. Terminal differentiation would also have major effects on cells that proliferate rapidly, such as stem cells during early development (Strickland and Sawey, 1980).

The relative contributions of both classes of mechanisms are likely linked to the reproductive strategy of the organism. Program senescence is characteristic of species with single massive reproductive episodes (e.g., periodic cicadas). Placental mammals have ample opportunity to undergo a variety of stochastic processes during their long reproductive and post-reproductive phases. The associated patterns of structural and functional decline can vary considerably, both qualitatively and quantitatively, and both between and within species.

It is beyond the scope of this report to describe and evaluate the many theories of aging that have been developed in recent decades. (See Warner et al., 1987, for a recent monograph on this topic.) For our purposes, however, it is useful to cite and summarize a few examples to illustrate how an appropriate theoretical framework might serve as a basis for exploring the effects of particular classes of environmental influences on specific aging processes, age-related diseases, or particular vulnerabilities of the elderly.

3.1.1. Deterministic Theories

3.1.1.1. Developmental Switches in Gene Expression

Senescence does not appear to be program in the same way as development, i.e., it is controlled by a series of interconnected gene actions whose primary outcome is a limited lifespan. Only under special conditions in organisms that reproduce only once in a lifetime (semelparent organisms) can senescence be assumed to be directly "program" Senescence does not appear to be controlled by a sequential, systematic switching on and off of new genes; in fact, the transcripts that are formed throughout the adult life of the organism hardly change (Rothstein, 1982).

This is not to say that modulation of transcriptional activity or gradual loss of tight control over gene transcription plays no role in senescence, and a detailed investigation of environmental influences that alter gene expression in ways that suggest an effect on certain aspects of the aging phenotype may be warranted. No examples are yet known, although agents such as amanitin, which interferes with transcription, and cyclohexamide, which interferes with translation, are of potential use.

3.1.1.2. Neuroendocrine-Cascade Theories

Finch and Landfield (1985) have examined a group of theories that can be categorized as neuroendocrine cascade theories. An excellent example is the glucocorticoid cascade hypothesis of aging proposed by Sapolsky et al. (1986b).

The basis of this hypothesis is the finding that the baseline concentration of plasma corticosterone in rats increases with age and that although the increase in plasma corticosterone in response to stress does not change with age, the return to baseline concentrations after the removal of stress is significantly delayed with age. The reason for the age-related changes is a gradual impairment of the negative feedback control of the glucocorticoid concentration in the plasma itself (Sapolsky et al., 1986a). The loss of sensitivity is initially related to the loss of corticosterone receptors in some hippocampal neurons and eventually to the loss of the hippocampal neurons themselves (Sapolsky et al., 1983a). In addition, it is the cumulative exposure to glucocorticoids that is responsible for the decline in glucocorticoid receptors and for the loss of the hippocampal neurons themselves (Sapolsky et al., 1986b). The end result is the appearance of hyperadrenocorticism, largely caused by the stresses of the rat's life. Hyperadrenocorticism could be responsible for many age-related problems, such as immunosuppression, muscle wasting, osteoporosis and glucose intolerance. There is evidence that hyperadrenocorticism underlies, at least in part, age-related diseases in rodents (Riley, 1981b; Sapolsky and Donnelly, 1985).

Although this theory deserves further experimental testing, a major problem is that the changes in adrenocortical function seen in rats with increasing age have not been found in most other species. There is no evidence for such an occurrence in normal human aging, although no systematic studies have been carried out. Such theories are of particular importance to toxicologists as they raise the possibility that global effects on aging follow exposure to certain environmental agents (e.g., stress, glucocorticoids and their analogs, agonists and antagonists of certain receptors, and specific neurotoxins).

3.1.2. Stochastic Theories

3.1.2.1. Intrinsic Mutagenesis Theory

Burnet (1974) summarized the arguments that cumulative damage to genetic material causes aging in mammals. According to this thesis, short-lived mammals are more susceptible to somatic cell mutations than long-lived mammals. This could be the case, for example, if the DNA polymerases of short-lived species were comparatively error-prone or if their various DNA repair mechanisms were comparatively inefficient. This theory is supported by the observation of a positive correlation between the longevity of species and the efficiency of cellular repair of DNA damage caused by ultraviolet light (Hart and Setlow, 1974; Francis et al., 1981).

However, there is controversy about the extent to which such gene mutations accumulate in the tissues of aging mammals (Horn et al., 1984; Trainer et al., 1984; Inamizu et al., 1986). However, various types of chromosomal mutations accumulate with aging (Crowley and Curtis, 1963; Curtis and Miller, 1971; Brooks et al., 1973; Martin et al., 1985). Chromosomal mutations can arise by several mechanisms, including chromosome breaks triggered by free radicals (Nichols and Murphy, 1976), rearrangements following gene amplification (Schimke et al., 1986), and insertional mutagenesis mediated by transposons (jumping genes) (Shapiro, 1983; Collins and Rubin, 1984).

Genomic instability could also arise through mechanisms not associated with the classical forms of somatic cell mutation. The latter, by definition, involve changes in the primary structure of the genetic material (including various rearrangements) as well as changes in the amount of genetic material. Stochastic changes in gene expression could, for example, be due to perturbations in chromatin configuration or DNA methylation patterns. This theory has obvious implications for categories of environmental factors (physical, chemical and viral mutagens) that could accelerate the aging process.

3.1.2.2. Protein-Synthesis Error

Orgel (1963, 1970) argued that errors in the synthesis of proteins involved in the machinery of protein synthesis, either at the transcriptional or translational level, have the potential to cause an overall exponential loss in the reliability of protein synthesis via a positive feedback loop. This loss could lead to an error catastrophe in which a large proportion of proteins in aged cells would be abnormal in structure and function. Since the abnormal proteins are thought to include various DNA-dependent DNA polymerases and DNA repair enzymes, the protein synthesis error catastrophe theory is one of the theories of aging that predict an accumulation of somatic mutations. In addition, the theory predicts a predominance of point mutations (missense and nonsense mutations) and an accumulation that exhibits exponential kinetics toward the end of the natural lifespan. Among the many host genetic loci that could modulate the rate of evolution of errors in protein synthesis, loci controlling the quality and quantity of scavenger proteases would be particularly important, as error catastrophe could be averted by preventing the inheritance of abnormal protein synthesis machinery in successive generations. Many experiments have attempted to support or refute this mechanism of aging, but none can be considered definitive, particularly because few studies have examined the problem in post-replicative cells in vivo (e.g., neurons). However, the bulk of the evidence strongly argues against the general validity of the theory (Gallant, 1981; Rothstein, 1982; Filion and Laughrea, 1985).

From the toxicologist's point of view, this theory would provide a rationale for studying the effects of agents such as amino acid analogs, some of which are found in large concentrations in plants. For example, the concentration of canavanine (an arginine analog) is about 1.5% of the dry weight of alfalfa sprouts and alfalfa seeds (a common natural or organic food) (Bell, 1960) and is toxic to primates (Malinow et al., 1982). Any chemical agent that interferes with the fidelity of protein synthesis would be worthy of further investigation, for example, antibiotics such as streptomycin that interfere with ribosome function and toxins that may interfere with protease function.

3.1.2.3. Free Radicals

Harman first proposed the theory of free radicals as the cause of aging in 1954 (revised by Harman, 1981). Free radicals are constantly generated in living systems by the action of ionizing radiation and a variety of non-enzymatic and enzymatic reactions. In mammals, the main source of free radicals is the consumption of oxygen by the mitochondria for oxidative metabolism; the superoxide radical is an example of the type of free radicals that are generated (Nohl and Hegner, 1978).

The damage caused by these radicals includes oxidative changes in long-lived molecules such as DNA or collagen (LaBella,

1965; Harman, 1981), oxidative degradation of mucopolysaccharides (Matsumura et al., 1966), formation of lipofuscin (Norkin, 1966) and changes in biological membrane characteristics (Hegner, 1980). However, cells have defense mechanisms that protect them from free radical damage, such as antioxidants (e.g., tocopherols and carotenes) (Klebanoff, 1980) and peroxidases and superoxide dismutases (Fridovich, 1977), as well as repair mechanisms, e.g., for DNA (Nichols and Murphy, 1977).

Although the free radical theory is provocative, there is a lack of hard evidence to support it. One approach to testing the theory has been to study the effects of dietary antioxidants on longevity in rodents. In some of the studies, life expectancy was increased, but not lifespan (Harman, 1981). In addition, many of the studies were flawed in that they did not measure food intake or that food intake was reduced (Masoro, 1985).

Further evidence for the free radical theory is the claim that life-prolonging food restriction lowers metabolic rate (Harman, 1981). However, more recent work has shown that food restriction can extend lifespan without reducing metabolic rate (McCarter et al., 1985). However, it is conceivable that food restriction could reduce the flux of active oxygen species independently of metabolic rate. In any case, the free radical theory has important implications for the study of environmental influences on aging, particularly the potential of food and chemical substances to alter the flux of active oxygen species.

3.1.2.4. Posttranslational Glycation of Proteins and DNA

Cerami (1985) suggested that glucose is a mediator of aging. He proposed that the loss of biological function due to the non-enzymatic reaction of glucose with proteins and nucleic acids (the glycation of proteins and nucleic acids), leading to advanced glycosylation end products, is a fundamental mechanism of aging.

Glycation of proteins and nucleic acids begins with the reaction of an amino group with the aldehyde group of glucose to form a Schiff base. Once formed, the unstable Schiff base of glucose can undergo an Amadori rearrangement to form a more stable product, the Amadori product (Mortensen and Christophersen, 1983). The Amadori product can undergo a series of dehydration steps and rearrangements to yield brown fluorescent pigments (Monnier and Cerami, 1981), referred to by Cerami (1985) as advanced glycosylation end products. The end products cross-link proteins and nucleic acids, causing a loss of biological function (Cerami, 1985). The chemical nature of advanced glycosylation end products has not been fully elucidated, but one appears to be 2-(2-furoyl)-4(5)-(2-furanyl)-1H-imidazole (Pongor et al., 1984). The rate of formation of advanced glycosylation end products increases with increasing glucose concentration and duration of glucose exposure (Monnier et al., 1984).

Although this theory of aging is intriguing, there is little solid evidence to support it. Cerami noted that the complications of diabetics are often cited as a paradigm of aging. Of course, these complications could be related to other changes in glucose metabolism or insulin action and not to glycation reactions themselves. Nevertheless, Cerami's glycation theory should be tested further. One starting point is the use of compounds such as aminoguanidine that prevent protein cross-linking by glucose (Brownlee et al., 1986). Another approach is the judicious application of the food restriction paradigm (Masoro, 1985).

3.1.2.5. Thymic Involution as a Pacemaker of Immunosenescence

The morphological and functional regression of the thymus gland is a particularly early and conspicuous precursor of immunological aging in humans and indeed in all mammalian species studied to date (mostly rodents). In humans, the loss of cellular mass of the thymus begins with sexual maturity and is completed at around 50 years of age, when the thymus has only 5–10% of its maximum mass. The conspicuous regression of the thymus gland in the first half of life can therefore be largely linked to the altered form and function of the immune system in the second half of life. These changes are well documented in humans and laboratory animals. The changes in T lymphocytes are particularly remarkable. Two functions of the thymus gland are known: the production of a family of polypeptide hormones and the maturation of T lymphocyte precursors from the bone marrow. The thymic hormones are important for the differentiation of pre- and post-thymic lymphocytes. In humans, the activity of thymic hormones in serum is maintained from birth until the age of 20–30 years and then decreases (Weksler, 1986). In healthy, normal people over the age of 60, thymus hormone can no longer be detected. It is assumed that the low activity of thymus hormone in serum is due to the presence of inhibitors (Weksler, 1986).

Immature lymphocytes from the bone marrow enter the cortex of the thymus gland. With increasing age, fewer immature lymphocytes enter the thymus and the gland loses its ability to promote the differentiation of these cells (Weksler, 1986). Possibly as a result of these events, immature T lymphocytes are found in increased numbers in the blood of older people (Weksler, 1986). Thus, with increasing age, the activity of thymic hormones in the serum decreases and the proportion of immature lymphocytes in the thymus and peripheral blood increases. Environmental influences that have the potential to influence these processes at a young age, either centrally (e.g., specific neurotoxins) or peripherally (e.g., exposure of the thymus to ionizing radiation), are expected to have far-reaching effects on the patterns of immunosenescence in later years.

3.2. Biomarkers of Age or Aging

A biomarker of aging is a biological event or measurement of a biological sample that is considered to be an estimate or predictor of one or more aging processes. The concept has attracted much attention in recent years and has been the subject of two extensive publications (Reff and Schneider, 1982; Ludwig and Masoro, 1983). More recently, biomarkers of aging were discussed at a 1986 workshop on this topic sponsored by the Task Force on Environmental Cancer and Heart and Lung Disease (Baker and Rogul, 1987). The fascination with the concept of biomarkers of aging stems from their immense potential utility (e.g., in the context of this report, to assess the effects of environmental agents on aging processes) and from the superficial suggestion that they are easy to develop. To illustrate the latter idea, consider physiological systems as potential markers. Most physiological systems change with age, and the extent and speed of these changes vary from person to person.

So why is there controversy about the biomarkers of aging? The main reason is that the nature of aging itself is unknown. Even the number of primary aging processes is controversial. Some researchers believe that there is only one primary aging process and that all other aging processes are secondary or even more distant. Most believe that there are multiple primary aging processes, none of which have been clearly identified. And a few believe that aging is not the result of a primary process at all, but is due to subtle changes in the interaction of the components of homeostatic regulatory processes. Because we know so little about the nature of aging, there is no central standard by which we can judge the validity of the many proposed biomarkers of aging. Another aspect of the controversy is related to the various uses that are being considered for biomarkers of aging. The uses can be divided into the following categories: Estimating the chronological age of an individual, estimating the biological or physiological age of an individual, predicting the onset of an age-related disease, predicting imminent death, and predicting the lifespan of a species. Each of these uses should be considered in terms of its relevance to aging.

A biomarker used to estimate chronological age is only of value if the age is unknown. The most important, if not the only, use of such a biomarker is to estimate the age of animals in a colony of animals of unknown age. A good biomarker for this purpose appears to be the racemization of amino acids in structural proteins that are shielded from metabolic turnover (Bada and Brown, 1980).

The problems of biomarkers proposed for estimating the biological or physiological age of an individual are related to the fact that different systems of the same individual may age independently (e.g., graying of hair is unrelated to age-related deafness) and that the rate of aging of an individual may not be constant (Costa and McCrae, 1980). Of course, most researchers interested in determining physiological age have recognized the pitfalls of making assessments based on a single physiological system and have moved to examining multiple systems simultaneously, using either multiple regression analysis (Furukawa et al., 1975) or profile analysis (Borkan, 1978). Costa and McCrae (1985) have pointed out that there is no evidence that such analyzes provide better information about functional age than chronological age itself. Biomarkers used to predict the onset of an age-related disease are generally considered to be risk factors for the disease in question. Elevated arterial blood pressure is a risk factor for stroke (Kannel, 1985), and the ratio of blood concentrations of total cholesterol or arterial low-density lipoprotein to high-density lipoprotein is a risk factor for coronary disease (Gotto, 1986).

These risk factors are at least partially associated with stroke and coronary heart disease, respectively, because they promote the atherosclerotic process (McGill, 1977). However, the relationship between atherosclerosis and aging is not clear. That is, do aging and atherosclerosis merely share the same time frame or are they causally linked? The uncertainty is similar for other age-associated diseases. Therefore, it is questionable whether the predictors of the onset of age-related diseases are valid biomarkers of aging. Predictors of impending death have been considered as biomarkers of aging. For example, impaired lung function predicts a higher mortality rate in the next 4–20 years than in individuals without this impairment (Beaty et al., 1982). But cardiovascular disease and cancer, not lung disease, are the main causes of death. Does this mean that impaired lung function is a biomarker of aging, or is it merely a predictor of two diseases, cancer and cardiovascular disease?

It is not yet possible to answer this question, but the changes in mortality in the United States over the last 150 years suggest the latter. For example, life expectancy and average length of life in the United States have increased significantly since 1840 (U.S. Bureau of the Census, 1984). Most of the increase in life expectancy is due to the control of infectious diseases through technology and medicine, not the aging process. The change in mortality characteristics is an indicator of the extent to which protection from environmental hazards has enabled the population to age. It is consistent with this view that while life expectancy in the United States has increased significantly over the past 150 years, the life span of Americans has not changed. This is a strong indication that changes in mortality characteristics may have little to do with the aging process.

Species lifespan predictors can serve as valid biomarkers of aging. Changes in lifespan are likely due to changes in the rate of aging. It is possible that the lifespan of a species can only be extended by slowing down the aging processes. Only a few manipulations are known to extend lifespan (Sacher, 1977). Low environmental temperatures, food restriction, and genetic manipulations have this effect in poikilotherms, and food restriction has this effect in rodents, the only mammals in which lifespan extension by manipulations has been rigorously demonstrated. Food restriction in rodents delays many age-related physiological changes and age-related diseases (Masoro, 1985), and these are all potential biomarkers of aging. The challenge is to determine whether a particular physiological or disease-related process affected by food restriction is indeed a biomarker of aging or whether it is otherwise related to food restriction. To address this question, we need to make more than one manipulation that affects the lifespan of a particular species. That is, if a physiological or disease-related process can be similarly delayed by multiple manipulations that extend the lifespan of a species, this would strongly suggest that the physiological or disease-related process in question is a biomarker for aging. Therefore, research to identify such manipulations should be a high priority if valid biomarkers of aging are to be developed. Such biomarkers are essential to test the effects of environmental factors on the aging process.

3.3. Altered Susceptibility of the Aged

In many ways, older people show greater individual variation in biological responses than younger people. These variations probably have a greater influence on their intrinsic susceptibility to the effects of toxic substances than physiological aging and preclude generalizations about their susceptibility. Nevertheless, both the increased incidence of disease in the older population and the normal physiological changes that occur with aging even in the absence of disease may make this population more susceptible to environmental exposures. Although few studies have been conducted on the altered response to environmental exposures in aging people, they show that older people tend to respond differently to drugs, both qualitatively and quantitatively, than younger people and have a higher incidence of adverse or idiosyncratic drug reactions (Conrad and Bressler, 1982). It is therefore reasonable to assume that older people would also react differently to other environmental factors. For example, "natural experiments" "such as the air pollution incidents in London, the Meuse Valley in Belgium, and Donora, Pennsylvania, have shown that the elderly – probably due to the normal age-related decline in cardiopulmonary function – and other people with pre-existing diseases of the cardiopulmonary system were the most susceptible. Since the response to pathogens depends on the immune response, the susceptibility of older people to diseases caused by pathogens is increased by the age-related decline in immune function.

One of the most important factors affecting the elderly population is the fact that multiple illnesses are the rule rather than the exception. Past injuries, illnesses and surgeries can be overlaid by a variety of chronic conditions such as cataracts, pernicious anemia, osteoarthritis, osteoporosis, arteriosclerosis and diabetes. Malignant diseases, stroke, Parkinson's disease, dementia and femur fractures occur more frequently in older people. In addition, chronic diseases in the elderly often lead to other complications such as thromboembolism, dehydration, urinary tract infections, pressure sores, hypostatic pneumonia and immobility contractures.

Older people often react differently to the disease, both physically and psychologically. In geriatric patients, the infection is often accompanied by mild tachycardia and mental confusion or other non-specific symptoms. Fever, leukocytosis, lymphadenopathy and lymphangitis may be minimal or absent. Older people appear to be less sensitive to pain and more stoic. Angina pectoris is often atypical, and painless myocardial infarction is more common in the elderly than in younger patients. In addition to the obvious diseases that are so common in older people, there are also important and sometimes subtle physiological changes that accompany the normal aging process. For example, age-related changes in the physiological processes that control the absorption, distribution, metabolism and excretion of drugs have been shown in some cases to affect drug responsiveness in older people and can also be expected to influence response to other toxic substances.

Physiological changes associated with age often alter susceptibility to health impairments, and a person's ability to withstand various environmental influences is often compromised as a result. Many of these changes are well documented, and not all are unique to older people. For example, changes in the immune system occur throughout the life cycle that affect a person's ability to fight off disease. The unfolding of the thymus is probably the most striking anatomical change in the immune system associated with aging. It begins with sexual maturity and is completed by the age of 45–50. The striking increase in influenza mortality in older people is a consequence of this decline in host defense. Aging is also associated with significant changes in the nervous system, which can lead to previously hidden neurotoxic disorders coming to light. It is generally assumed that altered neuronal function only occurs when structural and functional redundancy is depleted. A Parkinsonian state, for example, only occurs after a considerable loss of neurons in the substantia nigra. This can occur both as a result of aging processes and after exposure to certain chemical substances (e.g., N-methyl-4-phenyl-1,2,3,6-tetrahydropyridine, MPTP).

The various changes in the anatomy and function of human skin that are now known to occur with age can increase the susceptibility of older people to chemical and physical environmental influences. For example, the altered barrier function of the stratum corneum (thick layer) of the skin in older people can increase the percutaneous absorption of drugs and other chemicals (Roskos et al., 1986). The important role of the epidermis in the detoxification of percutaneously absorbed chemicals has only recently been recognized (Das et al., 1986) and has not yet been studied in relation to age. The decrease in skin vascular area (Gilchrest et al., 1982a; Montagna and Carlisle, 1979) and vasoreactivity (Gilchrest et al., 1982a; Grove et al., 1981) in aged skin could slow the dermal clearance of topically absorbed substances (Kligman, 1979) and reduce the thermoregulatory capacity of the body. These effects would contribute to hypothermia and heat stroke at extreme temperatures (Besdine, 1980).

The age-related loss of epidermal Langerhans cells (Gilchrest et al., 1982b) is thought to impair the recognition of foreign antigens in the skin, possibly including malignantly altered cells. The well-documented loss of melanocytes (pigment cells) — 10–20% of the remaining cell population per decade (Gilchrest, 1979) — is thought to reduce the body's protection against harmful UV radiation. In combination with the age-related decline in immunocompetence (Schneider and Reed, 1985), this loss could predispose older people to photocarcinogenesis. A decrease in the vitamin D precursor in the epidermis and a reduction in photoconvertibility combined with a lack of dairy products in the diet and a lack of regular sun exposure can easily lead to vitamin D deficiency (MacLaughlin and Holick, 1985) and clinically significant osteomalacia in the elderly (Nordin et al., 1980). Finally, the well-documented age-related decline in sensory perception, including pain perception (Procacci et al., 1974), undoubtedly makes older people more susceptible to certain types of environmental injury.

A Closer Look

Biomarkers of Aging

Biomarkers of aging are measurable indicators that reflect the biological processes of aging and predict the functional capacity and longevity of organisms. These biomarkers help to distinguish between chronological age (actual age in years) and biological age (the physiological condition of an individual).

Key biomarkers include telomere length, which shortens with each cell division and is associated with cellular aging and senescence. Another critical biomarker is DNA methylation patterns, specifically epigenetic clocks, which track age-related changes in gene expression. Additionally, levels of specific proteins such as C-reactive protein (CRP) and interleukin-6 (IL-6) are indicators of systemic inflammation, often increased in aging individuals.

Mitochondrial function is also a significant biomarker, with declining efficiency and increased oxidative stress contributing to the aging process. Biomarkers like insulin-like growth factor-1 (IGF-1) and the hormone dehydroepiandrosterone (DHEA) reflect metabolic and endocrine changes related to aging.

Studying these biomarkers aids in understanding the mechanisms underlying aging, developing anti-aging interventions, and predicting age-related diseases. Advances in this field hold promise for personalized medicine, enabling targeted strategies to enhance health span and lifespan. By identifying and monitoring these biomarkers, researchers can better assess the effectiveness of interventions aimed at mitigating the impacts of aging.

Summary

- Theories of aging aim to explain the biological, psychological, and social processes that contribute to the aging phenomenon. Broadly, these theories can be categorized into biological, psychological, and sociological perspectives. Biological theories include the wear and tear theory, which suggests that cells and tissues wear out over time, and genetic theories, which propose that aging is programmed into our DNA. Psychological theories focus on mental and emotional changes, with the disengagement theory suggesting that aging involves a gradual withdrawal from social roles and relationships, while the continuity theory posits that individuals maintain their previous habits and lifestyle. Sociological theories, such as the activity theory, emphasize the importance of ongoing social engagement and activity for healthy aging. Together, these theories provide a comprehensive framework for understanding the multifaceted nature of aging.

References

1. Aboderin, I. (2004). Modernization and ageing theory revisited: Current explanations of recent developing world and historical Western shifts in material family support for older people. *Ageing & Society, 24*(1), 29–50.
2. Achenbaum, W. A., & Stearns, P. N. (1978). Old age and modernization. *The Gerontologist, 18*(4), 307–312.
3. Adelmann, P. K. (1994). Multiple roles and psychological well-being in a national sample of older adults. *Journal of Gerontology, 49*(6), S277–S285.
4. Atchley, R. C. (1989). A continuity theory of normal aging. *The Gerontologist, 29*(2), 183–190.
5. Baum, W. (1980). Therapeutic value of oral history. *International Journal of Aging & Human Development, 12*(1), 49–53.
6. Bengtson, V. L., Dowd, J. J., Smith, D. H., & Inkeles, A. (1975). Modernization, modernity, and perceptions of aging: A cross-cultural study. *Journal of Gerontology, 30*(6), 688–695.
7. Bishop, A. J., Martin, P., & Poon, L. (2007). Happiness and congruence in older adulthood: A structural model of life satisfaction. *Aging & Mental Health, 10*(4), 445–453.
8. Bishop, A. J., Martin, P., MacDonald, M., & Poon, L. (2010). Predicting happiness among centenarians. *Gerontology, 56*(1), 88–92.
9. Bishop, A. J., Martin, P., Poon, L., & Johnson, M. A. (2011). Exploring positive and negative affect as key indicators of life satisfaction among centenarians: Does cognitive performance matter? *Journal of Aging Research, 2011*, 1–10.
10. Boyle, P. A., Barnes, L. L., Buchman, A. S., & Bennett, D. A. (2009). Purpose in life is associated with mortality among community-dwelling older persons. *Psychosomatic Medicine, 71*(5), 574–579.
11. Butler, R. N. (1964). The life review: An interpretation of reminiscence in the aged. In R. Kastenbaum (Ed.), *New Thoughts on Old Age* (pp. 265–280). Springer.
12. Carnes, B. A., Olshansky, S. J., & Hayflick, L. (2012). Can human biology allow most of us to become centenarians? *The Journals of Gerontology Series A: Biological Sciences and Medical Sciences, 68*(2), 136–142.

13. Carstensen, L. L. (2006). The influence of a sense of time on human development. *Science, 312*(5782), 1913–1915.

14. Carstensen, L. L., Isaacowitz, D. M., & Charles, S. T. (1999). Taking time seriously: A theory of socioemotional selectivity. *American Psychologist, 54*(3), 165–181.

15. Chen, K., Baek, M. J., Kim, K., Park, Y. H., & Kim, S. (2016). The validity and reliability of the mini-mental state examination-2 for detecting mild cognitive impairment and Alzheimer's disease in a Korean population. *PLoS ONE, 11*(10), e0163792.

16. Clarke, A., & Warren, L. (2007). Hopes, fears and expectations about the future: What do older people's stories tell us about active ageing? *Ageing & Society, 27*(4), 465–488.

17. Collins, M., & Bloom, R. (1991). The role of oral history in accounting. *Accounting, Auditing & Accountability Journal, 4*(1), 80–97.

18. Cornwell, B., Laumann, E. O., & Schumm, L. P. (2008). The social connectedness of older adults: A national profile. *American Sociological Review, 73*(2), 185–203.

19. Cumming, E., Dean, L. R., Newell, D. S., & McCaffrey, I. (1960). Disengagement—A tentative theory of aging. *Sociometry, 23*(1), 23–35.

20. Dalby, P. (2006). Is there a process of spiritual change or development associated with ageing? A critical review of research. *Aging & Mental Health, 10*(1), 4–12.

21. Dendinger, V. M., Adams, G. A., & Jacobson, J. D. (2005). Reasons for working and their relationship to retirement attitudes, job satisfaction and occupational self-efficacy of bridge employees. *International Journal of Aging & Human Development, 61*(1), 21–35.

22. Dilworth-Anderson, P., & Cohen, M. D. (2009). Theorizing across cultures. In M. Silverstein, V. L. Bengtson, N. M. Putney, & D. Gans (Eds.), *Handbook of Theories of Aging* (pp. 487–498). Springer.

23. Elo, S., & Kyngäs, H. (2008). The qualitative content analysis process. *Journal of Advanced Nursing, 62*(1), 107–115.

24. Franklin, N. C., & Tate, C. A. (2008). Lifestyle and successful aging: An overview. *American Journal of Lifestyle Medicine, 3*(1), 6–11.

25. Fung, H. H., & Carstensen, L. L. (2004). Motivational changes in response to blocked goals and foreshortened time: Testing alternatives to socioemotional selectivity theory. *Psychology and Aging, 19*(1), 68–78.

26. Gignac, M. A., Cott, C., & Badley, E. M. (2002). Adaptation to disability: Applying selective optimization with compensation to the behaviors of older adults with osteoarthritis. *Psychology and Aging, 17*(4), 520–524.

27. Gondo, Y. (2012). Longevity and successful ageing: Implications from the oldest old and centenarians. *Asian Journal of Gerontology & Geriatrics, 7*(1), 39–43.

28. Hahn, E. A., & Lachman, M. E. (2014). Everyday experiences of memory problems and control: The adaptive role of selective optimization with compensation in the context of memory decline. *Aging, Neuropsychology, and Cognition, 22*(1), 25–41.

29. Hjelmborg, J. V., Iachine, I., Skytthe, A., Vaupel, J. W., McGue, M., Koskenvuo, M., Kaprio, J., Pedersen, N. L., & Christensen, K. (2006). Genetic influence on human lifespan and longevity. *Human Genetics, 119*(3), 312–321.

30. Holtsberg, P. A., Poon, L. W., Noble, C. A., & Martin, P. (1995). Mini-mental state exam status of community-dwelling cognitively intact centenarians. *International Psychogeriatrics, 7*(3), 417–427.

31. Hutnik, N., Smith, P., & Koch, T. (2012). What does it feel like to be 100? Socio-emotional aspects of well-being in the stories of 16 centenarians living in the United Kingdom. *Aging & Mental Health, 16*(6), 811–818.

32. Jewell, A. J. (2014). Tornstam's notion of gerotranscendence: Re-examining and questioning the theory. *Journal of Aging Studies, 30*, 112–120.

33. Knapp, M. R. J. (1977). The activity theory of aging an examination in the English context. *The Gerontologist, 17*(6), 553–559.

34. Lang, F. R. (2001). Regulation of social relationships in later adulthood. *The Journals of Gerontology Series B: Psychological Sciences and Social Sciences, 56*(6), P321–P326.

35. Lansford, J. E., Sherman, A. M., & Antonucci, T. C. (1998). Satisfaction with social networks: An examination of socioemotional selectivity theory across cohorts. *Psychology and Aging, 13*(4), 544–552.

36. Leonard, W. P., Jazwinski, M., Green, R. C., Woodard, J. L., Martin, P., Rodgers, W. L., Johnson, M. A., Hausman, D., Arnold, J., Davey, A., et al. (2007). Methodological considerations in studying centenarians: Lessons learned from the Georgia centenarian studies. *Annual Review of Gerontology & Geriatrics, 27*, 231–264.

37. Ljungquist, B., Berg, S., Lanke, J., McClearn, G. E., & Pedersen, N. L. (1998). The effect of genetic factors for longevity: A comparison of identical and fraternal twins in the Swedish twin registry. *The Journals of Gerontology Series A: Biological Sciences and Medical Sciences, 53A*(6), M441–M446.

38. Lockenhoff, C. E., & Carstensen, L. L. (2004). Socioemotional selectivity theory, aging, and health: The increasingly delicate balance between regulating emotions and making tough choices. *Journal of Personality, 72*(6), 1395–1424.

39. Maddox, G. L., Jr. (1964). Disengagement theory: A critical evaluation. *The Gerontologist, 4*(2), 80–82.

40. Martin, P. (2008). Personality and coping among centenarians. In L. W. Poon & T. T. Perls (Eds.), *Annual Review of Gerontology & Geriatrics* (Vol. 27, pp. 89–106). Springer.

41. Menec, V. H. (2003). The relation between everyday activities and successful aging: A 6-year longitudinal study. *The Journals of Gerontology Series B: Psychological Sciences and Social Sciences, 58*(2), S74–S82.

42. Nimrod, G., & Kleiber, D. (2007). Reconsidering change and continuity in later life: Toward an innovation theory of successful aging. *International Journal of Aging & Human Development, 65*(1), 1–22.

43. Olshansky, S. J., Goldman, D. P., Zheng, Y., & Rowe, J. W. (2009). Aging in America in the twenty-first century: Demographic forecasts from the MacArthur Foundation Research Network on an Aging Society. *Milbank Quarterly, 87*(4), 842–862.

44. Ouwehand, C., de Ridder, D. T. D., & Bensing, J. M. (2007). A review of successful aging models: Proposing proactive coping as an important additional strategy. *Clinical Psychology Review, 27*(7), 873–884.

45. Perls, T. (2003). Understanding the determinants of exceptional longevity. *Annals of Internal Medicine, 139*(6), 445–449.

46. Poon, L. W., Martin, P., Bishop, A., Cho, J., da Rosa, G., Deshpande, N., Hensley, R., MacDonald, M., Margrett, J., Randall, G. K., et al. (2010). Understanding centenarians' psychosocial dynamics and their contributions to health and quality of life. *Current Gerontology and Geriatrics Research, 2010*, 1–13.

47. Poulain, M. (2010). On the age validation of supercentenarians. In *Supercentenarians* (pp. 3–30). Springer.

48. Reichstadt, J., Sengupta, G., Depp, C. A., Palinkas, L. A., & Jeste, D. V. (2010). Older adults' perspectives on successful aging: Qualitative interviews. *American Journal of Geriatric Psychiatry, 18*(6), 567–575.

49. Rhoads, E. C. (1984). Reevaluation of the aging and modernization theory: The Samoan evidence. *The Gerontologist, 24*(3), 243–250.

50. Schroots, J. J. F. (1996). Theoretical developments in the psychology of aging. *The Gerontologist, 36*(6), 742–748.

51. Silverstein, M., Bengtson, V. L., Putney, N. M., & Gans, D. (2009). Theories about age and aging. In M. Silverstein, V. L. Bengtson, N. M. Putney, & D. Gans (Eds.), *Handbook of Theories of Aging* (pp. 3–24). Springer Publishing Company.

52. Silverstein, M., Burholt, V., Wenger, G. C., & Bengtson, V. L. (1998). Parent child relations among very old parents in Wales and the United States: A test of modernization theory. *Journal of Aging Studies, 12*(4), 387–409.

53. Tallmer, M., & Kutner, B. (1969). Disengagement and the stresses of aging. *The Gerontologist, 9*(2), 70–75.

54. Thomson, A. (1998). Fifty years on: An international perspective on oral history. *Journal of American History, 85*(2), 581–595.

55. Tornstam, L. (1999). Gerotranscendence and the functions of reminiscence. *Journal of Aging Identity, 4*(3), 155–166.

56. Tornstam, L. (2011). Maturing into gerotranscendence. *Journal of Transpersonal Psychology, 43*(2), 166–180.

57. Urry, H. L., & Gross, J. J. (2010). Emotion regulation in older age. *Current Directions in Psychological Science, 19*(6), 352–357.

58. Utz, R. L., Carr, D., Nesse, R., & Wortman, C. B. (2002). The effect of widowhood on older adults' social participation: An evaluation of activity, disengagement, and continuity theories. *The Gerontologist, 42*(4), 522–533.

59. Vaupel, J. W. (2010). Biodemography of human ageing. *Nature, 464*(7288), 536–542.

60. Wang, J. D., & Lêng, C. H. (2016). Daily home gardening improved survival for older people with mobility limitations: An 11-year follow-up study in Taiwan. *Clinical Interventions in Aging, 11*, 947–959.

61. Wang, J. J., Lin, Y.-H., & Hsieh, L.-Y. (2011). Effects of gerotranscendence support group on gerotranscendence perspective, depression, and life satisfaction of institutionalized elders. *Aging & Mental Health, 15*(5), 580–586.

62. Wang, K., Duan, G. X., Jia, H. L., Xu, E.S., Chen, X. M., & Xie, H. H. (2015). The level and influencing factors of gerotranscendence in community-dwelling older adults. *International Journal of Nursing Sciences, 2*(2), 123–127.

63. Xie, B., & Bugg, J. M. (2009). Public library computer training for older adults to access high-quality internet health information. *Library & Information Science Research, 31*(3), 155–162.

Chapter 4

TOXICOLOGY AND THE AGING PROCESS: A CRITICAL EXAMINATION

Contents

Introduction

Toxicology is a scientific discipline that possesses a dual nature. Toxicology is the scientific investigation of how environmental agents cause harm to living organisms. It involves determining the extent of toxicity and the associated risk to human populations exposed to these agents. There is no text provided. Toxicology relies heavily on the comparison of experimental findings with extensive databases obtained by subjecting numerous chemicals and types of radiation to standardized test protocols.

To examine the potential impact of environmental agents on the aging process and the heightened vulnerability of elderly individuals to toxicity, it is necessary to analyze the similarities between the mechanisms of aging and the mechanisms of toxicity caused by known harmful substances. Furthermore, it is necessary to identify tests that can be used to screen environmental agents for their ability to interact with aging processes or pose a greater risk to the elderly. Once potential agents that may interact with each other are identified, they need to be assessed in animal models that accurately represent human responses. The chosen species must not only be suitable in terms of aging but also accurately reflect the human response to any specific chemical being tested. Both the identification of shared mechanisms and the development of testing systems need to occur within the framework of the current databases.

Certain individuals perceive aging as a noxious procedure, and in fact, certain age-related functional alterations resemble toxic processes. The process of aging is closely linked to disruptions in the body's ability to maintain balance and the overall health of organs and cells. Many of the changes that occur during aging are similar to those caused by exposure to toxic substances. Therefore, the process of aging could potentially be linked to changes in metabolic states that result in the production of harmful molecules by the body or disruptions in the normal regulation of concentrations of different natural substances within the body. Studies in toxicology have revealed that even substances that are considered unlikely can cause tissue damage when their concentrations deviate significantly from normal levels.

The importance of nutrition highlights the value of viewing aging as a harmful outcome. Both a deficiency and an excess of vitamin B6 can result in neurological damage, which can appear similar to the changes that occur with aging.

Exploring aging as a toxic process is valuable because it is likely the main cause or a contributing factor in all age-related diseases. Moreover, the process of aging cannot be easily halted and is consistently observed in any experiment involving whole animals. Therefore, any harmful processes caused by external factors can interact with the aging process, and the potential impact of this interaction would be more significant with long-term exposures or toxic effects that occur over a significant portion of one's lifetime.

Can chemical or physical agents mimic the toxic process of aging? The comprehensive response to the question is extensively covered in this discussion. However, the concise answer is that numerous agents in the environment can, when administered in high doses, cause pathological alterations and physiological decline that resemble those seen in elderly individuals. This represents a constrained type of imitation, as a specific agent typically only induces a small number of aging characteristics in a single tissue (or possibly a few). Only a limited number of agents, such as ionizing radiation, can cause harm to the entire body.

The lack of universal replication of aging through toxic substances, even within a specific tissue, is a significant observation that should not be exaggerated. A toxic substance may cause molecular damage that resembles the damage caused by aging. However, toxicology has observed that the expression of molecular or cellular harm at the tissue level is not strictly exclusive to the toxic substance. Various agents that are hypothesized to cause similar types of harm at the cellular or molecular level occasionally result in distinct types of harm at the tissue level. On the other hand, various harmful substances can sometimes cause similar pathological effects. This means that different agents can activate the processes that lead to certain effects.

Age-related degeneration affects all bodily tissues. To fully understand the wide-ranging impacts of aging, it is necessary to adopt a comprehensive toxicological approach. It is important to carefully assess databases for long-term whole-animal bioassays. These evaluations are used to analyze the effects of extended exposure to low concentrations of toxic substances, including those that are environmentally significant. They are a crucial tool for quantifying risk.

Greater emphasis should be placed on neurotoxicology and immunotoxicology. A significant number of environmental agents have not undergone testing to determine their potential neurotoxic and immunotoxic effects. Consequently, a considerable portion of the elderly population exhibits neurological and immunological deficits of unknown origin.

From a toxicological standpoint, two primary issues are of utmost concern when examining the connection between the environment and the aging process. The mechanisms underlying aging remain elusive, making it challenging to employ toxicologic techniques for identifying disruptions in the fundamental biological processes associated with aging. Furthermore, the empirical approach is hindered due to the absence of comparative data that can be used to verify any proposed test aimed at identifying agents that specifically impact the process of aging or individuals who are elderly.

An effective strategy for addressing both issues is to investigate the underlying mechanisms of aging and identify compounds that specifically target the aging process or older individuals. A significant amount of effort has been dedicated to the former, while substantial resources would be required for the latter. The primary objective of this report is to suggest a cost-effective and scientifically rigorous strategy for addressing both problems.

Furthermore, three additional types of inquiries need to be investigated in relation to the correlation between chemical toxicity and aging:

- How can agents that could potentially interact with the aging processes to accelerate the onset of pathological effects or decrease resilience in older individuals be identified? Undoubtedly, the conventional long-term bioassay is capable of identifying significant pathological changes that occur with age. However, it remains uncertain whether this method can accurately replicate the exposures that naturally occur in the human environment but are absent in the controlled laboratory setting of the surrogate animal.

How can we identify acute or subacute exposures that occur in utero, during development, or during maturity and sensitize the exposed individuals to other agents? In multistage carcinogenesis, exposure to a cancer initiator can make animals more sensitive to a cancer promoter that they may encounter later. The issue of whether comparable mechanisms contribute to any of the diverse range of pathological effects observed in the elderly is exceedingly challenging to investigate using conventional toxicological tests.

- How can environmental agents, specifically pharmaceuticals that pose a higher risk for the elderly, be recognized? The majority of toxicity assessments are conducted on young animals. Therefore, a more precise inquiry would be whether testing conducted on young animals can accurately forecast the reaction of older animals. If the reactions of young and old animals to a specific substance are similar in nature but vary in degree, the utilization of a safety factor could allow for the adjustment of data obtained from young animals to predict the potential risks in old animals. If there is a difference in the mechanism of action, it would not be possible to make such an extrapolation. In that case, it would be necessary to conduct tests using older animals, which would be costly and lack comparative data.

This chapter provides an overview of the fundamental principles of toxicology, including absorption, distribution, metabolism, and elimination of substances. It also discusses the impact of chemicals on the body in relation to age, the mechanisms of toxicity at different levels of physiological organization, and the significance of pharmacogenetics, biomarkers, and toxicity testing.

Orientation and Directional Terms:

Term	Definition	Illustration
Toxicology	The branch of science concerned with the nature, effects, and detection of poisons and the treatment of poisoning.	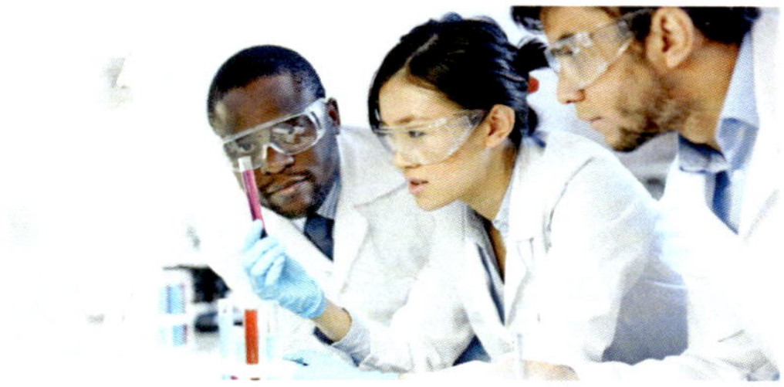
Pharmaceutical agents	Substances used in the diagnosis, treatment, or prevention of diseases and for restoring, correcting, or modifying organic functions.	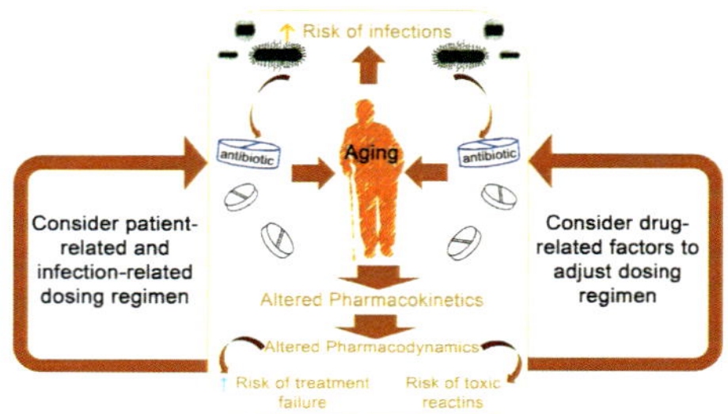
Nonhepatic tissues	Tissues in the body that are not part of the liver.	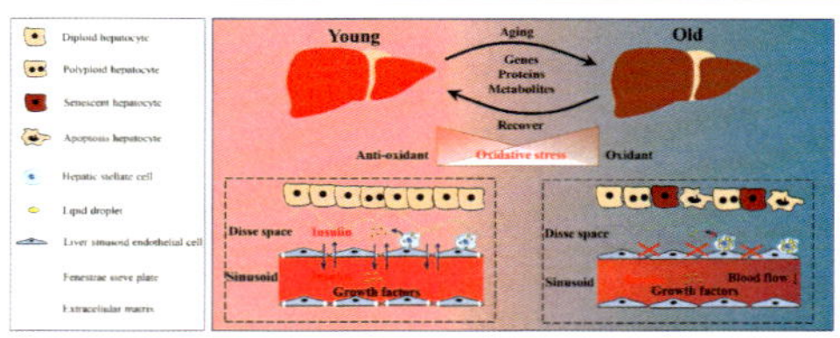
Neuroactive drugs	Substances that affect the nervous system by altering the function of neurons, influencing processes such as mood, cognition, and behavior.	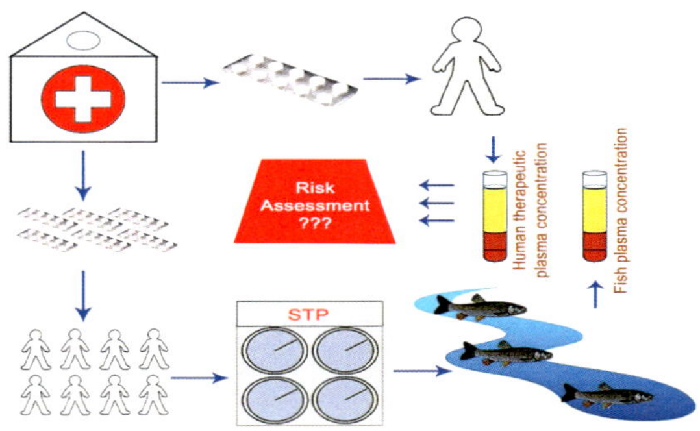
Tubular function	The function of the renal tubules in the kidneys, which involves the reabsorption and secretion of substances to form urine.	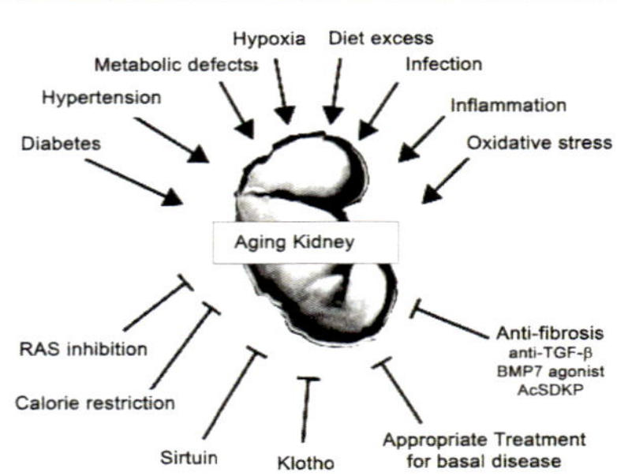

4.1. Chemical Fate and Effect

Chemicals can enter the body through inhalation, ingestion, or skin contact. They have the ability to exert their effects either directly at the specific location of contact, or they can be assimilated, enter the circulatory system, and be conveyed to exert their effects at different locations. Biological transformation and excretion or accumulation at different locations are how toxic agents are removed from the bloodstream. The liver plays a significant role in metabolizing harmful substances, but enzymes in other organs such as the kidneys, lungs, gastrointestinal tract, skin, and other tissues can also break down toxicants. Certain toxic substances tend to accumulate in specific organs or tissues, potentially resulting in toxic effects. The majority of toxic substances are excreted through the urine by the kidney or through the bile by the liver. However, certain volatile toxicants can be eliminated through exhaled air by the lungs.

The majority of research regarding the impact of old age on the absorption, distribution, metabolism, and elimination of chemicals has primarily concentrated on pharmaceuticals, rather than on toxic environmental substances. The biotransformation pathways responsible for the conversion of drugs also play a role in converting toxic chemicals into less toxic or, in some cases, more toxic forms. Therefore, data on drugs can provide valuable insights into toxicological concerns. Several comprehensive reviews of geriatric pharmacology, including studies by Greenblatt et al. (1982), Schmucker (1978, 1985), and Vestal and Dawson (1985), provide information on aging and drug disposition. Unlike pharmaceutical agents, which have data derived from studies involving both animals and humans, almost all the data on toxicants have been exclusively obtained from experimental animals. Moreover, as stated in a monograph authored by Calabrese (1986), the available evidence from human studies and a significant portion of the animal studies pertain to newborn and juvenile individuals. The potential impact of age on the detoxification of carcinogens, the conversion of procarcinogens to carcinogens, and the interaction of carcinogens with potential inducing agents is particularly noteworthy.

Birnbaum (1987) recently conducted a review on age-related alterations in the metabolism of carcinogens in young and old animals. The author concluded that the existing data on this topic were limited and contradictory. The outcomes of metabolic studies are contingent upon factors such as the substrate used, the species being studied, the gender of the subjects, and even the specific strain being examined. There has been a lack of investigation into the alterations that occur with age in the monooxygenase components of nonhepatic tissues. Therefore, while it may be tempting to speculate that age-related alterations in the metabolism of carcinogens could play a role in the higher occurrence of cancer in older individuals, this explanation is overly simplistic. The biotransformation of certain compounds may vary with age in a particular tissue, but these variations may not lead to an increased concentration or prolonged activity of carcinogenic chemicals or reactive metabolites at susceptible target sites.

While some animal studies have indicated that aging does not lead to a decline in the ability of oxidative metabolism to react to inducers like barbiturates, polycyclic hydrocarbons, and steroids, clinical investigators have not focused much on this question. Age can cause changes in various toxicokinetic measures, such as absorption, distribution, renal and biliary excretion, as well as toxicodynamic determinants of tissue sensitivity, in addition to metabolism. Therefore, the heightened susceptibility to carcinogens in older individuals may arise from the intricate interplay of numerous processes that have not been thoroughly examined in either human or animal studies.

Understanding the impact of age on how drugs are absorbed, distributed, metabolized, and eliminated can help us better comprehend why there are changes in how our bodies respond to chemicals in general. When studying age differences in pharmacodynamics, it is important to consider the potential variations in pharmacokinetics. Studies have consistently found that older individuals are more susceptible to the sedative effects of neuroactive drugs like diazepam, as well as the pain-relieving effects of narcotics such as morphine. On the other hand, the responsiveness of the heart to isoproterenol and its antagonist propranolol seems to decrease with age. Furthermore, there is compelling evidence indicating that the cellular biochemical responses to certain drugs are modified as individuals age.

4.1.1. Absorption

Absorption is the primary mechanism through which toxic substances are transported across the membranes of the body. The primary sites for the absorption of toxic substances are the skin, lungs, and gastrointestinal tract. Various toxic substances can penetrate the skin and enter the bloodstream. The skin's permeability can be heightened by chemical or physical injury, as well as other factors. The lung absorbs toxic substances in the form of gases, solid particles, or liquid aerosols. The rapid and complete absorption of substances occurs due to the extensive surface area and the proximity of the blood supply to the inhaled air in the alveoli of the lungs. Various environmental pollutants infiltrate the food chain and are assimilated through the gastrointestinal tract. Several variables can influence the absorption of toxic substances in the gastrointestinal tract, such as the movement of the digestive system, the specific characteristics of the toxic substance, and the contents present in the gastrointestinal tract.

Several physiological changes that occur with advancing age are likely to impact the absorption process in the gastrointestinal tract. The effects encompass an elevation in gastric pH, a decrease in intestinal blood flow, a reduction in the number of absorbing cells, a decline in gastrointestinal motility, and a deceleration of gastric emptying. An elevation in gastric pH can potentially impact the ionization and solubility of certain substances. However, there is limited information available regarding the spectrum of pH levels that may be observed in the elderly population, as well as the consequences of heightened pH on the bioavailability of substances. Elderly individuals experience a decline in gastrointestinal motility and delayed emptying, which is likely to result in a decrease in the absorption rate.

Several studies have demonstrated a rise in the duration it takes for the drug to reach its highest concentration in the blood after being taken orally. The clinical significance of this is minimal as there was no difference in the extent of absorption between young and old subjects. Despite limited data, the majority of studies on drug absorption in older individuals show no significant impact of age on the speed and amount of absorption.

4.1.2. Distribution

Once a toxic substance enters the bloodstream, it can be distributed throughout the body. Only unbound toxicants, which are not attached to plasma proteins, can enter other locations. The process of binding is especially worrisome for toxicologists and medical scientists, as toxic substances that are attached to these proteins can be replaced by other chemical agents. Once released, these substances can then travel to specific organs and cause harm there.

Toxicants are distributed based on their capacity to traverse cell membranes and their attraction to different parts of the body. Toxicants exhibit significant variation in these two characteristics. Certain substances have limited distribution because they do not easily pass through cell membranes. Others attach to different locations within the body, such as adipose tissue, liver, kidneys, or bone. The primary toxic effect of a toxic substance may occur at the site of binding, although this is not always the case. Binding sites frequently function as reservoirs that aid in safeguarding the body against toxic effects.

Various age-related changes can modify the distribution volume of substances throughout the body. Body composition is a highly significant factor. The amount of water in the entire body, both in absolute terms and as a percentage of body weight, decreases by 10–15% from the ages of 20 to 80. Additionally, the proportion of lean body mass to body weight decreases with age, while the amount of body fat increases. These alterations are expected to result in elevated blood concentrations of substances that primarily distribute in body water or lean body mass. Changes in body fat can lead to the buildup and extension of the effects of substances that dissolve easily in fat.

Furthermore, a decline in serum albumin levels in older individuals results in increased availability of substances that have an affinity for serum albumin, such as the anticonvulsant phenytoin, to freely spread into body tissues. On the other hand, the levels of serum a1-acid glycoprotein are higher in older individuals, which leads to a decrease in the binding of weak basic drugs like the antidepressant imipramine and the antiarrhythmic drug lidocaine to plasma proteins. Therefore, changes in plasma-protein binding could potentially be a reason for the altered pharmacokinetics observed in elderly individuals, as the concentration of free-drug plays a crucial role in drug distribution and elimination. Existing data indicate that disease and immobility have a more significant impact on albumin concentration than age alone.

4.1.3. Metabolism and Elimination

Certain chemical agents that enter the body can persist as intact molecules, while others undergo biological transformations through metabolic processes. Metabolic processes may encompass uncomplicated and reversible chemical or physical interactions that predominantly impact the transportation within the body and across membranes. Alternatively, metabolic processes can significantly modify the chemical composition of the toxic substance, resulting in the formation of a more potent or less potent compound. Metabolic processes can aid in the removal of substances from the body.

It has been beneficial to categorize metabolic processes into two distinct types. The first category encompasses oxidation, reduction, or hydrolysis processes that predominantly modify or introduce functional (reactive) groups to the molecule in consideration. The second process involves the chemical reactions of existing or newly formed functional groups on the molecule with different endogenous chemicals, such as amino acids, sulfate, and glucuronic acid. These reactions result in the formation of conjugates or new chemicals. The biosynthesis of these products frequently modifies the lipid or water solubility and ionization properties in a manner that facilitates their release and elimination.

The primary pathways for excretion of chemical agents from the body include renal elimination via urine, hepatic elimination via bile into feces, and pulmonary elimination via exhaled air. Minor routes encompass excretions from the body, such as perspiration, tears, saliva, mucus, digestive fluids, and milk, as well as hair, nails, and shed epithelial tissue. As previously stated, factors such as age and disease state can disrupt kidney function or biliary excretion in the liver, thereby impacting the toxicity of chemicals in the body.

The excretory mechanisms of the kidney involve the process of filtration occurring in the glomeruli, as well as the processes of secretion and reabsorption taking place in the renal tubules. The elimination through the kidneys depends on factors such as the blood flow to the kidneys, the size of the molecule in relation to the size of the glomerular filter, the physicochemical properties of the molecule that affect its transport across the membrane, and the presence of enzymatic or other systems that can enhance secretion and reabsorption. Chemicals that attach to large molecules, like plasma proteins, may not be removed through filtration and can remain in the body for extended periods of time.

The liver plays a crucial role in eliminating ingested chemicals, as it receives the majority of blood from the gastrointestinal tract before it enters the general circulation. The liver possesses distinctive capabilities to metabolize a chemical using its enzymatic systems and subsequently excrete the resulting metabolites into the bile. Bile is discharged into the intestines, where it can undergo additional modifications and reabsorption or be excreted in the feces. Liver injury frequently impacts biliary function, leading to impairment of this pathway for elimination.

Pharmacokinetic measurements can be used to study the removal of chemicals from the body. These measurements typically involve analyzing the concentration of a chemical or its metabolites in the blood over time. This information typically offers a reliable approximation of the quantity of the chemical accessible for toxic effects. Nevertheless, the storage of the chemical in tissue depots or the toxicity of unmeasured, activated, intermediate chemical forms can occasionally be of greater significance.

The metabolic and elimination processes can be changed in older individuals, but there is only indirect evidence of altered drug metabolism in the liver of humans. Autopsy studies have shown that the liver's mass relative to body weight decreases after middle age, and that liver blood flow decreases as age increases. Age does not have a significant impact on the metabolism of certain drugs, particularly those that undergo conjugation in the liver. Nevertheless, the impact of age on drug metabolism rates, specifically for drugs that undergo oxidation in the liver, seems to be inconsistent. The considerable differences in drug metabolism among individuals are more likely attributable to a combination of genetic and environmental factors. The existing data suggest that age does not have an impact on the inhibition of drug metabolism, as shown by studies conducted by Divoll et al. (1982) and Vestal et al. (1987). However, the available data on the vulnerability of elderly individuals to the induction of hepatic drug metabolism are limited and contradictory. Some studies, such as those conducted by Salem et al. (1978) and Twom-Barina et al. (1984), indicate a decrease in the extent of induction in the elderly, while others, like Crowley et al. (1986) and Pearson and Roberts (1984), show no age differences. Additional research is needed to explore the impact of age on the initiation and suppression of drug metabolism, as well as other interactions with drugs.

Cigarette smoke contains polycyclic hydrocarbons, which are powerful stimulators of certain forms of cytochrome P-450 enzymes. Most cross-sectional studies have shown that cigarette smoking is linked to reduced biotransformation induction in the elderly compared to young individuals. The determination of whether this phenomenon is inherent to the aging process or is caused by selective mortality can only be achieved through longitudinal studies, which have not yet been conducted. However, it is important to consider the potential for significantly decreased ability of certain elderly patients to process and remove drugs when prescribing medications for them. This can be achieved by either decreasing the dosage of potent drugs with low therapeutic indexes or closely monitoring patients to ensure the effectiveness of prescribed medications and early detection of undesirable drug-related side effects (Figure 4.1).

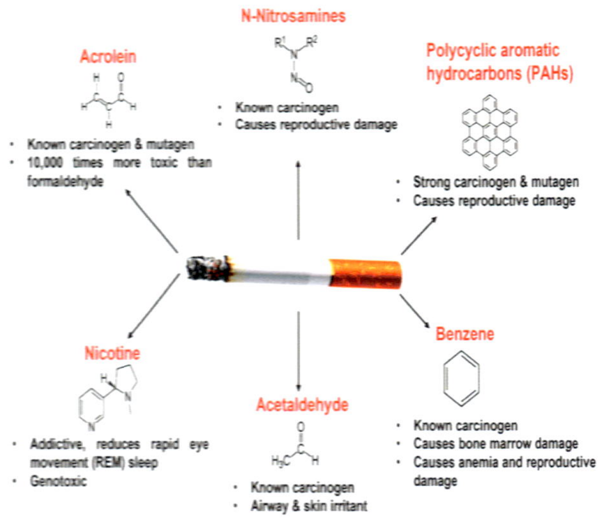

Figure 4.1. *Cigarette smoke contains more than 4000 chemicals that exert cytotoxic, mutagenic, and carcinogenic effects.*

Source: Agraval H, Chu HW. Lung organoids in smoking research: Current advances and future promises. Biomolecules. 2022; 12(10):1463. https://doi.org/10.3390/biom12101463.

Research conducted on aging laboratory animals has demonstrated a decrease in the activity of liver enzymes, leading to a reduced ability to process drugs and a decrease in the stimulation of liver enzymes. The majority of the data has been obtained from experiments conducted on rats and mice. It should be noted that the observed age-related changes may not apply to all species, strains, and sexes, as these factors are significant variables in rodent studies. Research conducted on liver tissue from nonhuman primates has not demonstrated a notable decrease in the levels of cytochrome P-450 or the specific function of NADPH cytochrome c (P-450) reductase, as reported by Schmucker and Wang in 1987. Similarly, limited in vitro studies conducted with human liver tissue have demonstrated that age does not have an impact on microsomal drug-metabolizing activity (Woodhouse et al., 1984). The results are inconsistent with those obtained in rodents, and to a certain degree, they are also inconsistent with in vivo studies conducted in humans. (No studies have been conducted on nonhuman primates in a live setting.) However, it is important to note the challenges in applying findings from experiments on animals to humans, and the necessity of clinical research to assess how drugs and chemicals are metabolized in humans.

Alcohol is a significant chemical compound that is extensively utilized as a pharmaceutical substance by individuals of nearly all age groups. Alcohol is evenly dispersed throughout the entire volume of water in the body. The volume of distribution of this substance decreases with age in both rodents and humans (Wiberg et al., 1971; Vestal et al., 1977). The decrease leads to higher blood concentrations in the elderly compared to the young, even when equivalent doses are given. Short-term alcohol consumption hinders, while long-term consumption promotes the process of breaking down drugs through oxidation in a healthy liver. The primary oxidation of alcohol occurs through the action of alcohol dehydrogenase, an enzyme found in the cytoplasm of the liver cells. Additionally, a smaller amount of oxidation is carried out by the hepatic microsomal enzyme system. While older individuals may be more susceptible to the behavioral and cognitive impacts of alcohol, research has not shown any variations in alcohol metabolism based on age in humans (Vestal et al., 1977). Research conducted by Wiberg et al. (1970) has demonstrated that age affects the process of alcohol metabolism in rats.

The dietary composition plays a crucial role in determining how drugs are metabolized and their potential for causing harm (Alvares et al., 1979; Campbell and Hayes, 1974). The majority of studies have been carried out on laboratory animals (Campbell and Hayes, 1974). Research conducted on individuals without health issues has demonstrated that a diet low in carbohydrates and high in protein (Kappas et al., 1976), as well as consuming charcoal-broiled beef (Kappas et al., 1978), can enhance the metabolism of antipyrine and theophylline. Additionally, the consumption of Brussels sprouts and cabbage (Pantuck et al., 1979) can increase the metabolism of antipyrine and phenacetin. Charcoal-grilled beef contains benzo[a]pyrene and other polycyclic hydrocarbons, as discovered by Lijinsky and Shubik in 1964. These substances have been found to enhance the metabolism of benzo[a] pyrene in the liver and placenta of rats, as observed by Harrison and West in 1971. According to Wattenberg (1971), Brussels sprouts, cabbage, turnips, broccoli, cauliflower, and spinach stimulate the activity of benzo[a] pyrene hydroxylase in rats. (Loub et al., 1975; Pantuck et al., 1976).

It is necessary to investigate the potential differences between the elderly and younger adults in their response to changes in carbohydrates, protein, polycyclic hydrocarbons, cruciferous vegetables, and other components of their diet. There has been some focus on clinical conditions caused by a lack of essential nutrients. Administering ascorbic acid to elderly patients with a deficiency of this compound resulted in an elevation of antipyrine plasma clearance. However, there were no initial differences in baseline values between patients with and without the deficiency, and ascorbic acid treatment had no impact on the nondeficient group (Smithard and Langman, 1978). A separate study conducted by Trang et al., in 1982 found that alterations in dietary ascorbic acid had no impact on caffeine metabolism in older individuals. Insufficient evidence exists to support the claim that poor nutrition and dietary habits directly cause the intricate alterations observed in hepatic drug metabolism in older individuals (Cusack and Denham, 1984).

Unlike hepatic function, reduced renal function is prevalent and can be readily quantified in older individuals. Research has shown that the process of aging has an impact on both glomerular function and tubular function. The glomerular filtration rate, as determined through the measurement of inulin or creatinine clearance, has the potential to decrease by up to 50%. The renal plasma flow decreases by approximately 2% annually. The decrease in renal function reduces the rate at which drugs that are excreted unchanged by the kidney are eliminated. Reducing the maintenance doses of drugs, such as aminoglycoside antibiotics and cardiac glycoside digoxin, is frequently required in clinical medicine to avoid toxicity.

The variability of renal function decline is evident, as some individuals demonstrate minimal or no observable decline (Lindeman et al., 1985). Hence, it is imperative in clinical practice to assess plasma levels of potentially harmful medications and modify dosages accordingly to attain therapeutic concentrations. Not only do geriatric patients, but also fetuses, neonates, and children exhibit rates of drug elimination that deviate from those observed in typical adults and can vary significantly depending on the specific drug and individual. Antipyrine and phenylbutazone elimination in children aged 1–8 years was approximately twice as rapid as in typical adults, as demonstrated by Alvares et al. in 1975. Eight children who did not show any clinical symptoms of acute or chronic lead poisoning, but had biochemical manifestations, had similar rates of antipyrine and phenylbutazone elimination as normal children. However, two children who showed both clinical and biochemical signs experienced longer plasma antipyrine half-lives. The half-lives of children returned to the typical range after the implementation of chelation therapy. Other studies have found similar outcomes, revealing that children experience faster elimination of diazoxide (Pruitt et al., 1973), phenobarbital (Garretson and Dayton, 1970), and clindamycin (Kauffman et al., 1972) compared to adults.

Human fetuses and neonates have a significantly lower ability than children or adults to remove drugs from their bodies. However, unlike certain rodents, human fetuses and neonates do show some level of measurable drug-metabolizing activity in the liver (Rane and Sjoqvist, 1972; Pelkonen et al., 1973). Premature infants exhibit lower rates of drug elimination compared to full-term healthy newborns. Plasma indomethacin half-lives were 2 and 24 hours in two premature infants (Friedman et al., 1978), while the average value was 4.7 hours in full-term healthy newborns (Traeger et al., 1973) and 2–3 or 7.2 hours in healthy adults (Hucker et al., 1966; Duggan et al., 1972; Palmer et al., 1974). The notable variations in the rates at which premature infants, full-term newborns, children, and adults eliminate substances from their bodies have practical importance when determining the correct dosages. Furthermore, they suggest the necessity of examining the pharmacokinetic and pharmacodynamic mechanisms of numerous drugs across different age cohorts.

All the aforementioned characteristics are crucial when examining the impact of environmental chemicals on the aging process. If the impact of chemicals on the aging process imitates other health effects in humans, it is unlikely that all individuals in an exposed population will respond uniformly. The extensive genetic diversity within the human population guarantees that individuals with similar levels of exposure to environmental chemicals will still exhibit varying responses.

4.2. Mechanisms of Toxicity at the Molecular, Cellular, and Tissue Level

Toxic agents employ a wide range of mechanisms to exert their actions. The mechanisms differ among particular agents and among different doses of the same agent. The mechanisms of toxic action can be defined by the dosage at which the fundamental toxic effect is triggered and by the specificity of that effect. This characterization is particularly applicable when studying aging, as it describes the decline in physiological systems that occurs with age and the lack of specificity in terms of affected cells and tissues. This characterization has been observed in elderly individuals, although the precise mechanism of aging remains unknown.

4.2.1. Molecular Action

Toxic agents can cause harm by generating destructive chemical species that target specific components of biological molecules. To investigate the toxic mechanisms that are common to aging and specific toxic agents, it is important to consider agents with a wide-ranging impact, as aging has a broad effect on all tissues. Various mechanisms can lead to a wide range of actions. An equally desirable outcome would be the identification of agents that have a specific molecular mechanism of action that can influence a particular aspect of the senescent phenotype. This would enable a more detailed analysis of the underlying mechanisms.

Damage can be caused to a particular molecule, which can then lead to a wide range of harmful effects due to its changed function. An instance of DNA damage with pleiotropic consequences serves as an example. General toxic effects can also occur due to the action of agents that cause molecular damage by producing a harmful species. Ionizing radiation and various chemical agents can generate free radicals either through direct means or via intrinsic metabolic processes. Free radicals, either directly or through a series of reactions, can interact with various biomolecules or cause different types of damage that can have varying effects on living organisms.

Moreover, different tissues can have varying levels of susceptibility to exposure, with each tissue being affected at different magnitudes. When ionizing radiation, such as X-rays, is used, it creates different types of ions and radicals in the tissue that is exposed to it. Excessive doses of X-rays (over 100 Gy) can rapidly or within a few hours cause the central nervous system to fail in humans who are not protected. At lower doses of radiation (10 Gy), the primary harmful effect is the suppression of the growth and division of the stem cells located in the gut crypts. This suppression causes the lining of the intestines to become exposed and results in death within a few days. At lower doses of 1 Gy, X-rays not only disrupt the hematopoietic system but also elevate the incidence of cancer in populations exposed to radiation. When exposed to X-rays at doses below 1 Gy, there is an increased risk of both cancer and heritable mutations. However, cancer is considered to be the more significant risk. Both epidemiologic and animal studies have observed the responses to lower exposures. According to previous research (Lindop and Rotblat, 1961; National Research Council, 1972; Sasaki and Kasuga, 1981), X-rays have been found to cause a reduction in lifespan, along with other harmful effects. Therefore, they serve as an example of an agent that generates a nonselective toxic free radical, which subsequently assaults vulnerable biomolecules. The biological response, however, can vary depending on the specific tissues involved, with the dominant effect being determined by the dose of exposure.

The preceding example involves another principle of toxicology, namely the principle of limiting toxicity. Animals that are exposed to extremely high doses of X-rays would also experience additional harmful effects unless these effects are mitigated by the more severe and immediate consequences. When examining the potential impact of any harmful substance on the process of aging and older individuals, it is important to regard the resulting reaction as one component of a sequence of toxic effects. This reaction is influenced by factors such as the amount of exposure, the method of exposure, the length of exposure, the species affected, and the duration of observation.

Other noxious substances are likely to exhibit greater specificity in their initial actions and subsequent consequences. For example, carbon monoxide attaches to hemoglobin, diminishes the ability to transport oxygen, and causes toxicity.

One additional factor to consider regarding the molecular-level damage that may lead to the various symptoms observed during aging is whether a particular harmful effect can manifest in broader ways. A hypothesis suggests that a particular action of a specific tissue can lead to multiple detrimental processes in different tissues. While changes in molecules that regulate processes can have various effects or impact different tissues (such as in diabetes), there has not been any observed instance of a response that is as extensive as the manifestations of aging.

4.2.2. Cellular Effects

Toxic mechanisms can affect cells in two main ways: firstly, if a sufficient number of cells of a specific type in a tissue are altered by exposure, it can lead to the failure of specific tissue functions. Secondly, toxic stress on a single cell can result in toxic effects such as cancer, heritable mutation, and teratogenesis. Aging can be understood as a phenomenon where the majority of cells in various tissues undergo noticeable changes. Therefore, it is reasonable to view aging as a process that leads to the deterioration of most cells in a particular tissue.

Several aging studies have shown that the cell is the fundamental component of aging, and that the decline of cells leads to the deterioration of tissues, organs, and organisms. Despite efforts in aging research to identify the specific molecular damage or alteration responsible for cellular aging, a definitive molecular cause has not yet been established. Therefore, when looking for harmful substances that imitate the process of aging, it is suitable to make comparisons at the cellular and tissue level.

4.2.3. Tissue-Level Effects

The toxic effects in intact animals are typically identified and studied at the tissue level, as changes in tissue structure or function are frequently observed. The particularity of the situation could be attributed to the presence of harmful stress at the location of contact (such as the lungs, skin, or gastrointestinal tract), at the location of metabolic activity (such as the liver, brain, or kidney), or within vulnerable target cells. Understanding the etiology of toxic mechanisms at the cellular and molecular levels is crucial for comprehending their effects on tissues.

In the case of ionizing radiation, the lining of the gut fails to perform its barrier function because the stem cells responsible for proliferation do not function properly, leading to the shedding of the intestinal mucosa. The inability of the stem cells to multiply is thought to result from the impact of X-ray-induced free radicals on their chromatin, which leads to the inhibition of cell division. Therefore, when examining the toxic effects that are mechanistically linked to aging, the primary objective is to determine the sequence of events that occur from molecular alterations to their consequences at the cellular, tissue, and organismal levels.

4.3. Pharmacogenetics

During studies on drug metabolism and drug disposition in humans, significant variations in drug response and the capacity to metabolize and eliminate drugs have been observed. Various disparities arise from environmental factors, some from age-dependent (developmental) factors, others from genetic factors, and many from intricate interactions among these factors. Pharmacogenetics is the scientific investigation of genetic factors that explain variations in drug metabolism and drug response among individuals. Pharmacogenetics is significant in toxicology as it uncovers how certain individuals, due to their genetic makeup, experience toxic effects when exposed to foreign substances at doses that are easily tolerated by others.

The focus lies on the correlation between genetic variations in metabolic rates among individuals and the production of potentially harmful biotransformation products of a drug or chemical. Historically, the hepatic drug-metabolizing enzyme system has been considered a detoxification system. This is because it transforms lipid-soluble compounds, which could otherwise persist in the body indefinitely, into more polar metabolites that can be easily eliminated through urine. Recently, it has been acknowledged that this enzyme system can generate potentially harmful and extremely reactive byproducts that bind with large molecules in tissues, such as DNA, leading to tissue death, immune reactions, and genetic alterations (Sipes and Gandolfi, 1986). The regulation and control of tissue damage may be influenced by qualitative variations in drug metabolism pathways among subjects, as well as quantitative variations in the activities of the enzymes responsible for catalyzing these reactions and pathways. Hence, variations in genetic makeup among individuals can make certain individuals more susceptible and others less susceptible to the harmful effects of various reactive metabolites.

As genetic entities are thoroughly examined, the impact of age on their expression frequently becomes evident. The manifestation of a phenotype, and consequently the altered susceptibility to chemical agents through genetic modification (either increased or decreased), may only arise when an individual possessing genes that predispose them to a specific type of toxicity is initially exposed to the harmful environmental chemical. This occurrence might not take place until later stages of life. Older individuals are more frequently prescribed drugs compared to younger individuals, therefore the likelihood of experiencing drug toxicity related to pharmacogenetics is expected to rise with age. Furthermore, certain conditions that are determined by genetics only manifest themselves later in life, such as Huntington's chorea, certain types of neuromuscular disease, and diabetes mellitus.

Various factors have been thoroughly examined and identified as contributing to the significant differences between individuals in their disposition and response to xenobiotics in humans (Figure 4.2).

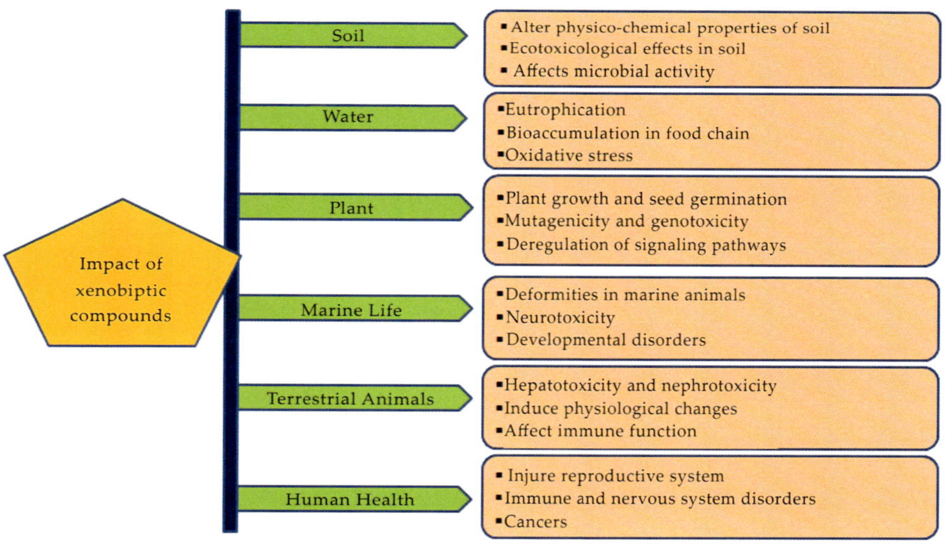

Figure 4.2. This diagram illustrates the known or suspected environmental factors that can modify the genetically determined rates at which drugs are eliminated from the body.

Source: Miglani R, Parveen N, Kumar A, Ansari MA, Khanna S, Rawat G, Panda AK, Bisht SS, Upadhyay J, Ansari MN. Degradation of xenobiotic pollutants: An environmentally sustainable approach. Metabolites. 2022; 12(9):818. https://doi.org/10.3390/metabo12090818.

The factors influencing drug metabolism include gender, timing of drug administration, disease presence, hormonal and nutritional status, stress levels, exposure to substances that activate or inhibit hepatic microsomal drug-metabolizing enzymes (including long-term use of various drugs), the condition of the heart, liver, kidneys, and endocrine organs, as well as age (Conney et al., 1971; Gillette, 1971; Vesell, 1982b).

Over the last two decades, researchers have identified genetic factors that have a direct impact on how humans respond to and process xenobiotics. These findings have been documented by several authors including La Du (1972), Omenn and Gelboin (1984), Omenn and Motulsky (1978), Vesell (1969, 1971, 1973, 1984), and Weinshilboum (1984). A total of 60 factors have been identified, and there are likely even more factors yet to be discovered. Genetic factors can be the primary or exclusive cause of interindividual differences in certain individuals under specific circumstances. When the age, sex, diet, and exposure to environmental chemicals that activate or inhibit the hepatic drug-metabolizing enzyme system are the same among human subjects, there are still significant differences in how individuals respond to and process xenobiotics. A significant number of these variations are genetically determined. Approximately 20% of patients in educational medical institutions in the United States seek treatment specifically for adverse drug reactions. Furthermore, a range of 5–30% of patients in these hospitals experience at least one such reaction (Cluff et al., 1965). Older patients experience drug adverse reactions more frequently and with greater severity compared to younger patients (Hall, 1982). The variability in how individual patients respond to drugs is a significant factor contributing to adverse reactions, such as drug toxicity. This variability is a major concern in the field of medicine.

Table 4.1 enumerates an example of studied pharmacogenetic conditions. Almost every individual experiences a toxic reaction due to the buildup of drugs caused by a significant decrease in the enzymatic conversion of the original drug into metabolites that are not pharmacologically active. The enzyme's function is abnormal due to a specific mutation in the gene responsible for its synthesis. The conditions like most other inborn errors of metabolism, are typically inherited as autosomal recessive traits. Therefore, the affected individuals receive a mutated version of a gene from both of their parents who do not show any physical abnormalities.

Table 4.1. Main Drugs Whose Metabolism Can Significantly Change Due to Cyp2c9 Gene Variations

Drug	Therapeutic Area	Clinical Impact
S-warfarin	Cardiovascular diseases	When usual doses of warfarin are used, in PMs, the risk of internal bleeding is greatly increased. Drug dose should be established according to CYP2C9 polymorphism genotype. IMs should use 65% of the standard initial dose; PMs 20%. Drug monitoring is recommended to establish maintaining doses.
Phenytoin	Neurology	PMs are at greater risk of developing CNS adverse effects as well as serious cutaneous adverse reactions when given usual dosages of phenytoin. It is recommended to start with recommended doses and reduce maintaining doses by about 50%.

Some NSAIDs (ibuprofen, celecoxib, meloxicam, piroxicam, flurbiprofen, mefenamic acid)	Diseases with inflammation	In PMs, increased risk of gastrointestinal ulcers, serious cardiovascular events, hypertension, acute renal failure, and worsening of preexisting heart failure. In these patients, it is recommended to initiate treatment at 25–50% of the traditional dose or use NSAIDs not metabolized by CYP2C9 (acetylsalicylic acid, ketorolac, naproxen, sulindac).
Some hypoglycemic drugs (glipizide, tolbutamide)	Diabetology	These drugs are a substrate of the genetically polymorphic enzyme CYP2C9. However, the pronounced differences in pharmacokinetics due to the variants did not significantly affect plasma insulin and glucose concentrations. No dose variations are needed.

Source: Principi N, Petropulacos K, Esposito S. Impact of pharmacogenomics in clinical practice. Pharmaceuticals. 2023; 16(11):1596. https://doi.org/10.3390/ph16111596.

There are variations in the gene frequencies of several pharmacogenetic conditions across different geographical regions. Age-related effects have also been observed for the acetylase polymorphism. However, further investigations are required to study the impact of age on other pharmacogenetic factors.

The historical account of the identification of an age-related impact on the gene frequency of the acetylation polymorphism is highly enlightening, as it exemplifies the meticulousness required in investigating such age-related effects. In the initial observations conducted by Evans et al. (1960), the significance of age was not acknowledged. Subsequent examination of a limited group of individuals appeared to validate that observation (Farah et al., 1977). However, in 1983, Evans conducted a reassessment of his initial data and documented that both age and sex have an impact on plasma isoniazid concentrations (Iselius and Evans, 1983). A study conducted in 1984 found that older individuals had a significantly higher proportion of slow acetylators. However, the study did not report any information regarding the distribution of slow acetylators based on sex (Gachalyi et al., 1984). The study conducted in 1985 confirmed the influence of age on the acetylator phenotype, but it was found to be limited to males (Paulsen and Nilsson, 1985). The higher occurrence of the slow-acetylator phenotype as people get older is particularly noteworthy, as this phenotype is also linked to a significantly higher vulnerability to developing bladder cancer when exposed to arylamines and hydrazines in industrial settings over a long period of time (Cartwright et al., 1982). A study by Ayesh et al. (1984) has suggested a connection between susceptibility to cancer and a specific genetic trait related to the metabolism of debrisoquin. The study found that patients with bronchogenic carcinoma were more likely to be extensive metabolizers of debrisoquin compared to age- and sex-matched controls.

An implication of the variations observed among individuals who are considered to be within the normal range is that a specific amount of a drug given through a specific method can be harmful in one person, beneficial in another, and have no pharmacological impact in a third individual. The presence of these disparities poses a significant obstacle for a physician who needs to tailor treatment, particularly for medications with narrow therapeutic ranges.

It is necessary to identify the mechanism responsible for the large differences in how drugs are processed by individuals, as this has important implications for therapy. Identifying individuals is challenging due to the significant variation in both genetic makeup and environmental factors among human beings. However, in laboratory animals such as rats and mice, heterogeneity can be regulated. It is possible to manipulate each variable separately, allowing for the study of the quantitative impact of each variable on the differences in drug disposition between individuals. Additionally, it is possible to create dose-response curves. Over the past ten years, extensive research has uncovered numerous variables that can influence the way drugs are processed and distributed in the body. Pharmacogenetic conditions in humans can be classified into two categories: pharmacokinetic conditions, which impact how the body processes drugs, and pharmacodynamic conditions, which impact how drugs affect the body (Vesell, 1973).

Due to their rarity and limited impact on drug toxicity, the majority of the monogenetic conditions mentioned above likely have a minimal role in the significant issue of adverse drug reactions. However, there is another advancement in pharmacogenetics that indicates genetic variations that directly impact the way the body processes foreign substances are a significant factor in frequently observed types of drug toxicity. The presence of significant interindividual variations in response to phenylbutazone, bishydroxy-coumarin, antipyrine, halothane, ethanol, phenytoin, nortriptyline, or salicylate was not observed among unrelated individuals. However, these variations were absent in pairs of monozygotic twins, but were present in most, though not all, pairs of dizygotic twins (Vesell, 1973). The degree of variation in rates of drug elimination among unrelated individuals was 30-fold for nortriptyline, 10-fold for bis-hydroxycoumarin, 6-fold for phenylbutazone and antipyrine, 3-fold for halothane, and 2-fold for ethanol.

Attributing specific portions of the overall variation in drug disposition among individuals to particular environmental factors is challenging due to the presence and impact of multiple environmental factors, each with varying abilities to modify the genetically determined baseline rate of drug disposition. Partitioning the total variation in drug elimination among large heterogeneous populations is made more complex by the strong correlation between seemingly pure environmental factors, such as smoking and diet, and other environmental and genetic factors.

Several environmental, developmental, nutritional, or endocrine factors can impact the rate at which an individual metabolizes a drug. These factors are interconnected as they are frequently correlated with one another in a specific subject, rather than existing independently. Indeed, these factors frequently interact dynamically to alter the fundamental rates at which drugs are absorbed, distributed, metabolized, excreted, or interact with receptors in a subject. The impact of each of these factors on drug response can be intricate and may vary over time, even within the same individual (Vesell, 1980, 1982a,b).

4.4. Biological Markers

A biological marker, also known as a biomarker, is a measurable characteristic, such as a biochemical, cellular, structural, or functional indicator, that signifies a specific event or condition in a biological system or sample. Biological markers in humans, animals, or other organisms can be used to measure exposure to or damage caused by a foreign substance by indicating the amount of the substance in the body, the amount stored in the body, the amount reaching a specific tissue, or the early signs of a harmful effect.

The development of biologic markers originated from cancer research aimed at identifying the influence of external agents or host factors in the development of human cancer. Perera and Weinstein (1982) provided a definition for molecular cancer epidemiology, which involves the integration of analytic epidemiology and molecular techniques to identify carcinogens in human tissues, cells, or fluids, as well as to quantify early morphologic, biochemical, or functional reactions to carcinogens. Lower and Kanarek (1982) defined molecular epidemiology as the quantification of molecular attributes associated with neoplastic disease.

Following the publication of those initial papers, numerous symposia and workshops have been organized to investigate the application of biologic markers in the field of disease prevention. The primary objective of marker research is to enhance the predictive correlation between exposure, dose, and response. Gaining a more comprehensive comprehension of the function of markers will aid in disease prevention by accurately evaluating the level of risk, identifying groups or individuals at high risk, and offering early detection of disease.

The utilization of cellular and molecular markers, which span from initial exposure to the progression of disease, has the potential to be a highly effective tool in the field of environmental health sciences. Markers that indicate the existence of internal or biologically impactful doses or the early stages of disease can be valuable in identifying hazards. This process involves establishing a causal link between an environmental agent and a harmful effect. Markers can also be employed to establish the correlation between dosage and response, especially when dealing with the small doses that are pertinent to the majority of environmental chemicals. Markers play a crucial role in determining the level of human exposure in populations, individual exposure levels, and the percentage of individuals who are highly responsive or deviate from the norm within the human population (Fowle, 1984).

The utilization of biological markers has given rise to several significant ethical concerns (Ashford, 1986). One concern is that biologic screening may lead to a shift in focus from monitoring the environment to monitoring humans in the workplace. There is apprehension regarding the potential use of a susceptibility marker to disqualify individuals from employment. This raises concerns that instead of prioritizing the removal of toxic chemicals from the workplace, efforts may shift towards identifying and excluding susceptible populations. Markers can be categorized along a time continuum based on their role in indicating susceptibility, exposure, internal dose circulation, biologically effective dose (or dose at receptor site), and potential or actual health impairment.

Markers of susceptibility are indicators of individual or population physiological variations that influence how individuals respond to environmental agents, regardless of their level of exposure. These differences encompass variations in receptors, metabolism, immunoglobulins, organ reserve capacity, and other factors that result in modified responses to environmental agents. These variations can be influenced by factors such as sex, age, physiological state, and even diet. One example is that the lack of the enzyme α-1-antitrypsin indicates a higher likelihood of developing chronic obstructive pulmonary disease.

Markers of exposure are biological indicators or circumstances that provide information about external exposure, internal absorbed dose, or dose at the receptor site or site of toxic action. Indicators of internal dose, which measure the quantity of a substance that is taken in by an organism, encompass various pharmacokinetic traits such as blood circulation, permeability of capillaries, mechanisms of transport, quantity of receptor sites, metabolism of the substance, and method of administration. Other factors to consider are the data on the structure and stability of the material, the peak or cumulative circulating dose, and the half-life (Gibaldi and Perrier, 1982). Biological indicators of the amount of effective dose include features of the target organ, such as the speed at which it metabolizes and detoxifies substances, any pre-existing vulnerabilities, and its ability to handle additional stress.

Indicators of possible health damage include initial biological reactions, such as changes in the functioning of specific or non-specific tissues soon after being exposed. Subsequently, in response to a harmful substance or following the buildup of large amounts, indicators of health deterioration arise, such as changes in the functioning of the affected tissue, which can be seen as an early stage of disease.

Exposure to environmental pollutants can result in the absorption of a biologically potent dose, which can ultimately cause either reversible or irreversible harm. Various markers can be utilized in distinct ways to ascertain exposure, dosage, or health deterioration. Nevertheless, markers of these categories are not consistently distinguishable from one another. Hence, distinguishing between indicators of exposures and indicators of effects can frequently be challenging.

Due to the body's limited range of biochemical or cellular responses to injury, an effect marker may not always indicate a specific pollutant.

4.5. Evaluation of Toxicity

Toxicity testing serves two main objectives: firstly, to analyze and identify the general or specific toxic properties of a given chemical or physical agent, and secondly, to evaluate a wide range of agents in order to assess their potential for causing specific toxic effects. Decisions regarding the nature and scope of testing are influenced by both practical and scientific factors. Every decision involves a scientific assessment that relies on established toxic mechanisms and data obtained from tests conducted on numerous chemicals using specific protocols. The testing of any specific agent is limited by practical constraints on resources and time. Conducting comprehensive testing of an agent across a diverse set of standard protocols can incur costs amounting to tens of millions of dollars. Only a small number of agents possess enough theoretical or practical significance to warrant such expenditures.

Toxicity-testing protocols can be categorized into screening or auxiliary tests and whole-animal tests. Screening or auxiliary tests are typically brief assessments created to detect the capacity to cause specific toxic effects. Whole-animal tests, whether short term or long term, aim to definitively determine the presence or absence of toxicity and quantitatively assess the level of risk.

The utility of screening tests is determined by two characteristics. The primary consideration is whether the biological process being examined by a test is the same as the process responsible for the harmful effect under consideration. Is mutation, as observed in the Salmonella typhimurium test, both necessary and sufficient for all types of carcinogenesis for which the test is used as a screen? The response to this particular inquiry regarding the Ames assay is likely negative; additional mechanisms that are not identifiable through this examination are also pertinent to the development of cancer. Nevertheless, the Ames assay is a valuable test due to its second characteristic: predictive value.

Predictive value refers to the capacity of a test to anticipate the result of another test or a human response. The probabilistic measure quantifies the correlation between the result of the basic test and the "truth" determined by whole-animal testing. The predictive value is not influenced by the fundamental biology. However, if a short-term test has the ability to accurately replicate essential biological processes and accurately predict the response of the entire organism, it can be considered close to the ideal.

When creating screening tests to identify substances that speed up the aging process, it is important to consider the following criteria: – Does the proposed test accurately replicate the fundamental biological processes of aging?

Does the proposed test have the ability to identify substances that hasten the aging process when tested on entire organisms?

These questions highlight the challenges of developing screening tests for substances that speed up or interact with the aging process.

Experiments that involve studying the entire animal, especially over a long period of time, provide the most accurate predictions of how humans will respond and the quantitative risks involved. The species selected for testing should accurately reflect the toxic responses observed in human populations, as well as accurately replicate the absorption, metabolism, and distribution of the chemical agent being tested. While it is true that all animals experience aging, it is important to note that not every species can serve as an appropriate substitute for studying how humans respond metabolically to a specific substance. The choice of species for comprehensive, extended-term testing pertaining to aging must meet the dual requirements of the gerontologist and the toxicologist. Furthermore, the specific species to be used by the toxicologist will vary depending on the particular substance being tested.

Due to practical constraints, laboratory tests are typically conducted using relatively small animal populations. Environmental agent tests are typically conducted at significantly higher dosages than what human populations are typically exposed to. Information obtained from these tests needs to be extrapolated in order to forecast how humans will respond to the doses they encounter in their surroundings. To make this extrapolation, it is necessary to measure (or at least predict or assume) the shape of the dose-response curve. Toxic effects are typically categorized based on the presence of a threshold dose, below which no toxic effects are expected, or the occurrence of toxic effects in only a small fraction of exposed animals at low doses. It is crucial to take into account this significant differentiation when examining toxic interactions in relation to aging. Quantifying the correlation between dosage and the decrease in lifespan is a challenging task. Life-shortening dose-response curves are intricate and cannot be easily extended to low doses through simple extrapolation. A potential method to test the hypothesis that radiation exposure causes premature aging would involve showing that the development of all diseases occurs earlier to the same degree, and this advancement is proportional to the extent of the reduction in lifespan (National Research Council, 1980b).

Another important factor to consider is the extrapolation from laboratory conditions to real-world environments. Traditionally, laboratory tests have primarily focused on evaluating the toxic effects of individual agents. However, it is important to note that the human environment consists of multiple agents that can potentially interact with each other. Furthermore, there is scant evidence to suggest that agents interact at the low concentrations commonly observed in the environment. However, it is crucial to acknowledge the potential for such interactions. The toxic effects of multiple agents are currently being examined, and the findings may inform future studies on age-related effects. (Yunes, 2018; Czarnywojtek et al., 2021)

A Closer Look

Neuroactive drugs

Neuroactive drugs play a crucial role in addressing the complex neurological changes that accompany aging. As individuals grow older, they often experience cognitive decline, neurodegenerative diseases like Alzheimer's, and changes in mood and behavior. Neuroactive drugs encompass a broad spectrum of pharmaceuticals that target these neurological processes, aiming to enhance cognitive function, alleviate symptoms of neurodegeneration, and improve overall quality of life.

One key category of neuroactive drugs includes acetylcholinesterase inhibitors, such as donepezil and rivastigmine, commonly prescribed for Alzheimer's disease. These drugs work by increasing the availability of acetylcholine, a neurotransmitter crucial for memory and learning, thus temporarily improving cognitive function in affected individuals. Another class, NMDA receptor antagonists like memantine, regulates glutamate activity in the brain, which is important for memory and cognitive processes disrupted in Alzheimer's.

Beyond Alzheimer's, neuroactive drugs are also utilized for managing depression and anxiety in older adults. Selective serotonin reuptake inhibitors (SSRIs) and serotonin-norepinephrine reuptake inhibitors (SNRIs) are commonly prescribed antidepressants that help regulate mood by affecting neurotransmitter levels in the brain.

However, the use of neuroactive drugs in aging populations requires careful consideration due to potential side effects and interactions with other medications commonly taken by older adults. Dosing adjustments and monitoring are essential to mitigate risks and maximize therapeutic benefits. Moreover, ongoing research aims to develop new neuroactive compounds that target specific mechanisms of aging-related neurological decline, promising advancements in personalized medicine approaches for older adults.

Therefore, neuroactive drugs represent a critical tool in managing the neurological challenges of aging, offering potential improvements in cognitive function, mood regulation, and overall quality of life for older individuals facing age-related neurological conditions.

Summary

- As we age, our bodies undergo a multitude of changes that can affect our susceptibility to toxins and our ability to metabolize them. "Toxicology in the Context of Aging" explores the complex relationship between aging and toxicology, highlighting the ways in which age-related physiological changes can impact our response to toxins.
- One of the primary concerns in aging is the decline of organ function, particularly in the liver and kidneys, which are responsible for detoxifying and eliminating toxins from the body. As these organs slow down, the body's ability to process and remove toxins is impaired, making older adults more vulnerable to toxic effects.
- Additionally, age-related changes in the body's composition, such as increased fat mass and decreased muscle mass, can alter the distribution and storage of toxins. This can lead to a buildup of toxins in the body, further exacerbating their harmful effects.
- The chapter also deals with the effects of age on the body's natural defense mechanisms, including the immune system and antioxidant defenses. As we age, these defenses can become compromised, making us more susceptible to oxidative stress and cellular damage.
- Furthermore, the chapter examines the impact of aging on the brain and nervous system, which can affect our cognitive function, behavior, and mood. Exposure to toxins can have a profound impact on these systems, leading to neurodegenerative diseases and other age-related disorders.

References

1. Aichinger, G. (2021). Natural dibenzo-α-pyrones: Friends or foes? *International Journal of Molecular Sciences, 22*(23), 13063.
2. An, B. H., Jeong, H., Kim, J. H., Park, S., Jeong, J. H., Kim, M. J., & Chang, M. (2019). Estrogen receptor-mediated transcriptional activities of spent coffee grounds and spent coffee grounds compost, and their phenolic acid constituents. *Journal of Agricultural and Food Chemistry, 67*(30), 8649–8659.
3. Autrup, H., Barile, F. A., Berry, S. C., Blaauboer, B. J., Boobis, A., Bolt, H., & Domingo, J. L. (2020). Human exposure to synthetic endocrine disrupting chemicals (S-EDCs) is generally negligible as compared to natural compounds with higher or comparable endocrine activity. How to evaluate the risk of the S-EDCs? *Environmental Toxicology and Pharmacology, 78*, 103396.
4. Balló, A., Busznyákné Székvári, K., Czétány, P., Márk, L., Török, A., Szántó, Á., & Máté, G. (2023). Estrogenic and non-estrogenic disruptor effect of zearalenone on male reproduction: A review. *International Journal of Molecular Sciences, 24*(5), 1578.
5. Barbaud, A., & Lafforgue, C. (2021). Risks associated with cosmetic ingredients. *Annales de Dermatologie et de Vénéréologie, 148*(1), 77–93.
6. Cano, R., Pérez, J. L., Dávila, L. A., Ortega, Á., Gómez, Y., Valero-Cedeño, N. J., & Díaz Albornoz, M. P. (2021). Role of endocrine-disrupting chemicals in the pathogenesis of non-alcoholic fatty liver disease: A comprehensive review. *International Journal of Molecular Sciences, 22*(9), 4807.

7. Caserta, D., De Marco, M. P., Besharat, A. R., & Costanzi, F. (2022). Endocrine disruptors and endometrial cancer: Molecular mechanisms of action and clinical implications, a systematic review. *International Journal of Molecular Sciences, 23*(6), 2956.

8. Chen, Y., Li, T., Ji, H., Wang, X., Sun, X., Miao, M., & Yuan, W. (2021). Associations of maternal soy product consumption and urinary isoflavone concentrations with neonatal anthropometry: A prospective cohort study. *Environmental Pollution, 274*, 115752.

9. Cooke, P. S., Heine, P. A., Taylor, J. A., & Lubahn, D. B. (2001). The role of estrogen and estrogen receptor-a in male adipose tissue. *Molecular and Cellular Endocrinology, 178*(1–2), 147–154.

10. Czarnywojtek, A., Jaz, K., Ochmańska, A., Zgorzalewicz-Stachowiak, M., Czarnocka, B., Sawicka-Gutaj, N., & Florek, E. (2021). The effect of endocrine disruptors on the reproductive system—Current knowledge. *European Review for Medical and Pharmacological Sciences, 25*(22), 26450.

11. de Moraes, A. C. N., Caires, F. O., Imperio, G. E., Nóbrega, R. H., Ortiga-Carvalho, T. M., & de Magalhães, V. F. (2022). Cylindrospermopsin disrupts estrous cycle and increases spermatogenesis in mice. *Reproductive Sciences, 29*(11), 2876–2884.

12. Desmawati, D., & Sulastri, D. (2019). Phytoestrogens and their health effect. *Open Access Macedonian Journal of Medical Sciences, 7*(3), 495–499.

13. Erguc, E. I., Tascioglu-Aliyev, A., Entezari, B., & Gurer-Orhan, H. (2021). The role of biotransformation in the activity of endocrine disruptors. *Current Drug Metabolism, 22*(8), 628–644.

14. Eustache, F., Bennani Smires, B., Moison, D., Bergès, R., Canivenc-Lavier, M. C., Vaiman, D., & Auger, J. (2020). Different exposure windows to low doses of genistein and/or vinclozolin result in contrasted disorders of testis function and gene expression of exposed rats and their unexposed progeny. *Environmental Research, 190*, 109975.

15. Fan, Y., Qian, H., Wu, Z., Li, Z., Li, X., Zhang, Y., & Wang, X. (2022). Exploratory analysis of the associations between urinary phytoestrogens and thyroid hormones among adolescents and adults in the United States: National Health and Nutrition Examination Survey 2007–2010. *Environmental Science and Pollution Research, 29*(3), 2974–2984.

16. Fan, Y., Tao, C., Li, Z., Huang, Y., Yan, W., Zhao, S., & Wang, X. (2023). Association of endocrine-disrupting chemicals with all-cause and cause-specific mortality in the U.S.: A prospective cohort study. *Environmental Science & Technology, 57*(5), 2877–2886.

17. Frayn, K. N., Karpe, F., Fielding, B. A., Macdonald, I. A., & Coppack, S. W. (2003). Integrative physiology of human adipose tissue. *International Journal of Obesity, 27*(7), 875–888.

18. Fucic, A., Mantovani, A., Vena, J., Bloom, M. S., Sincic, N., Vazquez, M., & Aguado-Sierra, J. (2023). Impact of endocrine disruptors from mother's diet on immuno-hormonal orchestration of brain development and introduction of the virtual human twin tool. *Reproductive Toxicology, 117*, 108357.

19. Gao, Y., Zhao, Y., Zhang, H., Zhang, P., Liu, J., Feng, Y., & Sun, Z. (2019). Pubertal exposure to low doses of zearalenone disrupting spermatogenesis through ERα related genetic and epigenetic pathways. *Toxicology Letters, 315*, 31–38.

20. Garritty, C., Gartlehner, G., Nussbaumer-Streit, B., King, V. J., Hamel, C., Kamel, C., & Stevens, A. (2021). Cochrane Rapid Reviews Methods Group offers evidence-informed guidance to conduct rapid reviews. *Journal of Clinical Epidemiology, 130*, 13–22.

21. Garritty, C., Hamel, C., Hersi, M., Butler, C., Monfaredi, Z., Stevens, A., & Moher, D. (2020). Assessing how information is packaged in rapid reviews for policy-makers and other stakeholders: A cross-sectional study. *Health Research Policy and Systems, 18*(1), 112.
22. Grgic, D., Betschler, A., Früholz, R., Novak, B., Varga, E., & Marko, D. (2022). Estrogenic in vitro evaluation of zearalenone and its phase I and II metabolites in combination with soy isoflavones. *Archives of Toxicology, 96*(10), 3385–3402.
23. Hawkins, J., Hires, C., Dunne, E., & Baker, C. (2020). The relationship between lavender and tea tree essential oils and pediatric endocrine disorders: A systematic review of the literature. *Complementary Therapies in Medicine, 49*, 102288.
24. Heras-González, L., Latorre, J. A., Martinez-Bebia, M., Espino, D., Olea-Serrano, F., & Mariscal-Arcas, M. (2020). The relationship of obesity with lifestyle and dietary exposure to endocrine-disrupting chemicals. *Food and Chemical Toxicology, 136*, 110983.
25. Imai, H., Nishikawa, H., Suzuki, A., Kodama, E., Iida, T., Mikura, K., & Sugisawa, C. (2022). Secondary hypogonadism due to excessive ingestion of isoflavone in a man. *Internal Medicine, 61*(22), 2899–2903.
26. Jing, S., Liu, C., Zheng, J., Dong, Z., & Guo, N. (2022). Toxicity of zearalenone and its nutritional intervention by natural products. *Food & Function, 13*(22), 10374–10400.
27. Kabir, E. R., Rahman, M. S., & Rahman, I. (2015). A review on endocrine disruptors and their possible impacts on human health. *Environmental Toxicology and Pharmacology, 40*, 241–258.
28. Kinkade, C. W., Rivera-Núñez, Z., Gorcyzca, L., Aleksunes, L. M., & Barrett, E. S. (2021). Impact of Fusarium-derived mycoestrogens on female reproduction: A systematic review. *Toxins, 13*(6), 373.
29. Kiyama, R. (2019). Estrogenic activity of coffee constituents. *Nutrients, 11*(6), 1401.
30. Komsky-Elbaz, A., Kalo, D., & Roth, Z. (2022). New evidence for deleterious effects of environmental contaminants on the male gamete. *Animal Reproduction Science, 246*, 106886.
31. Křížová, L., Dadáková, K., Kašparovská, J., & Kašparovský, T. (2019). Isoflavones. *Molecules, 24*(6), 1076.
32. Lee, A. W., Poynor, V., & McEligot, A. J. (2022). Urinary phytoestrogen levels are associated with female hormonal cancers: An analysis of NHANES data from 1999 to 2010. *Nutrition and Cancer, 74*(2), 2748–2756.
33. Lephart, E. D. (2021). Phytoestrogens (resveratrol and equol) for estrogen-deficient skin—Controversies/misinformation versus anti-aging in vitro and clinical evidence via nutraceutical-cosmetics. *International Journal of Molecular Sciences, 22*(20), 11218.
34. Li, F., Zhao, X., Jiao, Y., Duan, X., Yu, L., Zheng, F., & Zhao, X. (2023). Exposure assessment of aflatoxins and zearalenone in edible vegetable oils in Shandong, China: Health risks posed by mycotoxin immunotoxicity and reproductive toxicity in children. *Environmental Science and Pollution Research, 30*(3), 3743–3758.
35. Men, Y., Zhao, Y., Zhang, P., Zhang, H., Gao, Y., Liu, J., & Sun, Z. (2019). Gestational exposure to low-dose zearalenone disrupting offspring spermatogenesis might be through epigenetic modifications. *Basic & Clinical Pharmacology & Toxicology, 125*(4), 382–393.

36. Messina, M., Mejia, S. B., Cassidy, A., Duncan, A., Kurzer, M., Nagato, C., & Barnes, S. (2022). Neither soyfoods nor isoflavones warrant classification as endocrine disruptors: A technical review of the observational and clinical data. *Critical Reviews in Food Science and Nutrition, 62*(17), 5824–5885.

37. Narciso, L., Catone, T., Aquilina, G., Attias, L., De Angelis, I., Iuliano, M. G., & Maranghi, F. (2017). The juvenile toxicity study as a tool for a science-based risk assessment in the children population group. *Reproductive Toxicology, 72*, 136–141.

38. Nasri, A., & Pohjanvirta, R. (2021). In vitro estrogenic, cytotoxic, and genotoxic profiles of the xenoestrogens 8-prenylnaringenine, genistein and tartrazine. *Environmental Science and Pollution Research, 28*(28), 27988–27997.

39. Oliveira, J. M., Oliveira, I. M., Sleiman, H. K., Dal Forno, G. O., Romano, M. A., & Romano, R. M. (2022). Consumption of soy isoflavones during the prepubertal phase delays puberty and causes hypergonadotropic hypogonadism with disruption of hypothalamic-pituitary gonadotropins regulation in male rats. *Toxicology Letters, 369*, 1–11.

40. Pallottini, V., Bulzomi, P., Galluzzo, P., Martini, C., & Marino, M. (2008). Estrogen regulation of adipose tissue functions: Involvement of estrogen receptor isoforms. *Infectious Disorders - Drug Targets, 8*(1), 52–60.

41. Patisaul, H. B. (2021). Endocrine disrupting chemicals (EDCs) and the neuroendocrine system: Beyond estrogen, androgen, and thyroid. *Advances in Pharmacology, 92*, 101–150.

42. Qasem, R. J. (2020). The estrogenic activity of resveratrol: A comprehensive review of in vitro and in vivo evidence and the potential for endocrine disruption. *Critical Reviews in Toxicology, 50*(6), 439–462.

43. Rami, Y., Ebrahimpour, K., Maghami, M., Shoshtari-Yeganeh, B., & Kelishadi, R. (2022). The association between heavy metals exposure and sex hormones: A systematic review on current evidence. *Biological Trace Element Research, 200*(12), 3491–3510.

44. Ramsey, J. T., Li, Y., Arao, Y., Naidu, A., Coons, L. A., DIaz, A., & Korach, K. S. (2019). Lavender products associated with premature thelarche and prepubertal gynecomastia: Case reports and endocrine-disrupting chemical activities. *The Journal of Clinical Endocrinology & Metabolism, 104*(12), 5393–5405.

45. Ramsey, J. T., Shropshire, B. C., Nagy, T. R., Chambers, K. D., Li, Y., Korach, K. S., & Korach, S. (2020). Essential oils and health. *Yale Journal of Biology and Medicine, 93*, 387–396.

46. Rashid, H., Alqahtani, S. S., & Alshahrani, S. (2019). Diet: A source of endocrine disruptors. *Endocrine, Metabolic & Immune Disorders Drug Targets, 20*(5), 633–645.

47. Rivera-Núñez, Z., Barrett, E. S., Szamreta, E. A., Shapses, S. A., Qin, B., Lin, Y., & Bandera, E. V. (2019). Urinary mycoestrogens and age and height at menarche in New Jersey girls. *Environmental Health, 18*(1), 24.

48. Salsano, S., Pérez-Debén, S., Quiñonero, A., González-Martín, R., & Domínguez, F. (2019). Phytoestrogen exposure alters endometrial stromal cells and interferes with decidualization signaling. *Fertility and Sterility, 112*(5), 947–958.e3.

49. Shi, T., Xu, L. L., Chen, L., He, J., Wang, Y. K., Chen, F., & Wu, Q. H. (2023). Acute exposure to microcystins affects hypothalamic-pituitary axes of male rats. *Environmental Pollution, 318*, 120843.

50. Singh, V. K., Pal, R., Srivastava, P., Misra, G., Shukla, Y., & Sharma, P. K. (2021). Exposure of androgen mimicking environmental chemicals enhances proliferation of prostate cancer (LNCaP) cells by inducing AR expression and epigenetic modifications. *Environmental Pollution, 272*, 116397.

51. Sleiman, H. K., de Oliveira, J. M., & Langoni de Freitas, G. B. (2021). Isoflavones alter male and female fertility in different development windows. *Biomedicine & Pharmacotherapy, 140*, 111448.

52. Solano, F., Hernández, E., Juárez-Rojas, L., Rojas-Maya, S., López, G., Romero, C., & Heidari, R. (2022). Reproductive disruption in adult female and male rats prenatally exposed to mesquite pod extract or daidzein. *Reproductive Biology, 22*(5), 100683.

53. Sridevi, V., Naveen, P., Karnam Venkat, S., Reddy, P. R., & Arifullah, M. (2020). Beneficiary and adverse effects of phytoestrogens: A potential constituent of plant-based diet. *Current Pharmaceutical Design, 27*(8), 802–815.

54. Szukiewicz, D. (2023). Insight into the potential mechanisms of endocrine disruption by dietary phytoestrogens in the context of the etiopathogenesis of endometriosis. *International Journal of Molecular Sciences, 24*(21), 12195.

55. Urbanek, K. A., Kowalska, K., Habrowska-Górczyńska, D. E., Kozieł, M. J., Domińska, K., & Piastowska-Ciesielska, A. W. (2023). Revealing the role of alternariol in the local steroidogenesis in human prostate normal and cancer cells. *International Journal of Molecular Sciences, 24*(17), 9513.

56. Walker, C., Boisvert, A., Malusare, P., & Culty, M. (2023). Impact of fetal exposure to endocrine disrupting chemical mixtures on FOXA3 gene and protein expression in adult rat testes. *International Journal of Molecular Sciences, 24*(3), 1211.

57. Walker, C., Garza, S., Papadopoulos, V., & Culty, M. (2021). Impact of endocrine-disrupting chemicals on steroidogenesis and consequences on testicular function. *Molecular and Cellular Endocrinology, 527*, 111215.

58. Wan, M. L. Y., Co, V. A., & El-Nezami, H. (2022). Endocrine disrupting chemicals and breast cancer: A systematic review of epidemiological studies. *Critical Reviews in Food Science and Nutrition, 62*(16), 6549–6576.

59. Wang, L. H., Chen, L. R., & Chen, K. H. (2021). In vitro and vivo identification, metabolism and action of xenoestrogens: An overview. *International Journal of Molecular Sciences, 22*(8), 4013.

60. Warth, B., Preindl, K., Manser, P., Wick, P., Marko, D., & Buerki-Thurnherr, T. (2019). Transfer and metabolism of the xenoestrogen zearalenone in human perfused placenta. *Environmental Health Perspectives, 127*(10), 107004.

61. Xue, P., Wang, Y., Chen, Y., Wu, X., Tang, Y., Ding, Y., & Liu, S. (2022). A case of peripheral precocious puberty may be caused by a diet containing phytosterols in a 20-month-old boy. *Hormone Research in Paediatrics, 95*(6), 484–491.

62. Yao, S., Wei, W., Cao, R., Lu, L., Liang, S., Xiong, M., & Ma, Y. (2021). Resveratrol alleviates zea-induced decidualization disturbance in human endometrial stromal cells. *Ecotoxicology and Environmental Safety, 207*, 111511.

63. Yu, L., Rios, E., Castro, L., Liu, J., Yan, Y., & Dixon, D. (2021). Genistein: Dual role in women's health. *Nutrients, 13*(9), 3048.

64. Yuan, G., Liu, Y., Liu, G., Wei, L., Wen, Y., Huang, S., & Cheng, J. (2019). Associations between semen phytoestrogens concentrations and semen quality in Chinese men. *Environment International, 129*, 136–144.

65. Yunes, J. S. (2018). Cyanobacterial toxins. In *Cyanobacteria: From Basic Science to Applications* (pp. 443–458). Elsevier.

66. Zhang, S., Mo, J., Wang, Y., Ni, C., Li, X., Zhu, Q., & Ge, R. S. (2019). Endocrine disruptors of inhibiting testicular 3β-hydroxysteroid dehydrogenase. *Chemico-Biological Interactions, 303*, 90–97.

67. Zoller, O., Brüschweiler, B. J., Magnin, R., Reinhard, H., Rhyn, P., Rupp, H., & Felleisen, R. (2015). Natural occurrence of bisphenol F in mustard. *Food Additives & Contaminants: Part A, 33*(1), 137–146.

Chapter

THE BIOLOGY OF AGING

5

Contents

Introduction

For a very long time, the process of aging has been a phenomenon that has left humanity bewildered. In the history of ancient Greek mythology, the story of Eos, a goddess who represents dawn, and her feelings for Tithonus, the younger brother of Laomedon, the king of Troy, has been an important subject of discussion. While Eos made a request to Zeus to bestow immortality upon Tithonus, she failed to make a request for eternal youth. Consequently, Tithonus was entering a state of contentment at that moment. Despite this, the constant progression of the natural process of aging continued unabated. Over the course of time, the individual's physical form gradually deteriorated to the point where it was nothing more than a rasping vocalization, and it eventually transformed into a cicada. Despite the passage of time, the question of whether or not aging is an inevitable process continues to be a constant concern. However, this is not always the case, as there are some organisms that do not show any signs of aging. One of the most notable of these is the Hydra, which is a small cnidarian that lives in freshwater environments. There is no evidence that the organism in question has reached senescence and possesses a neurological system that is only quite basic. The inexhaustible capacity of Hydra's stem cells to continually renew themselves is the source of the exceptional quality that Hydra possesses. It is important to note that the transcription factor FoxO is of significant significance in this regard.

In contrast to Hydra, it is important to note that the process of aging is something that all vertebrates go through, albeit at somewhat different rates. The lifespan of a mouse is considered to be between two and four years, whereas the Greenland shark has been known to live for more than four hundred years. When looking at mammals, there is a significant degree of variation in lifespan, which can vary by a factor of as much as one hundred. The maximum lifespan of the Etruscan shrew is approximately two years, whereas the bowhead whale is estimated to have a lifespan that is much longer than two centuries at the present time. Larger animals, on average, have a longer lifespan than smaller animals. This is a general trend.

Canine species have a lifespan that is noticeably longer than that of rodents, whereas pachyderms have a lifespan that is significantly longer than that of canines. As was mentioned earlier, there is a substantial disparity in the length of life spans among different species. For example, the lifespan of a mouse is typically between two and four years, whereas the naked mole rat, which is a creature of comparable size, can live for as long as thirty years. There is a significant difference in the rate of aging that occurs between different organisms, with some displaying a sped-up aging process while others displaying a slowed-down aging process. However, this assertion is true for each and every one of them. A decline in both physical and mental fitness, an increased susceptibility to age-related illnesses, and a significant increase in the risk of death are all characteristics of the aging process. When it comes to mortality in humans, the probability of death for a person who has reached the age of 80 is approximately 300 times higher than the probability of death for a person who has reached the age of 20. Providing a concise overview of significant themes in contemporary research on aging is the goal of this chapter. To add insult to injury, it is important to highlight the potential opportunities that may emerge from this area of research. These opportunities have the potential to lead to a significant extension of the human lifespan in a healthy state.

Orientation and Directional Terms:

Term	Definition	Illustration
DNA damage	Structural alteration to DNA, which can result from various factors such as environmental toxins, radiation, or errors in replication. It may lead to mutations and affect cell function.	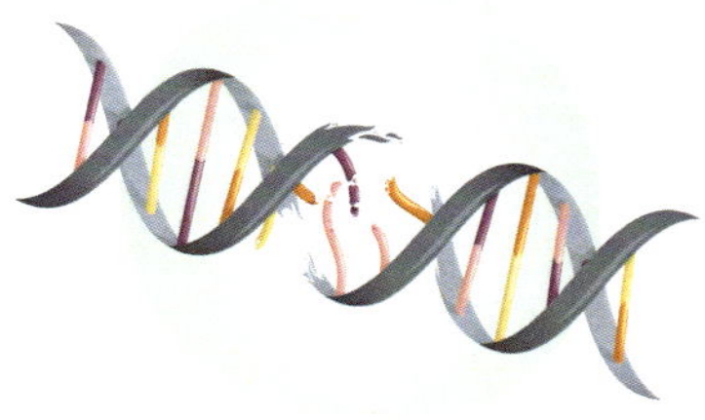
Lipid peroxidation	Oxidative degradation of lipids, where free radicals "steal" electrons from lipids in cell membranes, leading to cell damage and potentially contributing to various diseases.	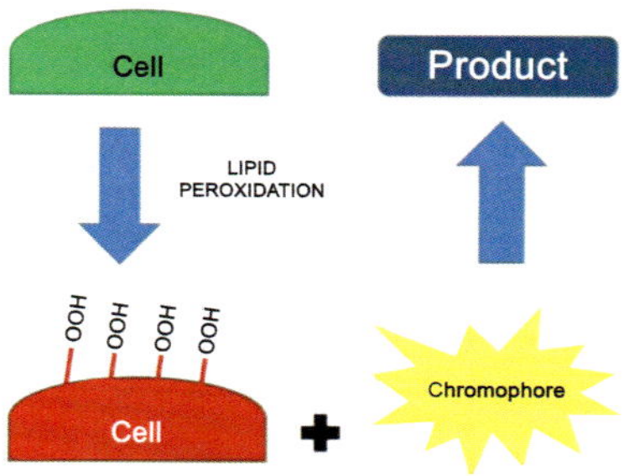
Protein oxidation	Process where proteins are chemically modified due to oxidative stress, altering their structure and function, potentially leading to cellular dysfunction and disease.	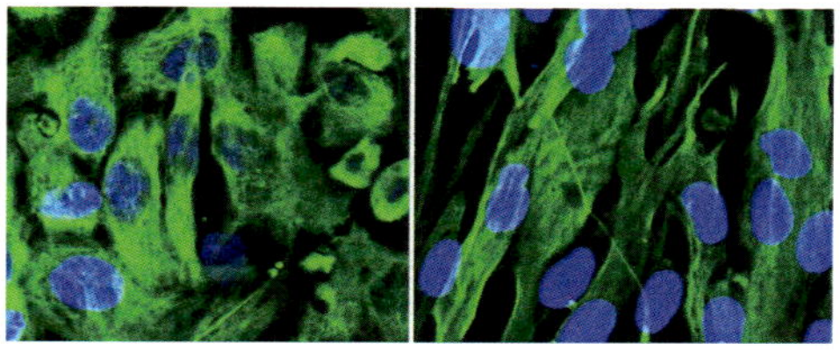
Multiple sclerosis	A chronic autoimmune disease where the immune system attacks the protective myelin sheath covering nerve fibers, leading to communication problems between the brain and the rest of the body.	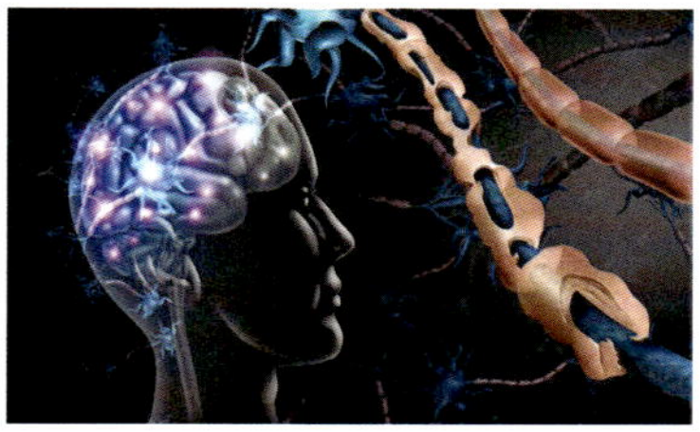
Osteoarthritis	Degenerative joint disease characterized by the breakdown of cartilage in joints, leading to pain, stiffness, and reduced mobility over time. It is often associated with aging and wear-and-tear on joints.	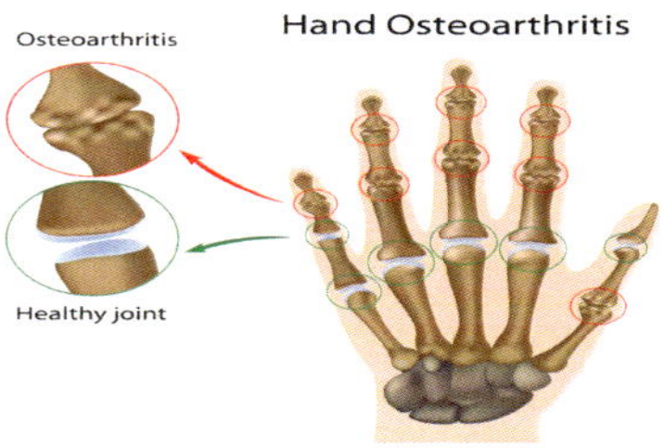

5.1. Theories of Aging

There have been a great number of hypotheses developed to explain the process of aging. In the year 1990, Zhores Medvedev compiled more than 300 different theories altogether. This has resulted in the introduction of many new ones. On the basis of this premise, one can conclude that the process of aging is extremely complex. Because of this, a complete comprehension of the aging process continues to elude us. "Program Theories," "Combined Theories," and "Damage Theories" are the three distinct categories that have delineated the categorization of various theories, which have been delineated in the most recent publication. These theories have been classified into three distinct categories.

According to the programmatic theories, the process of aging is predetermined by factors that are genetic for the individual. The theory of replicative senescence is one of the hypotheses that scholars have put forward. Haylick discovered in 1965 that living cells in a grown environment go through approximately forty to fifty divisions before reaching a permanent cell cycle stoppage, which means that they are unable to recover. During each and every instance of cellular replication, the length of telomeres gradually decreases, which led to the discovery of the reason for this phenomenon. A significant shortening of the telomeres results in the loss of the shelterin complex, which causes the cell to recognize a double-strand tear in the DNA at that location. This recognition sets off a response that causes DNA to lose its integrity permanently. On top of that, it has been found that cellular senescence can be brought on by many different stressors, such as oxidative stress and the upregulation of cellular oncogenes. Through the process of preventing the proliferation of damaged cells, cellular death is a powerful mechanism that effectively inhibits the development of tumors. It is commonly known as the secretory phenotype associated with senescence (SASP), and it is characterized by the fact that senescent cells undergo significant changes in their phenotype and begin the secretion of a wide variety of proteins, including cytokines and chemokines. In addition to phagocytes, neutrophils, and natural killer cells, which are responsible for the elimination of senescent cells, these amino acids attract immune cells.

On the other hand, the accumulation of aged cells is known to increase with age and is known to initiate pathological alterations in the particular organ. A mouse model has demonstrated that the elimination of senescent cells through the use of a living organism can prevent diseases in the lungs, kidneys, heart, and fat tissue. There is compelling evidence to suggest that senescent cells play a significant role in the decline in functionality of aging organs as well as the development of pathologies that are associated with aging. One possible interpretation of the appearance of senescent cells is that they exhibit a hostile pleiotropy. According to the theory of aging, also referred to as the "program," advantageous mutations occur during development, which are beneficial during the early stages of life but prove to be detrimental later in life. To be more specific, cells that undergo senescence as a result of damage can prevent the development of tumors in the early stages of life, but they give rise to detrimental effects in the later stages of its development. According to the "disposable soma theory," which is also referred to as the "program" theory, the supplies of a living thing are limited and must be distributed among the living thing and its reproductive functions.

In addition, it is important to consider whether the "neuroendocrine theory of aging" is the type of theory that is classified as "program theories." Specifically, the statement suggests that the process of aging is controlled by hormones that are comparable to those that are involved in puberty and menopause processes. Additionally, it is a well-known fact that organisms that reach sexual maturity at a rapid pace also have a lifespan that is relatively shorter than average. This rodent has a lifespan of two to four years and reaches sexual maturity within six to eight weeks. Its lifespan is also between two and four years. On the other hand, the Greenland shark has a life expectancy that exceeds 400 years, although it takes it approximately 150 years to reach sexual maturity. Experiments involving parabiosis have shown that aged mice can benefit from the rejuvenating effects of young mouse blood. This is an important finding. Alterations in gene expression oversight that occur during the aging process are the primary factor that affects genes, according to recent studies. In this context, the entities that are responsible for the process of expansion and growth are being under consideration. Without a doubt, the genome of an organism is the primary factor that determines its lifespan. Even though they are both exposed to the same environment, the lifespan of a human is significantly longer than that of a mouse. However, there is only one gene that is responsible for the active regulation of the aging process.

Within the context of the discussion on hypotheses regarding aging, the damage theories are examples of the opposite end of the spectrum. The idea that getting older is a free radical concept. According to the information that has been provided, reactive oxygen species (ROS) are produced as a result of oxidative phosphorylation, which takes place in the mitochondria. This process has the potential to cause damage to genetic material, lipids, and amino acids. Over the course of this discussion, we will briefly touch on the following topics:

1. **DNA Damage:** It is of the utmost importance to effectively repair DNA damage. If this problem is not addressed, it may lead to a more rapid progression of the aging process, as demonstrated by people who have been diagnosed with progeria (also known as Werner Syndrome). As a consequence of this, numerous DNA repair mechanisms can effectively rectify DNA damage. These mechanisms include the direct reversal route, mismatch restoration, base removal repair, nucleotide removal repair, homologous replication, and non-homologous ends joining. There are over one hundred different enzymes that are capable of repairing DNA damage and preventing it from significantly contributing to the aging process. However, as people get older, their effectiveness decreases. A significant factor that is likely to contribute to the aging process is the presence of broken double-strands of DNA.
2. **Lipid Peroxidation:** Reactive oxygen species (ROS) are primarily responsible for targeting unsaturated lipids that are in the membranes of cells. Peroxidation of lipids causes the cleavage of fatty acids, which in turn leads to the formation of highly reactive aldehydes. Because of their reactivity toward proteins and DNA, the aldehydes in question are responsible for modifications that are considered to be irreversible. Proteins that go through such modifications frequently suffer from functional impairment and have a tendency to aggregate, which presents a challenge for the process of cellular degradation,

particularly in the brain. Research has demonstrated that lipid peroxidation can be the initial step in the process of neurodegeneration.

3. **Protein Oxidation:** Scientists have found that reactive oxygen species (ROS) are responsible for the oxidation of proteins. To be more specific, the process of oxidation is focusing on amino acids that contain sulfur. It is possible to reverse the oxidation process beginning with the first stage through the use of enzymes, but the subsequent stages cannot be reversed. As a result of oxidative damage, proteins have a tendency to aggregate and denaturation, which presents a challenge for the mechanisms that are responsible for the degradation of cellular components. Recent years have seen an increase in the number of people who are interested in a modified version of the theory that free radicals are the cause of aging. A disruption in redox homeostasis, rather than reactive oxygen species (ROS), is the primary factor that is responsible for the aging process, as stated in the assertion.

The "Inflamm-Aging" theory is one of the hypotheses that have been proposed to explain the fundamental reasons behind the aging process. This theory proposes that the aging process can be traced back to a persistent, low-level sterile inflammation. An inflammatory component is present in many degenerative diseases that are associated with aging. These diseases include, but are not limited to, Parkinson's disease, Alzheimer's disease, artery disease, multiple sclerosis, osteoarthritis, bone loss, and type II diabetes. The debris of diseased cells and protein aggregates that have not been completely eliminated are frequently attributed to a variety of inflammatory responses. After the concept of inflame-aging was established, the conceptual foundation for the term "Garb-Aging" (which is derived from the words "garbage" and "aging") was established as a complement to the concept of inflame-aging. To this point, neither of the hypotheses presented above has been able to provide evidence that demonstrates their ability to provide a comprehensive explanation of the aging phenomenon. Recent years have seen the introduction of a novel perspective, which proposes that the process of aging can be defined as a gradual decline in both physical and physiological well-being, which can be attributed to the growing influence of factors that are detrimental to overall health. Following this theoretical framework, the production of biomolecules and the repair mechanisms that are present within a cell contain a certain amount of imperfection. Further, numerous chemical reactions take place between the many different types of biomolecules. There is some degree of difficulty in removing the compounds that result. Alongside the process of aging, there is a positive correlation between the accumulation of undesirable reaction byproducts and damage that has not been repaired, which is also referred to as deleterious. (Salthouse, 2010)

5.2. Hallmarks of Aging

To provide an alternative approach to explaining the phenomenon of aging, one alternative method is to provide an outline of the characteristics that are most significant to each individual. When compared to the conventional method, which is to rely on theoretical frameworks, this is an alternative approach. The fact that these are the characteristics that are typically associated with the process of getting older is something that is common knowledge!

5.2.1. Genomic Instability

The genetic material, DNA, is susceptible to a wide variety of harmful effects that originate from a variety of sources, including reactive oxygen species, peroxidation of lipids byproducts, mutagenic environmental factors, hydrolytic responses, ultraviolet radiation, and multiple other sources. It is typically impossible to undo these kinds of damages. In addition to the chemical modifications that can occur to DNA, there are also single- and double-strand ruptures, depurination, and various cross-linkages that can occur between bases. Changing the nucleotide bases by adding, removing, or replacing them can result in significant variations. These modifications, when taken as a whole, have the potential to induce epigenetic modifications, which in turn lead to changes in the activity of genes.

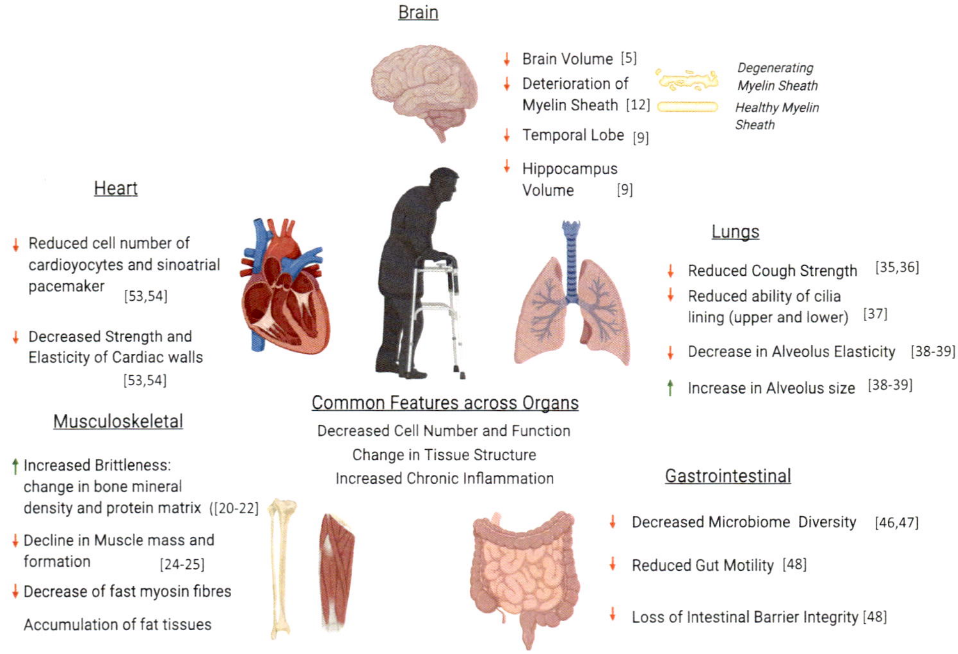

Figure 5.1. *A schematic presentation of causes of aging.*

Source: Xu, W., Wong, G., Hwang, Y.Y. et al. The untwining of immunosenescence and aging. Semin Immunopathol 42, 559–572 (2020). https://doi.org/10.1007/s00281-020-00824-x.

As progeria and other signs of aging syndromes demonstrate, it is of the utmost importance to repair the damage effectively. A marked acceleration of the aging process is the consequence of these diseases, which are characterized by abnormalities in the mechanisms within the DNA that provide restoration. In most cases, the process of repairing damage to DNA is carried out with a high degree of effectiveness. In spite of this, the effectiveness of the repair mechanisms has a tendency to decrease as the aging process progresses (Figure 5.1).

5.2.2. Telomere Attrition

Telomeres are specialized structures that reside at the end of chromosomes and serve the purpose of protecting against the deterioration or combination of chromosome finishes. During each cellular division, the telomeres undergo a process of shortening, and once they reach a critical length, the cells are unable to divide any further. Telomere attrition is a process that ultimately leads to replicative senescence at the end of the spectrum. A direct correlation exists between the degree of reduction and the likelihood of a variety of illnesses that are associated with aging. Researchers have discovered that having short telomeres can cause bone marrow failure, which in turn can result in anemia and immune senescence. In addition, they have been associated with the motility of the intestinal epithelium, which is important for intestinal function. At the same time, the presence of abbreviated telomeres has been associated with the early development of pulmonary fibrosis and emphysema, both of which are conditions that affect the respiratory system, as well as fibrosis in the hepatic system and osteoporosis.

In addition, the presence of abbreviated telomeres can exert an influence on gene expression through the potential implications of telomere length position for genes that are located nearby. We observed a delay in the normal process of aging that occurs in mice. A total of eleven mutations that lead to the inactivation of a single gene have been discovered in human beings. Age-related illnesses and accelerated aging are both linked to these mutations, which have a direct impact on the maintenance of telomeres. In telomere biological science, the Hoyeraal-Hreidarsson (HH) condition is a mental illness that is associated with telomeric duties. Gene mutations are the cause of this condition. People who are affected by this condition typically die during childhood, primarily as a result of hematopoietic insufficiency. The condition is distinguished by telomeres that are significantly or significantly shorter than normal. There is evidence to suggest that the rate of telomere shortening in slow-aging creatures in nature is slower than the rate at which their counterparts in fast-aging creatures experience this phenomenon (Tedone et al., 2014)

5.2.3. Epigenetic Alterations

Alterations to histone markings, changes to the location of nucleosomes, and RNAs that do not code for a protein are all examples of epigenetic modifications. There is a significant relationship between the modification of histones and the methylation patterns of CpG islands, which all affect the expression of genes. Among the 353 islands of CpG, there was found to be a correlation that was statistically significant between age and other factors. There have been observations made that during the process of aging, 193 CpGs go through the process of hypermethylation, while 160 CpGs go through the process of hypomethylation. The set-in question has been referred to as the genetic clock since it consistently experiences changes in its social standing in terms of methylation. With the help of the genetic clock, it is possible to estimate the biological age of an individual and to identify the signs of age-related functional decline.

In addition, there is compelling evidence that lifestyle factors, including dietary patterns, levels of physical activity, and educational attainment, have an effect on epigenetic time. Acetylation and methylation are two examples of the modifications that histones go through in addition to DNA. As people get older, the patterns of a number of methylation marks change or become different. On the other hand, in comparison to DNA methylation, the current depiction is relatively imprecise. Sirtuins have received a significant amount of attention up until this point.

Sirtuins are members of the class III family of histone deacetylases. They use NAD+ as a cofactor to catalyze the removal of acetyl groups in comparison to lysines before modifiable through the N-terminal tails that are present in them. The removal of the acetyl group from amino acids and the charged state of the amino acids in question increased their affinity for DNA binding. An arrangement of chromatin that is more compact and a reduction in the expression of genes are the results of this occurrence. Earlier studies have demonstrated that sirtuins can remove histone methyl groups, which in turn allows for an extension of the lifespan of an organism. There are currently seven sirtuins that are referred to, with SIRT1, SIRT6, and SIRT7 being specifically restricted in the nucleus. During the G/M phase of the cellular life cycle, SIRT2 is only found in the chromatin, and its presence is only found in the cytoplasm. This is the predominant location of SIRT2 within the cell. The mitochondria have been found to contain three different deacetylases, which are referred to as SIRT3, SIRT4, and SIRT5. Not only do sirtuins play a part in the process of histone deacetylation, but they also regulate a wide variety of other proteins. Because of this, they play a crucial role in regulatory networks that are important for the process of aging and for extending one's lifespan. It was observed that mice that exhibited mutations in singular sirtuin genes exhibited a variety of pathologies that were associated with metabolic dysfunction, carcinogenesis, and inflammatory processes.

5.2.4. Loss of Proteostasis

The synthesis of proteins is necessary, but they also require removal and degradation at some point in the future. Degradation of proteins by proteasomes and autophagy are the two primary mechanisms that are available for the elimination of impaired proteins. Molecular chaperones are also present within the structure of the cell (cell structure). The proper folding of proteins or the restoration of proteins that had been denatured in the past is one of the functions that these proteins facilitate. Chaperones can selectively navigate folded proteins in the direction of the proteasome in situations where refolding is not possible. The term "proteostasis" refers to a collection of processes that contribute to the preservation of a functional proteome. These processes include the synthesis of proteins, the degradation of proteins, folding of proteins, and the maintenance of the correct conformation. Most people agree that one of the most important factors that contributes to aging is the disruption of the proteostasis system. When people get older, they experience a decline in chaperone levels, a reduction in proteasomal activity, and an increase in autophagy. All of these characteristics occur simultaneously. Because of the reduction in cellular function described above, there is an accumulation of proteins that have been denatured, which leads to the formation of aggregates that are no longer able to be removed by the cell. There is evidence that aggregates have a detrimental impact on the function of cells and may even result in the death of cells, as seen in the nerve cells of people who suffer from Alzheimer's disease and Parkinson's disease.

Furthermore, studies have demonstrated that species that live for longer periods have a lower prevalence of denatured proteins compared to species that live for shorter periods. If we compare the activity of the proteasome in the long-lived naked mole rat to that of the only temporary mouse, we find that the activity of the proteasome is significantly higher in the latter. Particularly intriguing are experimental treatments that slow down the aging process by stimulating autophagy. Some examples of such treatments include reducing calorie intake, rapamycin, metformin, resveratrol, and spermidine. (Kirkwood and Kowald, 1997; Kirkwood, 2005) (Figure 5.2).

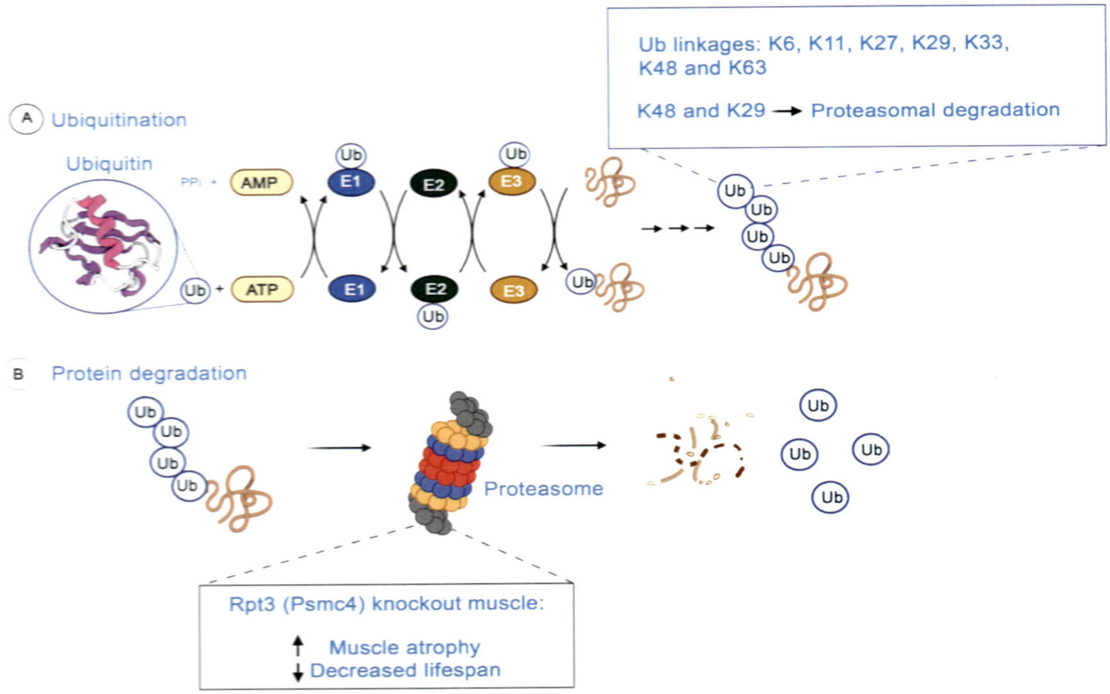

Figure 5.2. *The proteosome in Aging.*

Source: Hughes DC, Baehr LM, Waddell DS, Sharples AP, Bodine SC. Ubiquitin ligases in longevity and aging skeletal muscle. International Journal of Molecular Sciences. 2022; 23(14):7602. https://doi.org/10.3390/ijms23147602.

5.2.5. Deregulated Nutrient Sensing

The ability to sense nutrients is crucial for every cell. The principal sense of nutrient mechanisms that also serve as pathways for longevity include:

- The mTOR pathway,
- the (AMPK) AMP-activated kinase protein pathway
- the IGF-1 and insulin signaling pathways
- Sirtuins that depend on NAD+

In the same way that insulin does, IGF-1 is a growth factor that has an effect on a wide variety of cells and functions by way of the insulin and IGF-1 indicating (IIS) pathway. The down-regulation of this pathway is responsible for the increased lifespan. However, the activation of the mTOR pathway, which is responsible for promoting protein synthesis and growth, is not only facilitated by IGF-1 but also by EGF and increased protein levels. On the other hand, this process can be accompanied by a reduction in the activity of autophagy. AMP-activated protein kinase, also known as AMPK, is a protein that acts as a sensor and controls the regulation of cellular metabolic activity or the equilibrium state. An increase in the lifespan of bacteria, bacterium C. elegans, and drosophila, as well as an improvement in the health span of rats, has been associated with the activation of AMPK. Metabolic diseases can cause the deregulation of pathways of signaling that detect nutrient availability throughout the aging process.

5.2.6. Mitochondrial Dysfunction

Mitochondria, which are both the powerhouses of the cell and significant signaling hubs, play a crucial role in the process of aging. To generate ATP, which is for the production of energy, the reduction of oxygen to water takes place. When oxygen receives a single electron, it has the potential to produce reactive oxygen species (ROS) rather than water rather than water. This phenomenon served as a source of inspiration for Harman as early as 1956, which led to the introduction of his "Free Radical Theory of Aging," which he went on to develop further on multiple occasions.

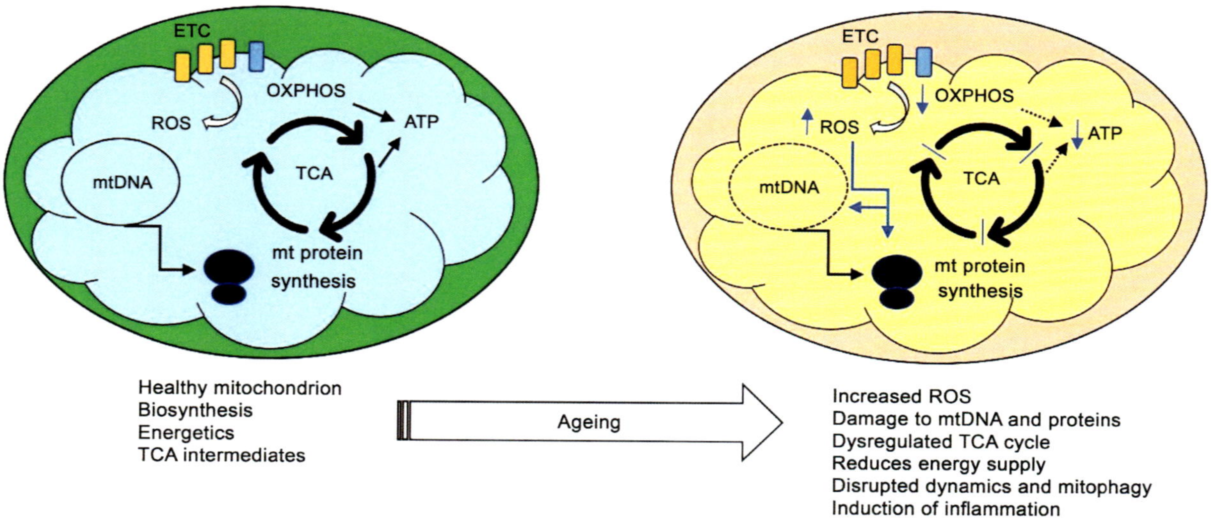

Figure 5.3. *Role of mitochondria in aging.*

Source: Webb M, Sideris DP. Intimate relations—Mitochondria and ageing. International Journal of Molecular Sciences. 2020; 21(20):7580. https://doi.org/10.3390/ijms21207580.

Furthermore, it has been demonstrated that reactive oxygen species (ROS) are responsible for inducing damage and can act as significant signaling molecules that can regulate a variety of pathways. For instance, it has been observed that reactive oxygen species (ROS) have the capability to initiate autophagy, more specifically mitophagy for that matter (Figure 5.3).

The concept of mitochondrial function encompasses the processes of biogenesis, which include nuclear fusion, nuclear fission, and mitophagy. When it comes to regulating the function and quality of mitochondria, dietary metabolism is an extremely important factor. Observations have shown that an abundance of nutrients can lead to the fragmentation of mitochondria through the process of fission, whereas a deficiency of nutrients can lead to the fusion and elongation of mitochondria. The functioning of mitochondria has been observed to be influenced by a variety of external factors, including hormones, nutrients, and physical exercise. There is evidence that suggests that multiple signaling pathways, such as mTOR, AMP-activated kinase, and sirtuins, are involved. As opposed to merely regulating a small number of target proteins, sirtuins play a significant role in the regulation of functional groups. These functional groups include the process of TCA, the utilization of fatty acids, the transport of electrons chain, and other related physiological processes. Therefore, they possess the ability to regulate signaling pathways using reactive oxygen species (ROS) and the elimination of harmful ROS. Moreover, they control the adaptability of the metabolic system. There is evidence that SIRT3 plays a role in facilitating the transition toward fatty acid oxidation in response to calorie restriction. One of the most important aspects of the aging process is the regulation of metabolic changes (also known as metabolic regulation).

Additionally, mitochondria that are not functioning properly contribute to inflammatory responses, which in turn contribute to the aging process. Damage to mitochondria is known to play a role in a variety of age-related conditions, including metabolic and cardiovascular disorders, neurodegenerative disorders, and sarcopenia or fibrosis in multiple organs. The aforementioned evidence demonstrates that the quality of mitochondria has a significant impact on the duration of the aging process (Bratic and Larsson, 2013).

5.2.7. Cellular Senescence

The permanent cessation of the cell's life cycle is the defining characteristic of the senescence process that occurs in cells. It can be deduced that the influence of cellular senescence is restricted to cells that are capable of undergoing division, such as stem cells, precursor cells, or cells that have not yet reached a state of terminal differentiation. This is because these cells are limited in their ability to undergo division. In vitro examination of cultured cells has revealed the occurrence of this phenomenon. It was found that their capacity for division is limited and that it stops after approximately forty to fifty instances of cellular division.

Telomere shortening, significant DNA damage, oxidative damage, oncogenic overexpression, mitochondrial dysfunction, and proteotoxicity are all potential factors that can result in a permanent stoppage of the cell cycle. Senescent cells are characterized by their altered morphologies, their increased size, and the significant structural changes that they have undergone in their chromatin and DNA. In addition to this, they begin secreting a great deal of proteins. In the context of senescence-associated secretory phenotype, the term "SASP" refers to the entirety of these proteins. A few examples of proteins that belong to this category include pro-inflammatory cells, chemokines, growth hormones, and matrix metalloproteases (MMPs). By inducing localized sterile inflammations, which are a significant contributor to the process of "inflame-aging," the cytokines that promote inflammation are responsible for inducing inflammation. Attracting immune cells that are capable of eliminating senescent cells is a common phenomenon. There is a hypothesis that suggests that a decrease in the effectiveness of the immune system is responsible for the disproportionate increase in senescent cells that is observed during the aging process. One of the most important characteristics of senescent cells is their ability to actively inhibit apoptosis. In order to facilitate a long-lasting cell cycle arrest at the gene expression level, the protein that is known as p16Ink4a acts as a kinase inhibitor of cyclin-dependent kinases four and six (CDK4 and CDK6) (Figure 5.4).

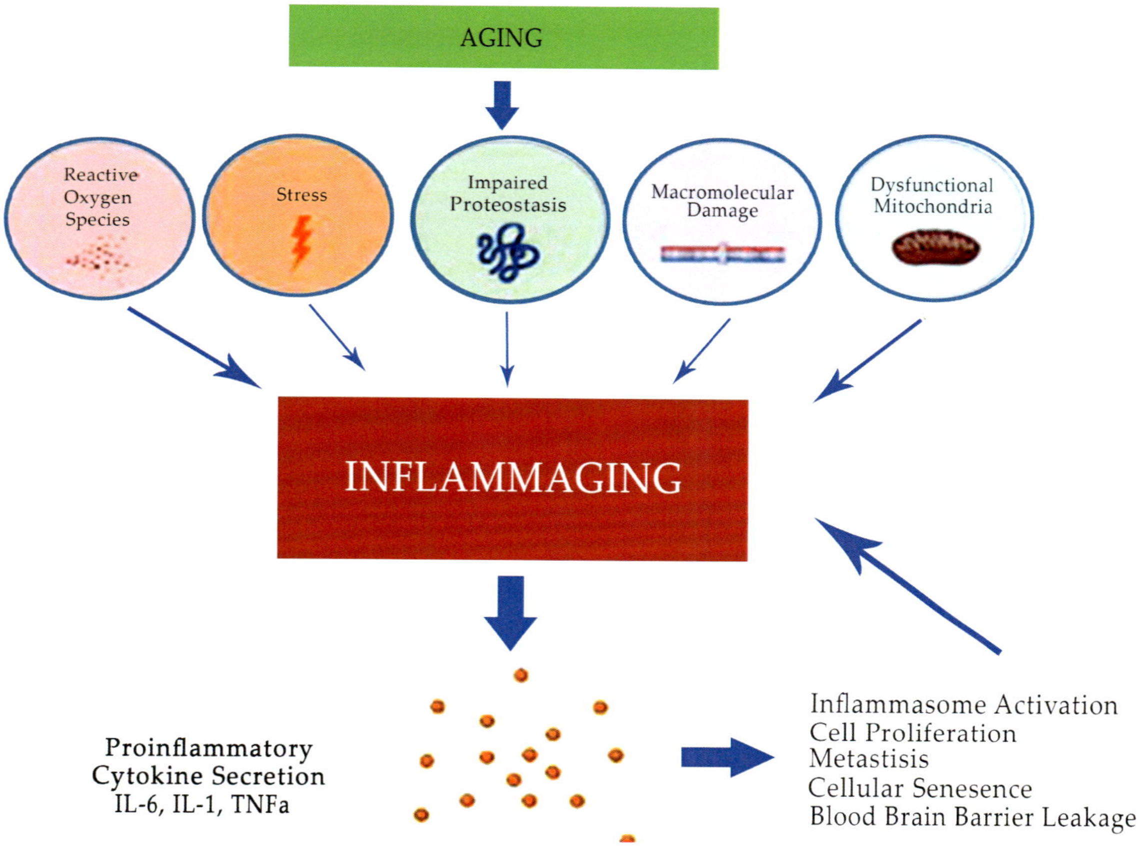

Figure 5.4. *Inflamm-aging.*

Source: By Myelinav – Own work, CC BY-SA 4.0, https://commons.wikimedia.org/w/index.php?curid=112923420.

When it comes to robust juvenile cells, the expression of p16Ink4a is either very low or completely absent. However, it goes through a significant increase in the number of cells that have gone through the process of senescence. The activation of a safeguard mechanism to inhibit unregulated cell proliferation, which has the potential to lead to the development of tumors, is one of the most important functions of senescence, which is perhaps the most important aspect of an organism. When it comes to the process of wound healing, senescent cells are an extremely important component. A surplus of cells is produced in the aftermath of an injury to facilitate the healing process of the wound. It is during the subsequent remodeling stage that a significant number of cells go through the process of senescence, which is followed by elimination by the immune system of the body. Since a considerable amount of time ago, researchers have been debating the potential influence that cellular senescence could have on how an individual ages. In the most recent years, researchers have established that the process of aging is responsible for cell death. Genetically modified rats can eradicate senescence cells, also known as p16Ink4a beneficial cells. The animals described above had a lower incidence of age-related illnesses, a longer period of time during which they were in good health, and a longer median lifespan during their lifetimes.

As a consequence of this, numerous interventions are currently being investigated to investigate the possibility of eradicating aging cells in the human body. It is possible that achieving success in this regard will significantly increase the amount of time that a human being can remain healthy. There is a significant relationship between the presence of senescent cells and the development of age-related degenerative pathologies. Senescent cells have a detrimental impact on the physiological processes of the organs in which they are located.

5.2.8. Stem Cell Exhaustion

There is widespread agreement that stem cells play an important role in maintaining the equilibrium of tissues and facilitating the process of regeneration. The depletion of stem cells is one of the most noticeable characteristics that mark the aging process. A decrease in the capacity to regenerate tissues is a consequence of the depletion of stem cells that occurs during the aging process. The premature depletion of stem cells is another characteristic of diseases that are associated with aging. Stem cells are typically smaller than other cell types and remain dormant throughout their evolution. Differentiating characteristics of the state in question include a slowed metabolic rate and a dearth of mitochondria. It is possible to stimulate stem cells to differentiate into transit-amplifying cells after they have been in a state of quiescence. These cells then generate a large number of cells that can either restore or regenerate the particular tissue that is being concerned. During the process of differentiation, cells go through a growth cycle that adapts them to their newly acquired function in a very specific manner.

The bone marrow, the intestines, and the epidermis of the skin are examples of tissues that have a cellular turnover rate that is significantly higher than average. There are some tissues, such as those found in the mind and the muscles, in which the activation of stem cells occurs more infrequently than in other tissues. For stem cells to continue to exist and remain in a state of quiescence, they must have a niche that encompasses their immediate surroundings. Proteins derived from the extracellular matrix and neighboring cells are essential components of the stem cell microenvironment. These proteins are responsible for the production of various amino acids, including Wnts, BMPs, EGF, and Notch. In order to complete the process, it is necessary to regulate a state of inactivity. Many factors contribute to the process of aging, such as the attrition of telomeres and the senescence of cells. It is possible to attribute stem cell degeneration to a number of different factors, such as DNA damage, epigenetic changes, nutrient sensing, and disrupted proteostasis, which also has an effect on other biological processes. Stem cells are characterized by their behavior of remaining in a quiescent state and exhibiting infrequent division. However, their niche is vulnerable to a wide variety of pro-aging influences that have the potential to affect stem cells. Satellite cells, also known as muscle stem cells, undergo significant proliferation in response to stimuli, but they only divide infrequently. They are responsible for the production of myoblasts, which are necessary precursor cells for the regeneration of muscle. It is possible to demonstrate the influence of the youthful niche by observing the increased capacity for regeneration that occurs as a consequence of transplanting aged cell satellites into younger muscle tissue (Figure 5.5).

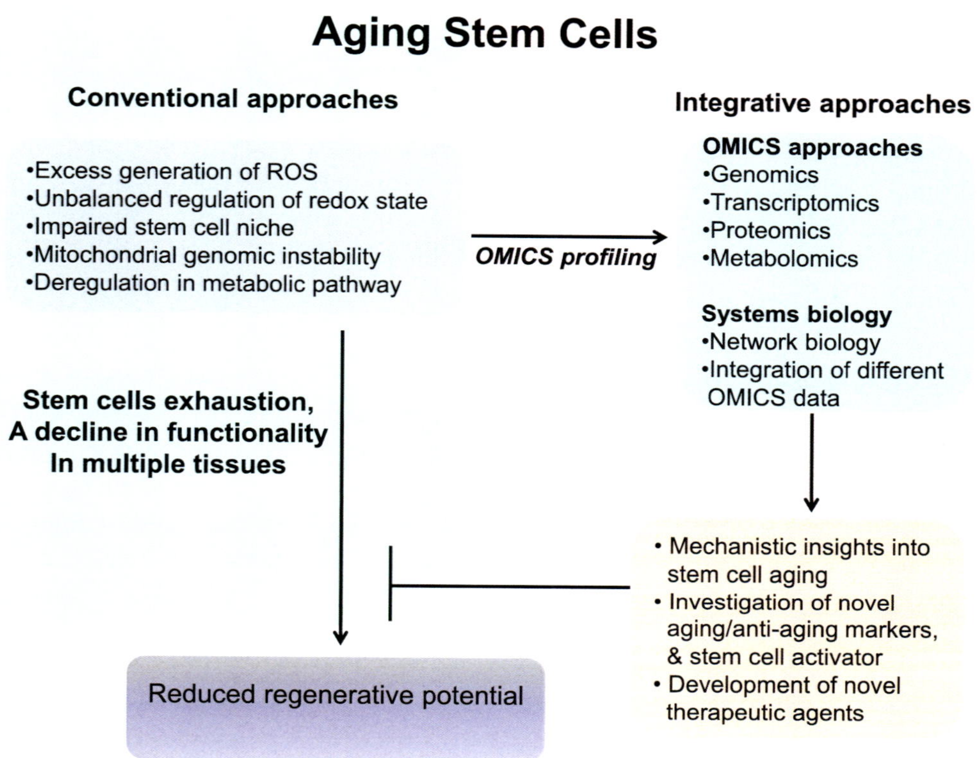

Figure 5.5. *Stem Cell Exhaustion.*

Source: Bae, SH., Kim, CH., Leblanc, P. et al. Perspectives of aging study on stem cell. Biomed Dermatol 1, 9 (2017). https://doi.org/10.1186/s41702-017-0007-2.

On the other hand, the opposite is true for transforming growth factor beta (TGF-beta1). This factor is a result of the environmental function of a specific habitat, and it reduces the ability of satellite cells to undergo the process of proliferation. Under certain circumstances that occur during the process of aging, the niche demonstrates an increase in the secretion of fibroblast growth factor (FGF2). The activation of stem cells causes them to undergo a transition from a quiescent state to a proliferative state. This leads to a reduction in the pool of satellite cells, which are essential for the process of regenerating muscular tissue. It is believed that the exhaustion of stem cells occurs as a consequence of the prolonged activation of the development hormone (GH)/insulin/insulin-like growth factor (IGF) axis.

There have been discoveries made regarding the presence of stem cells in specific regions of the adult brain. These regions include the dentate gyrus, which is a component of the hippocampus, which is a component of the region of the hypothalamus, and the subventricular region, which is the region of the left ventricle. Similar to the changes that take place in other tissues, the microenvironment of stem cells changes as one gets older, which results in a decrease in the population of neural stem cells. There is a correlation between the aging process and an increase in the level of TGF-beta1, which is responsible for the decrease in the number of stem cells and the inhibition of the growth of precursor cells. According to the findings of research, neurogenesis has been decreasing, while oligodendrogenesis has remained relatively stagnant.

It is also possible that the presence of clean micro-inflammation within the cerebral cortex could lead to a reduction in the number of neural stem cells, which would then lead to a decline in cognitive abilities.

The regenerative potential of a tissue or organ is dependent on many systemic variables, such as the number of stem cells that are present and the function of the cell niche. Through the utilization of parabiosis experiments, which involve the interconnection of an aged mouse with a younger counterpart, it has been demonstrated that the dysfunction of aged satellite cells within muscle tissue can be remedied. This was an important discovery. Reactivating those satellite cells is in fact a possibility. Similarly, it was possible to improve the effectiveness of embryonic stem cells or neurogenesis in brains that had reached an advanced age. The proteins that are responsible for this particular function are known as growth differentiation factor 11 (GDF11) and oxytocin. When it comes to the biological functionality of stem cells, there are a multitude of factors that govern their functioning. Metabolic changes and epigenetic alterations appear to be the most significant factors at the moment. The early depletion of adult neural stem cells is a consequence of excessive nutrient sensing, and the loss of origin cells from the epithelium of the airways in the mouse is the result of chronic stimulation of mTOR. Both of these processes occur simultaneously.

5.2.9. Altered Intercellular Communication

When it comes to the capacity of stem cells to regenerate, both intrinsic and extrinsic factors can exert independent influences. The maintenance of autophagy is an example of an endogenous factor that helps to determine the outcome of a particular situation. A lack of autophagy may be the cause of the ultimate senescence of satellite cells that occurs in people who are getting older.

The somatotrophic axis, and more specifically the growth hormone/insulin/IGF-1 pathway, is an external factor that plays a significant role in the regulation of development in mammals. Rodent models that have mutations that affect the synthesis of growth hormones, such as Ames dwarf mice, Snell dwarf mice, and GHRKO mice (GH receptor deletion), display a size reduction that is significantly greater than that of their wild-type counterparts.

Nevertheless, these mutants exhibit a mortality rate that is approximately 50% longer than average. Throughout the course of human development, some changes occur in the levels of growth hormone or insulin-like growth factor 1 (IGF-1) that are already in circulation. The second decade, which is characterized by the most prominent surge in development, is the time when growth reaches its highest point on the growth scale. After that, the concentration gradually decreases until it reaches a point where it reaches a plateau of decreased concentration in the sixth decade (Figure 5.6).

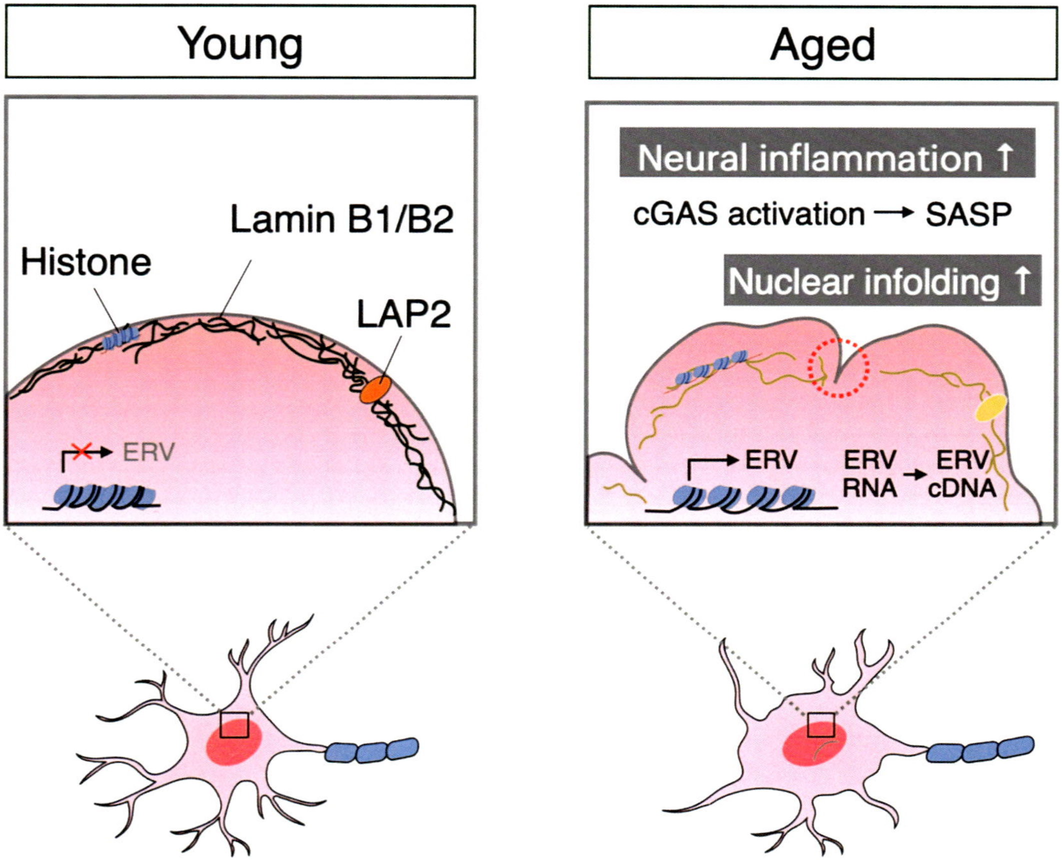

Figure 5.6. *Altered Communication during Aging.*

Source: Maeda C, Tsuruta F. Molecular basis of neuronal and microglial states in the aging brain and impact on cerebral blood vessels. International Journal of Molecular Sciences. 2024; 25(8):4443. https://doi.org/10.3390/ijms25084443.

There is a significant increase in the lifespan of individuals who possess genetic variants that result in a reduction in the activity of IGF-1. There is a correlation between an increased concentration of insulin-like growth factor 1 (IGF-1) and an increased risk for certain types of tumors. This correlation is positive. In addition, there is a modified interaction that takes place between myogenic progenitor cells and the microenvironment that surrounds them. Growth hormones are essential for the continued development of skeletal muscle, which is dependent on their presence. It has been believed that IGF-1 is responsible for the modulation of muscle progenitor cell differentiation, more specifically myoblasts, as well as the influence on satellite cells. On the other hand, an accelerated aging process in muscle stem cells has been identified as being caused by elevated levels of Wnt-proteins, such as Wnt3A. It has been determined that the protein klotho is an antagonist. This antagonist is associated with the W pathway. With increasing age, unfortunately, there is a decrease in the levels of klotho that are circulating in the body. After the deletion of the Klotho genes, the mice exhibited an acceleration of the aging process.

When it comes to maintaining the homeostasis of mineral metabolism, specifically phosphate levels, Klotho protein plays a crucial role. At the same time, Klotho can control the signaling pathways of either IGF-1 or Wnt. The absence of the Klotho genes in murine subjects results in a significant reduction in their longevity, with a lifespan of only two to three months, which is only 10% of their typical lifespan.

There is evidence that GDF11 can significantly boost the rate of regeneration in organisms that are getting older. In addition, the serum levels of GDF11 in elderly individuals are significantly lower than those of younger individuals. Research has shown that there is a higher level of regenerative action in a variety of bodily tissues, such as the bones, the brain, the skeleton, and the muscles of the heart.

In addition, a number of chemokines, specifically CCL2, CCL11, CCL12, and CCL19, were found through parabiosis tests. Furthermore, the association between these chemokines and decreased neurogenesis in elderly individuals has been established. In addition to TGF-beta1, IL-6, and TNF-alpha, other factors have the potential to accelerate the aging process and are known to increase in concentration over the course of an individual's lifetime.

These factors include, but are not limited to, TNF-alpha. Because it is responsible for inducing cognitive decline that is associated with aging, beta2 microglobulin is also considered to be a systemic factor in the aging process.

The production of plasminogen activation inhibitor 1 (PAI-1), which is considered to be a factor that contributes to the aging process, is a characteristic of senescent cells. Ultimately, the process leads to the accumulation of p16Ink4a, which ultimately results in the senescence of the cells. In order to accomplish its anti-wrinkle properties, kallistatin works by inhibiting oxidative stress in addition to inflammation. Additionally, it can reduce the production of miR21 in conjunction with miR-34a, which ultimately leads to a reduction in the aging process and the maturation of the vascular system. The human umbilical vein was used to isolate the protein that is now known as the tissue inhibitor for a protein called 2 (TIMP 2), which was obtained through the use of isolation procedures.

This protein is known for its anti-aging properties because it effectively rejuvenates the hippocampus, enhances synaptic plasticity, and ultimately leads to improved cognitive function. It is associated with several benefits.

Senescent cells secrete a variety of cytokines that promote inflammation, which alter how cells interact with one another. Inflammatory responses from substances that are known as cytokines.

In addition, it is important to note that the inflammasomes that are present in the cells of the innate immune system have the capability of being stimulated by DAMPs, which are molecular patterns that are associated with damage. Necrotic cells, amyloid particle fibers, high mobility group box 1 (HMGB1), heat shock proteins, cholesterol, and uric acid crystals are some of the components that together make up damage-associated molecular patterns (DAMPS).

DAMPS are a complex mixture of a variety of components. The stimulation of inflammatory cells, which results in the release of interleukins such as IL-1beta or IL-18 for example. Interleukins are responsible for inducing inflammatory responses in the tissue that is adjacent to them. These responses are a contributing factor in the development of age-related diseases such as Alzheimer's disease.

These exosomes provide an additional channel through which cells can communicate with one another. Extracellular vesicles are small structures that are bound to lipids and are released by cells. They are responsible for transporting proteins and working RNAs throughout the cell ecosystem.

The dissemination of these entities can occur through a variety of channels, including communication between cells and systemic distribution through circulation. In addition to facilitating communication between cells, these cellular mechanisms contribute to the cleaning up of harmful protein waste. The latter scenario is one in which microRNAs play a significant role in the majority of cases.

The amount of exosomes that are present in the bloodstream does not change significantly throughout the aging process. On the other hand, their composition demonstrates a higher degree of symptoms that are associated with inflammation. The results of recent studies have shown that they also play a role in the processes of aging and senescence of the body (Weinert and Timiras, 2003; Vlachopoulos et al., 2015).

5.3. Possible Therapeutic Interventions

5.3.1. Physical Exercise

One of the most straightforward and efficient ways to slow down the aging process is to participate in physical activity. On the other hand, it has been discovered that a lifestyle that is characterized by a lack of physical activity and prolonged periods of sitting has negative health effects that are comparable to those that are associated with smoking. Participating in strenuous physical activity is the most effective method for preserving the health of skeletal muscles and reducing the risk of developing sarcopenia and frailty as one ages.

Elderly people who participate in physical exercise experience improvements in both their physical and mental well-being. This is because physical exercise improves physiological factors such as the highest utilization of oxygen and decreased cholesterol levels in the bloodstream. Engaging in physical activity has the potential to significantly improve a variety of physiological parameters. The protective benefits for the circulatory system, on the other hand, appear to be approximately two times greater than the expected improvements based solely on these parameters.

As a result, there are a great deal of questions that have not yet been answered concerning the molecular mechanisms that are triggered by physical exercise. There is a wealth of evidence demonstrating the beneficial effects on the brain, particularly on cognitive development and neuronal growth in the hippocampus, which is an essential region for the processes involved in memory. Research has shown that engaging in physical activity can both increase the volume of the hippocampus and improve the functional connectivity of the brain.

To add insult to injury, research has demonstrated that engaging in physical activity can improve connectivity between the prefrontal cortex and the default mode network. It is important to point out that individuals with Alzheimer's disease who participate in physical exercise experience a significant improvement in their memory capabilities in this particular environment by engaging in physical activity (Wessner et al., 2000) (Figure 5.7).

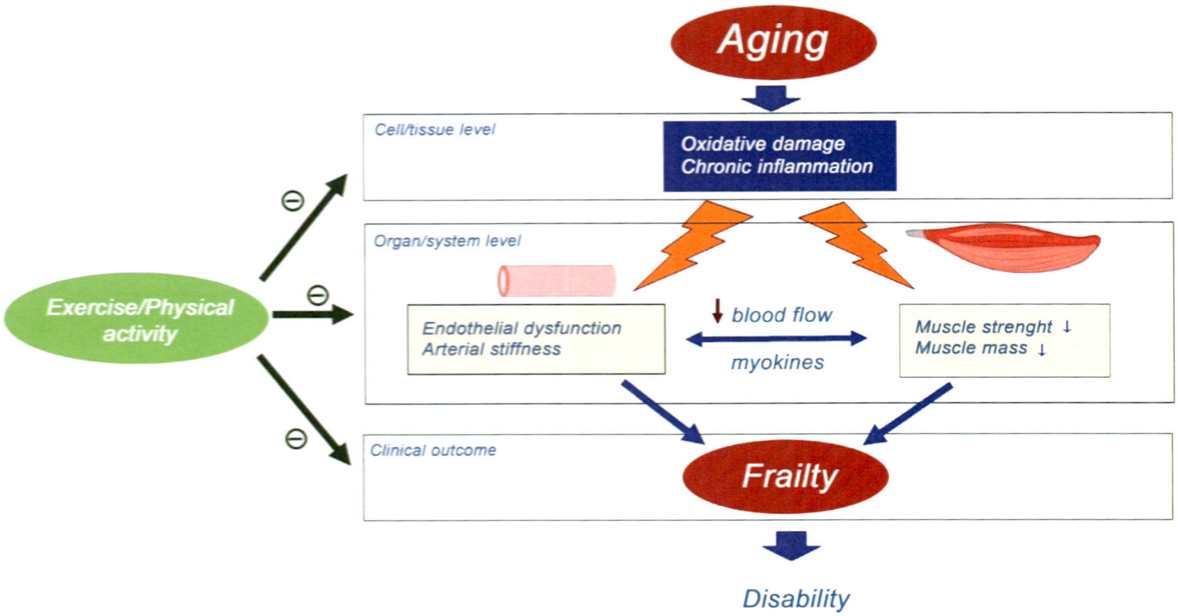

Figure 5.7. *Effect of Exercise on Aging and Longevity.*

Source: El Assar M, Álvarez-Bustos A, Sosa P, Angulo J, Rodríguez-Mañas L. Effect of physical activity/ exercise on oxidative stress and inflammation in muscle and vascular aging. International Journal of Molecular Sciences. 2022; 23(15):8713. https://doi.org/10.3390/ijms23158713.

5.3.2. Caloric Restriction/Dietary Restriction

As early as 1935, research conducted on rats suggested that a reduction in the amount of food consumed could increase the lifespan by as much as thirty percent. There have been multiple instances in which the study has been repeated, and the results indicate that animals have a longer lifespan and a reduction in impairments that are associated with aging. Research conducted in recent years has demonstrated that the amount of protein that is consumed may be more significant than the amount of calories that are consumed. Because of this, the term "dietary restriction" has effectively replaced the phrase "caloric restriction" in certain instances. It is important to consider the temporal pattern of food consumption, even though the quantity of food consumed itself is important. The animals that received a uniform food distribution throughout the day had no favorable outcomes, whereas those fed only once daily demonstrated positive effects. In addition, is there any evidence to suggest that fasting on alternate days leads to a 30% increase in lifespan?

There have been a great number of experiments carried out on this topic, and the results have occasionally been opposite of one another. Multiple authors have made it clear that they have placed a strong emphasis on the significance of carrying out experiments that involve testing a variety of different combinations of carbohydrates and proteins. Research has demonstrated that a ratio of one-tenth of a percent between carbohydrates and proteins results in the greatest longevity in mice. Particularly noteworthy is the fact that the Okinawan population has a protein-to-carbohydrate ratio of 9:85 in their eating habits. There is a significant amount of evidence that the people who live in Okinawa have the highest average lifespan of any people anywhere in the world. It is important to note that in addition to permanent food restriction, intermittent fasting has been shown to be effective in achieving the desired results. Both rats and mice, as well as humans, show significant improvements in their health. In particular, when practiced for two days a week and on alternate days, the results of intermittent fasting have been observed to result in a decrease in insulin levels, an increase in resistance to stress within both the brain and the heart, a reduction in inflammation, an improvement in autophagy, and an improvement in mitochondrial health and DNA repair. These outcomes have been observed to be associated with the practice of intermittent fasting.

Specifically with regard to the subject of DNA repair, the experiment that followed is particularly noteworthy. Mice that are lacking in the DNA removal repair gene Ercc1 have a phenotype that is characterized by an accelerated aging process, which is characterized by a significantly reduced lifespan of between four and six months. The average lifespan of an individual is increased by a factor of three when they are placed on a diet that restricts their caloric intake by thirty percent. Nutrient sensing pathways, specifically GH/insulin/IGF-1, mTOR, sirtuins, and AMPK, are accountable for determining whether or not an individual cell actually possesses the capacity to take in nutrients. In the process of regulating the metabolic response to aging, these pathways play an extremely important role.

5.3.3. The Somatotrophic Axis (GH/insulin/IGF-1)

As a result of the reduction in the signaling that occurs along the somatotrophic axis, the lifespan of the organism grows longer. In addition to the presence of genetic variations and functional changes within the IGF1R genes in the human population, this has also been demonstrated in animal models. Examples of this can be found in the human population. In the present day, researchers are investigating the possibility of developing medications that can block the communication of this pathway. But at this time, there is not a single drug that has been authorized for use in humans.

5.3.4. mTOR

It is widely acknowledged that the mTOR protein is an essential regulator of metabolism and aging. It is classified as a kinase that binds to serine, and it exhibits this property. Both mTORC1 and mTORC2 are examples of multiprotein complexes that contain it present in the body. In the process of stimulating growth and inhibiting autophagy, growth factors like insulin, IGF-1, amines, and sugar are responsible for activating mTOR, which in turn leads to the stimulation of growth.

Through its interaction with FKBP12, rapamycin can exert its inhibitory effect on mTOR. Researchers have found that inhibiting mTOR can lengthen the lifespan of a variety of organisms, including mice. Regrettably, the daily use of the substance is hindered by many negative effects, as was mentioned earlier by individuals who are in good health.

5.3.5. Sirtuins

There is evidence that sirtuins interact with various signaling pathways, such as IGF-1, mTOR, and AMPK. These signaling pathways are known to modulate a wide variety of proteins that are involved in the metabolism of energy, the repair of DNA, the survival of cells, the processes of inflammation, and the regeneration of tissue. According to research, SIRT1 is responsible for the modification of more than fifty proteins, in addition to the deacetylation of histones H1, H3, and H4. Sirtuin-activating substances (STACs) have received a great deal of attention ever since their discovery in 2003. To date, more than 14,000 STACs have been identified. The following should be considered two separate categories: compounds that trigger the activation of sirtuins and increase the concentrations of nicotinamide adenine dinucleotide (NAD+). The use of rodents in various applications. Several studies have shown that STACs have a beneficial effect on health during the aging process by protecting a variety of conditions. These conditions include diabetes, cardiovascular disease, dementia, and tumors.

5.3.6. AMP-Activated Protein Kinase (AMPK)

A heterotrimeric protein, the AMP-protein kinase is an essential enzyme that plays a role in the recognition of cellular energy. It is composed of three subunits, which determine its chemical structure. Upstream kinases are responsible for the phosphorylation of the conserved threonine in the alpha subunit enzyme domain, which in turn prompts AMPK to become active. The beta subunit is the one that is accountable for binding with both the alpha and gamma parts, and it also possesses an additional domain that enables it to detect glycogen. As a result of the presence of four binding sites within the gamma domain, which are capable of interacting with molecules of ATP, ADP, and AMP, AMPK can detect ratios of AMP to ATP as well as ADP to ATP. For an energy-sensing route that displays a large number of outputs and inputs, AMPK is considered to be the central component.

AMPK is responsible for the activation of glucose uptake, fatty acid oxidation, autophagy, and mitochondrial biogenesis. At the same time, it inhibits mTOR and the biosynthesis of protein and lipids. In light of this, it is an essential regulator of metabolic pathways, which includes the influence that these pathways have on age-related diseases. Throughout the course of aging, the inflammasome NLRP3 is responsible for regulation, which brings into question the role that inflammation plays in this process. With increasing age comes a decrease in the capacity of AMPK signaling, which has a detrimental effect on the maintenance of cell equilibrium. In light of these circumstances, it is clear that a substantial amount of research is being carried out to investigate the possibility of restoring or enhancing the activity of AMPK through the utilization of metformin or other nutraceutical substances, particularly polyphenols like resveratrol.

5.4. Pharmacological Substances

5.4.1. Metformin

A significant amount of time has passed since metformin was first utilized as a therapeutic intervention for the treatment of type 2 diabetes. It is the phosphorylation of AMPK that is responsible for the inhibitory effect that it has on the synthesis of glucose in the liver. As an additional point of interest, it has been observed that metformin acts as an inhibitor of both mTOR and complex I within the mitochondria electron transport chain. This results in a reduction in the production of reactive oxygen species (ROS). It has also been observed that metformin promotes autophagy, reduces inflammatory pathways and senescence, and increases longevity in animal models. All of these effects have been observed. In addition to demonstrating favorable effects in cases of cardiac arrest, severe liver disease, persistent renal failure, and multiple sclerosis, among other diseases, metformin has been found to improve the overall lifespan, as well as the potential for mitigating the risk of certain cancers. This information comes from several reports that have recently been published. Several researchers have referred to metformin as "the narcotics of the modern era." Metformin is a form of diabetes medication.

5.4.2. Rapamycin

The compound known as rapamycin has been extracted from the strain of microbe. Rapa Nui Island proved to be the location where these hygroscopic bacteria were found, and they were subsequently given their namesake. The use of this substance as an immunosuppressive agent is common practice in the process of reducing the likelihood of organ rejection following the transplantation procedure. The amino acid complex that is inhibited by this compound has been referred to as the "Target of rapamycin" and TOR during the research process. Many studies have demonstrated that the application of this substance to mice and other biological models that are displaying signs of aging results in a significant extension of their lifespan.

5.4.3. Resveratrol

Polyphenols are a form of secondary metabolites that are found in plants and are considered to be of significant importance. phenolic acids, lignin, flavonoids, and stilbenes are the four distinct groups that correspond to the compounds that are under consideration. Resveratrol, which is produced by a wide variety of plants and is most commonly found in wine, is the most notable component of stilbenes. According to the findings, the activation of SIRT1 by resveratrol has been demonstrated to mediate the effects of caloric restriction. In certain organisms, specifically mice, the administration of resveratrol has been observed to have the potential to extend lifespan; however, this benefit was only observed when the mice were fed a diet that was high in fat. In addition to this, resveratrol generates many advantageous effects in the areas of cardiovascular health, cancer, type 2 diabetes, inflammatory processes, and neurodegenerative disorders. It is possible that resveratrol could have therapeutic implications for the treatment of Alzheimer's disease due to its neuroprotective properties and its ability to induce autophagy. Bear in mind that resveratrol is responsible for many of its anti-inflammatory and antioxidant effects because it stimulates AMPK and SIRT1, which is an important fact to keep in mind. The fact that resveratrol inhibits phosphodiesterases, which are enzymes that degrade cAMP, and activates a wide variety of transcriptional factors that react to stimuli is another factor that helps to explain the complex range of effects that it has.

5.4.4. Spermidine

While polyamine spermidine promotes autophagy in a manner that is comparable to that of sildenafil and resveratrol, it does so through a particular chemical mechanism. In a manner analogous to that of resveratrol, the promotion of autophagy requires a modification in the acetyl condition of several proteins. Nevertheless, this occurs without the participation of SIRT1 (possibly as a result of the inhibition of acetylase activities). A number of studies have demonstrated that spermidine can lengthen the lifespan of mice and other "aging" model species. It comes as a surprise that as people get older, their consumption of this substance, which occurs in every cell, drops dramatically. In addition to its neuroprotective properties, spermidine is known to reduce the likelihood of developing cardiovascular diseases. Another benefit of spermidine is that it stimulates the production of cytokines, which in turn reduces inflammation and enhances lipid metabolism.

5.4.5. Vitamin D

Skeletal muscle and bone come together to form a physical unit that is characterized by the regulation of each other through the use of endocrine signals. The role that vitamin D plays in this regulatory network is extremely important. When vitamin D levels are adequate, they are effective in preventing the occurrence of sarcopenia as well as the accumulation of fat in muscles that is associated with aging.

Additionally, it has been observed that vitamin D is beneficial to cognitive abilities during the stage of life that is similar to that of an elderly person. Mice that are lacking in vitamin D receptors have a faster rate of aging than mice that are not lacking in these receptors. At the same time, the animal model utilized for Alzheimer's disease research demonstrates improved memory function and a decrease in certain markers associated with Alzheimer's pathology following the administration of vitamin D supplements. Alzheimer's disease patients have significantly lower levels of vitamin D in their bloodstream than the general population. To the fullest extent possible, vitamin D functions as a protective agent.

5.4.6. Soluble Proteins/Growth Factors

Due to the fact that it is simple to administer through uncomplicated infusions, the administration of soluble protein as a treatment for age-related diseases is an extremely appealing approach. As a result of the rejuvenating effect that GDF11 and oxytocin have demonstrated in aged mice, these two substances are among the most promising candidates. A specific group of proteins that were found to be elevated in the blood of centenarians was discovered as a result of a research investigation that was carried out to compare the health status of individuals who have lived beyond the lifespan of 100 years with those who are between the ages of 70 and 80 years. According to the findings of this investigation, there is a connection between the idea of "successful aging" and the presence of four particular proteins. These proteins are chemerin, fetuin-A, FGF19, and FGF21. There is evidence that FGF21 is a factor that contributes to an increase in longevity on a systemic level. As part of its function, this entity is responsible for regulating the metabolism of glucose and lipids, as well as maintaining the homeostasis of the tissues during times of stress. There is evidence that the overexpression of FGF21 can increase autophagy, which in turn can result in a lifespan extension of up to 40% in mice. Adiponectin is a promising candidate for promoting a healthy and longer lifespan with its ability to promote longevity. The expression and secretion of adiponectin are both carried out by adipocytes that are relatively small in size. The compound has been discovered to improve insulin sensitivity, that it possesses anti-atherosclerotic properties, and that it improves metabolic function in the liver, skeletal muscles, and fat tissue. There is evidence that adiponectin can activate AMPK and SIRT1, and as a result, it demonstrates properties that are comparable to those of an exercise mimetic agent. In conclusion, it is important to point out that it also activates catalase and super oxygen dismutase, which helps to reduce oxidative stress in organs that are involved in metabolic processes. Another factor that contributes to youthful characteristics is follistatin-like 1 (FSTL1), which, in conjunction with GDF11, encourages the regeneration of the heart by increasing the capacity of heart cells to survive. As a result of its capacity to either extend the lifespan of mice or demonstrate neuroprotective properties, the dissolved form of Klotho has been recognized as a potentially useful candidate. Because of this, it is a prospective option for potential therapeutic interventions in the context of a variety of diseases, including Alzheimer's disease and multiple sclerosis, amongst others.

5.4.7. Acetylcholinesterase Inhibitors

Many people believe that Alzheimer's disease (AD) is the most incapacitating illness that is associated with aging. In 2013, it was estimated that more than 44 million people around the world were affected by the disease. According to projections, this number is expected to increase to more than 135 million by the year 2050. Although there is no known cure for Alzheimer's disease, there are a limited number of pharmacological interventions that have the potential to improve the residents' quality of life. When it comes to pharmacological agents that have a moderate level of effectiveness in improving cognitive function, acetylcholinesterase inhibitors are the most notable. The degenerative conditions of cholinergic neurons are responsible for the decrease in acetylcholine levels that are observed in patients with Alzheimer's disease and Parkinson's disease-related dementia (PDD). In addition, cholinergic pathways are extremely important in the brain and spinal cord, as well as in the somatic and autonomic nervous systems. It has been demonstrated that increasing acetylcholine levels by blocking acetylcholine can improve cognitive function and confer advantageous outcomes on certain comorbidities that are commonly observed in patients who have Alzheimer's disease (AD) and Parkinson's disease (PD).

5.5. Selective Elimination of Senescent Cells

Inadequate immune clearance has been linked to the persistence of senescent cells, which has been implicated in the beginning stages of organ dysfunction and is a significant contributor to age-related pathologies. They have experienced a significant improvement in their physiological well-being as a result of the elimination of aging cells in murine models. An option that can be considered is the elimination of senescent cells in humans through the administration of drugs (stenosis) or the induction of death (apoptosis). By observing that senescent cells do not react to their very own pro-apoptotic SASP, it was possible to conclude that these cells have senescent-cell anti-apoptotic routes (SCAPs). This was the basis for the deduction. According to the findings, there are six different senescent cell-associated secretory phenotypes (SCAP) profiles. Following that, these SCAPs were subjected to screening to identify targets that were susceptible to senolytic medicine. Recent discoveries have led to the identification of many senolytic drugs, both synthetic and derived from plants. According to research, quercetin is an example of a compound that has demonstrated the demonstration of potential activity. It is important to note that the effectiveness of senolytic drugs varies by type of senescent cell, and that the utilization of a small number of drugs frequently results in a higher level of effectiveness. The ability of senolytic drugs to exert their effect intermittently, as opposed to requiring continuous administration, is one of the advantages that senolytic drugs have over pharmaceuticals. Idiopathic pneumonia (IPF), a severe respiratory condition, is one example of a condition that has become more optimistic as a result of the utilization of analytical medications for the management of ailments that have limited therapeutic alternatives. Using a synthetic peptide, which is considered to be a sophisticated method, scientists will demonstrate a novel technique for inducing death in cells that are getting older. The peptide that enters the cell (CPP) was derived from the sequence of the expression factor FOXO4 and serves the purpose of facilitating the removal of p53 from the nucleus. To initiate the process of programmed cell death, also known as apoptosis, the p53 protein binds to mitochondria rather than being located within the nucleus or other parts of the cell. An alternative method involves the elimination of senescent cells in a targeted manner through specialized antibodies or altered T cells.

5.6. Transplantation of Stem Cells

One of the most important aspects of stem cells is their capacity to promote the regeneration of all organs in the body and ensure that they are functioning correctly. To correct significant abnormalities, the transplantation of stem cells into particular tissues presents a potential avenue of treatment. The field of regenerative medicine is currently on the verge of presenting us with extraordinary opportunities. There is a wide variety of potential applications for multipotent mesenchymal embryonic stem cells.

However, it has been observed that as these cells age, their capacity to regenerate undergoes a significant decline, as stated in reference 179. These findings have been reported. It has been discovered that the induction of pluripotency can be accomplished by only four transcription parameters, namely OCT3/4, SOX2, and KLF4, in addition to MYC. This discovery has resulted in significant advancements in the field. It is possible to induce pluripotency in somatic cells, which will result in the development of stem cells that have characteristics that are characteristic of younger cells. Induced pluripotent stem cells, also known as iPSCs, are the cells that undergo this process. It is possible to obtain induced pluripotent stem cells (iPSCs) from human fibroblasts and then use them in a variety of tissues by following specific differentiation procedures. In clinical studies, the differentiation of specific cells from induced pluripotent stem cells (iPSCs) has been investigated as a potential treatment for a variety of medical conditions. These conditions include Alzheimer's disease, Parkinson's disease, injury to the spinal column, obesity, and congestive cardiac failure. When it comes to the rejuvenation of aged organs, the implementation of a strategy that involves stem cell therapy presents a comprehensive range of opportunities for future advancements. The effectiveness of stem cell transplantation is, however, significantly influenced by a number of different factors. The state of the stem cell niche is the most important factor in determining whether or not regenerative therapy will be successful. This is true regardless of the method that is used to generate substitute cells, whether it be through induced pluripotent stem cells (iPSCs) followed by differentiation steps or through direct transdifferentiation of ordinary somatic cells. In addition, the engraftment of transplanted cells is significantly influenced by numerous protein variables that are present in the bloodstream. More than that, the inflammatory mechanisms that are frequently upregulated during the process of aging have a significant impact on stem cells, as demonstrated by the impairment of satellite cell function. When it comes to essential requirements, the reduction of pro-inflammatory signaling is considered very important (Weinert and Timiras, 2003; Vlachopoulos et al., 2015).

A Closer Look

DNA Damage

DNA damage refers to physical or chemical alterations in the structure of DNA molecules, which can impair its normal function and lead to genetic mutations or cell death if not properly repaired. This damage can occur due to various factors such as exposure to radiation (UV, X-rays), environmental toxins, oxidative stress, or errors during DNA replication. Understanding DNA damage is crucial as it underpins many diseases, including cancer and aging.

There are several types of DNA damage:

- **Single-Strand Breaks (SSBs)**: Occur when one strand of the DNA double helix is severed. While less severe than double-strand breaks, if left unrepaired, they can cause errors during DNA replication.
- **Double-Strand Breaks (DSBs)**: Involve the simultaneous breakage of both strands of the DNA double helix. They are more serious and can lead to chromosomal rearrangements if repaired incorrectly.
- **Chemical Modifications**: Such as base modifications (e.g., methylation, oxidation) can alter the coding sequence or affect DNA-protein interactions, leading to malfunction.

DNA damage triggers cellular responses aimed at maintaining genomic integrity. Cells have evolved intricate repair mechanisms:

- **Direct Reversal**: Enzymes can directly reverse some forms of DNA damage without replacing nucleotides.
- **Base Excision Repair (BER)**: Corrects small base lesions caused by oxidation or alkylation.
- **Nucleotide Excision Repair (NER)**: Removes larger DNA lesions like UV-induced pyrimidine dimers.
- **Mismatch Repair (MMR)**: Corrects errors that escape DNA polymerase proofreading during replication.

Failure to repair DNA damage correctly can result in mutations, genomic instability, and ultimately, diseases like cancer. Moreover, persistent DNA damage accumulates with age, contributing to aging processes and age-related diseases.

Research in DNA damage and repair mechanisms not only sheds light on fundamental biological processes but also informs therapeutic strategies for diseases linked to DNA damage, such as cancer treatment modalities involving radiation or chemotherapy. Understanding and mitigating DNA damage are critical for advancing both basic biology and clinical medicine.

Summary

- Since the beginning of the 21st century, there have been various fields of study that have made significant progress in the field of research on aging.
- Epigenetics has the potential to improve health span, which is a topic that is receiving a lot of attention. Nevertheless, it is difficult to determine the full extent of this potential. In the field of regenerative medicine, the program of stem cells appears to be an approach that is highly realistic and presents exceptional opportunities.
- By increasing autophagy, it is possible to realize the potential for extending the health span of most individuals, provided that any adverse effects that are associated with this process are mitigated. The elimination of aging cells has the potential to produce a comparable impact on life expectancy and to mitigate the effects of age-related illnesses. If we consider everything, there is a good chance that in the not-too-distant future, a sizeable number of people will be able to receive assistance to achieve healthy aging.

References

1. Arai, Y., Martin-Ruiz, C. M., Takayama, M., Abe, Y., Takebayashi, T., Koyasu, S., Suematsu, M., Hirose, N., & von Zglinicki, T. (2015). Inflammation, but not telomere length, predicts successful ageing at extreme old age: A longitudinal study of semi-supercentenarians. *EBioMedicine, 2*, 1549–1558.
2. Borup, M. T., Trusina, A., & Andersson, A. M. (2008). Aging mechanism as the "down side" of adaptation: A network approach. *Journal of Theoretical Biology, 250*, 66–74.
3. Bratic, A., & Larsson, N. G. (2013). The role of mitochondria in aging. *Journal of Clinical Investigation, 123*, 951–957.
4. Briel, M., Ferreira-Gonzalez, I., You, J. J., Karanicolas, P. J., Akl, E. A., Wu, P., & Sharman, A. (2009). Association between change in high density lipoprotein cholesterol and cardiovascular disease morbidity and mortality: Systematic review and meta-regression analysis. *BMJ, 338*, b92.
5. Burkle, A., Moreno-Villanueva, M., Bernhard, J., Blasco, M., Zondag, G., Hoeijmakers, J. H., & Collino, S. (2015). Mark-age biomarkers of aging. *Mechanisms of Ageing and Development, 151*, 2–12.
6. Cesari, M., Fielding, R. A., Pahor, M., Goodpaster, B., Hellerstein, M., van Kan, G. A., & Isaac, M. (2012). Biomarkers of sarcopenia in clinical trials—recommendations from the international working group on sarcopenia. *Journal of Cachexia, Sarcopenia and Muscle, 3*, 181–190.
7. Chevanne, M., Calia, C., Zampieri, M., Cecchinelli, B., Caldini, R., Monti, D., & Caiafa, P. (2007). Oxidative DNA damage repair and parp 1 and parp 2 expression in epstein-barr virus-immortalized b lymphocyte cells from young subjects, old subjects, and centenarians. *Rejuvenation Research, 10*, 191–204.
8. Clerico, A., Fortunato, A., Ripoli, A., Prontera, C., Zucchelli, G. C., & Emdin, M. (2008). Distribution of plasma cardiac troponin I values in healthy subjects: Pathophysiological considerations. *Clinical Chemistry and Laboratory Medicine, 46*, 804–808.

9. Cohen, A. A., Milot, E., Li, Q., Bergeron, P., Poirier, R., Dusseault-Belanger, F., & Metter, E. J. (2015). Detection of a novel, integrative aging process suggests complex physiological integration. *PLoS ONE, 10*, e0116489.

10. Cooper, R., Kuh, D., Hardy, R., & Mortality Review Group; FALCon and HALCyon Study Teams. (2010). Objectively measured physical capability levels and mortality: Systematic review and meta-analysis. *BMJ, 341*, c4467.

11. Cruz-Jentoft, A. J., Baeyens, J. P., Bauer, J. M., Boirie, Y., Cederholm, T., Landi, F., & Schneider, S. M. (2010). Sarcopenia: European consensus on definition and diagnosis: Report of the European working group on sarcopenia in older people. *Age and Ageing, 39*, 412–423.

12. Cunningham, G. R. (2013). Andropause or male menopause? Rationale for testosterone replacement therapy in older men with low testosterone levels. *Endocrine Practice, 19*, 847–852.

13. De Hollander, E. L., Bemelmans, W. J., Boshuizen, H. C., Friedrich, N., Wallaschofski, H., Guallar-Castillon, P., & Rosengren, A. (2012). The association between waist circumference and risk of mortality considering body mass index in 65- to 74-year-olds: A meta-analysis of 29 cohorts involving more than 58,000 elderly persons. *International Journal of Epidemiology, 41*, 805–817.

14. Emerging Risk Factors Collaboration; Kaptoge, S., di Angelantonio, E., Lowe, G., Pepys, M. B., Thompson, S. G., & Danesh, J. (2010). C-reactive protein concentration and risk of coronary heart disease, stroke, and mortality: An individual participant meta-analysis. *The Lancet, 375*, 132–140.

15. Fenech, M. (1998). Important variables that influence base-line micronucleus frequency in cytokinesis-blocked lymphocytes—a biomarker for DNA damage in human populations. *Mutation Research, 404*, 155–165.

16. Fenech, M., & Bonassi, S. (2011). The effect of age, gender, diet and lifestyle on DNA damage measured using micronucleus frequency in human peripheral blood lymphocytes. *Mutagenesis, 26*, 43–49.

17. Forestier, E., Vinzio, S., Sapin, R., Schlienger, J. L., & Goichot, B. (2009). Increased reverse triiodothyronine is associated with shorter survival in independently-living elderly: The alsanut study. *European Journal of Endocrinology, 160*, 207–214.

18. Franceschi, C., Bonafe, M., Valensin, S., Olivieri, F., de Luca, M., Ottaviani, E., & de Benedictis, G. (2000). Inflamm-aging. An evolutionary perspective on immunosenescence. *Annals of the New York Academy of Sciences, 908*, 244–254.

19. Franzke, B., Halper, B., Hofmann, M., Oesen, S., Peherstorfer, H., Krejci, K., & Höglinger, O. (2014). The influence of age and aerobic fitness on chromosomal damage in Austrian institutionalised elderly. *Mutagenesis, 29*, 441–445.

20. Franzke, B., Neubauer, O., & Wagner, K. H. (2015). Super dnaging-new insights into DNA integrity, genome stability and telomeres in the oldest old. *Mutation Research Reviews in Mutation Research, 766*, 48–57.

21. Frassl, W., Kowoll, R., Katz, N., Speth, M., Stangl, A., Brechtel, L., & Luchner, A. (2008). Cardiac markers (BNP, NT-pro-BNP, troponin I, troponin T) in female amateur runners before and up until three days after a marathon. *Clinical Laboratory, 54*(3–4), 81–87.

22. Gallucci, M., Mazzuco, S., Ongaro, F., di Giorgi, E., Mecocci, P., Cesari, M., & Caraci, F. (2013).

Body mass index, lifestyles, physical performance and cognitive decline: The "Treviso Longeva (TRELONG)" study. *The Journal of Nutrition, Health & Aging, 17*(4), 378–384.

23. Garagnani, P., Giuliani, C., Pirazzini, C., Olivieri, F., Bacalini, M. G., Ostan, R., & Capri, M. (2013). Centenarians as super-controls to assess the biological relevance of genetic risk factors for common age-related diseases: A proof of principle on type 2 diabetes. *Aging, 5*(6), 373–385.
24. Giannoni, A., Giovannini, S., & Clerico, A. (2009). Measurement of circulating concentrations of cardiac troponin I and T in healthy subjects: A tool for monitoring myocardial tissue renewal? *Clinical Chemistry and Laboratory Medicine, 47*(10), 1167–1177.
25. Gobbens, R. J., van Assen, M. A., & Schalk, M. J. (2014). The prediction of disability by self-reported physical frailty components of the Tilburg Frailty Indicator (TFI). *Archives of Gerontology and Geriatrics, 59*(2), 280–287.
26. Goodpaster, B. H., Park, S. W., Harris, T. B., Kritchevsky, S. B., Nevitt, M., Schwartz, A. V., & Newman, A. B. (2006). The loss of skeletal muscle strength, mass, and quality in older adults: The health, aging and body composition study. *The Journals of Gerontology Series A: Biological Sciences and Medical Sciences, 61*(10), 1059–1064.
27. Halper, B., Hofmann, M., Oesen, S., Franzke, B., Stuparits, P., Vidotto, C., & Strasser, E. M. (2015). Influence of age and physical fitness on miRNA-21, TGF-beta and its receptors in leukocytes of healthy women. *Exercise Immunology Review, 21*, 154–163.
28. Hatse, S., Brouwers, B., Dalmasso, B., Laenen, A., Kenis, C., Schoffski, P., & Wildiers, H. (2014). Circulating microRNAs as easy-to-measure aging biomarkers in older breast cancer patients: Correlation with chronological age but not with fitness/frailty status. *PLoS ONE, 9*(10), e110644.
29. Hazane, F., Sauvaigo, S., Douki, T., Favier, A., & Beani, J. C. (2006). Age-dependent DNA repair and cell cycle distribution of human skin fibroblasts in response to UVA irradiation. *Journal of Photochemistry and Photobiology B: Biology, 82*(3), 214–223.
30. Horvath, S., Pirazzini, C., Bacalini, M. G., Gentilini, D., Di Blasio, A. M., Delledonne, M., & Monti, D. (2015). Decreased epigenetic age of PBMCs from Italian semi-supercentenarians and their offspring. *Aging, 7*(12), 1159–1170.
31. Huang, W.N., Perera, S., VanSwearingen, J., & Studenski, S. (2010). Performance measures predict onset of activity of daily living difficulty in community-dwelling older adults. *Journal of the American Geriatrics Society, 58*(4), 844–852.
32. Ibanez-Ventoso, C., & Driscoll, M. (2009). Micrornas in C. elegans aging: Molecular insurance for robustness? *Current Genomics, 10*(3), 144–153.
33. International Expert Committee. (2009). International expert committee report on the role of the a1c assay in the diagnosis of diabetes. *Diabetes Care, 32*(7), 1327–1334.
34. Inukai, S., & Slack, F. (2013). Micrornas and the genetic network in aging. *Journal of Molecular Biology, 425*(19), 3601–3608.
35. Janssen, I., Heymsfield, S. B., & Ross, R. (2002). Low relative skeletal muscle mass (sarcopenia) in older persons is associated with functional impairment and physical disability. *Journal of the American Geriatrics Society, 50*(5), 889–896.
36. Johnson, T. E. (2006). Recent results: Biomarkers of aging. *Experimental Gerontology, 41*(12), 1243–1246.

37. Junnila, R. K., List, E. O., Berryman, D. E., Murrey, J. W., & Kopchick, J. J. (2013). The gh/igf-1 axis in aging and longevity. *Nature Reviews Endocrinology, 9*(6), 366–376.

38. Kabagambe, E. K., Judd, S. E., Howard, V. J., Zakai, N. A., Jenny, N. S., Hsieh, M., & Cushman, M. (2011). Inflammation biomarkers and risk of all-cause mortality in the reasons for geographic and racial differences in stroke cohort. *American Journal of Epidemiology, 174*(3), 284–292.

39. Keller, A., & Meese, E. (2016). Can circulating miRNAs live up to the promise of being minimal invasive biomarkers in clinical settings? *Wiley Interdisciplinary Reviews: RNA, 7*(1), 148–156.

40. Kirkwood, T. B. (2005). Understanding the odd science of aging. *Cell, 120*(4), 437–447.

41. Kirkwood, T. B., & Kowald, A. (1997). Network theory of aging. *Experimental Gerontology, 32*(4–5), 395–399.

42. Kistorp, C., Raymond, I., Pedersen, F., Gustafsson, F., Faber, J., & Hildebrandt, P. (2005). N-terminal pro-brain natriuretic peptide, c-reactive protein, and urinary albumin levels as predictors of mortality and cardiovascular events in older adults. *JAMA, 293*(13), 1609–1616.

43. Koster, A., Ding, J., Stenholm, S., Caserotti, P., Houston, D. K., Nicklas, B. J., & Newman, A. B. (2011). Does the amount of fat mass predict age-related loss of lean mass, muscle strength, and muscle quality in older adults? *The Journals of Gerontology. Series A, Biological Sciences and Medical Sciences, 66*(8), 888–895.

44. Lakoski, S. G., Le, A. H., Muntner, P., Judd, S. E., Safford, M. M., Levine, D. A., & Cushman, M. (2011). Adiposity, inflammation, and risk for death in black and white men and women in the United States: The reasons for geographic and racial differences in stroke (regards) study. *The Journal of Clinical Endocrinology and Metabolism, 96*(6), 1805–1814.

45. LaPak, K. M., & Burd, C. E. (2014). The molecular balancing act of p16(ink4a) in cancer and aging. *Molecular Cancer Research, 12*(2), 167–183.

46. Lewington, S., Clarke, R., Qizilbash, N., Peto, R., Collins, R., & Prospective Studies Collaboration. (2002). Age-specific relevance of usual blood pressure to vascular mortality: A meta-analysis of individual data for one million adults in 61 prospective studies. *The Lancet, 360*(9349), 1903–1913.

47. Llewellyn, D. J., Lang, I. A., Langa, K. M., Muniz-Terrera, G., Phillips, C. L., Cherubini, A., & Melzer, D. (2010). Vitamin D and risk of cognitive decline in elderly persons. *Archives of Internal Medicine, 170*(13), 1135–1141.

48. Lobo, R. A. (2013). Where are we 10 years after the women's health initiative? *The Journal of Clinical Endocrinology & Metabolism, 98*(5), 1771–1780.

49. Lovell, M. A., & Markesbery, W. R. (2007). Oxidative DNA damage in mild cognitive impairment and late-stage Alzheimer's disease. *Nucleic Acids Research, 35*(21), 7497–7504.

50. Lowe, D., Horvath, S., & Raj, K. (2016). Epigenetic clock analyses of cellular senescence and aging. *Oncotarget, 7*(7), 8524–8531.

51. Malavolta, M., Cipriano, C., Costarelli, L., Giacconi, R., Tesei, S., Muti, E., & Mocchegiani, E. (2008). Metallothionein downregulation in very old age: A phenomenon associated with cellular senescence? *Rejuvenation Research, 11*(2), 455–459.

52. Martin-Ruiz, C., Dickinson, H. O., Keys, B., Rowan, E., Kenny, R. A., & von Zglinicki, T. (2006). Telomere length predicts poststroke mortality, dementia, and cognitive decline. *Annals of Neurology, 60*(2), 174–180.

53. Martin-Ruiz, C., Jagger, C., Kingston, A., Collerton, J., Catt, M., Davies, K., & von Zglinicki, T. (2011). Assessment of a large panel of candidate biomarkers of aging in the Newcastle 85+ study. *Mechanisms of Ageing and Development, 132*(9–10), 496–502.

54. McGregor, R. A., Poppitt, S. D., & Cameron-Smith, D. (2014). Role of micrornas in the age-related changes in skeletal muscle and diet or exercise interventions to promote healthy aging in humans. *Aging Research Reviews, 17*, 25–33.

55. Mullner, E., Brath, H., Toferer, D., Adrigan, S., Bulla, M. T., Stieglmayer, R., & Wagner, K. H. (2013). Genome damage in peripheral blood lymphocytes of diabetic and non-diabetic individuals after intervention with vegetables and plant oil. *Mutagenesis, 28*(2), 205–211.

56. Mushtaq, G., Greig, N. H., Anwar, F., Zamzami, M. A., Choudhry, H., Shaik, M. M.,... Kamal, M. A. (2016). miRNAs as circulating biomarkers for Alzheimer's disease and Parkinson's disease. *Medicinal Chemistry, 12*(3), 217–225.

57. Olivieri, F., Bonafe, M., Spazzafumo, L., Gobbi, M., Prattichizzo, F., Recchioni, R., & Procopio, A. D. (2014). Age- and glycemia-related miR-126-3p levels in plasma and endothelial cells. *Aging, 6*(9), 771–787.

58. Ouchi, N., Parker, J. L., Lugus, J. J., & Walsh, K. (2011). Adipokines in inflammation and metabolic disease. *Nature Reviews Immunology, 11*(2), 85–97.

59. Park, D. C., & Yeo, S. G. (2013). Aging. *Korean Journal of Audiology, 17*(2), 39–44.

60. Poehls, J., Wassel, C. L., Harris, T. B., Havel, P. J., Swarbrick, M. M., Cummings, S. R., & Kanaya, A. M. (2009). Association of adiponectin with mortality in older adults: The Health, Aging, and Body Composition Study. *Diabetologia, 52*(4), 591–595.

61. Prospective Studies Collaboration; Lewington, S., Whitlock, G., Clarke, R., Sherliker, P., Emberson, J., & Collins, R. (2007). Blood cholesterol and vascular mortality by age, sex, and blood pressure: A meta-analysis of individual data from 61 prospective studies with 55,000 vascular deaths. *The Lancet, 370*(9602), 1829–1839.

62. Prospective Studies Collaboration; Whitlock, G., Lewington, S., Sherliker, P., Clarke, R., Emberson, J., & Peto, R. (2009). Body-mass index and cause-specific mortality in 900,000 adults: Collaborative analyses of 57 prospective studies. *The Lancet, 373*(9669), 1083–1096.

63. Rodier, F., Kim, S. H., Nijjar, T., Yaswen, P., & Campisi, J. (2005). Cancer and aging: The importance of telomeres in genome maintenance. *International Journal of Biochemistry & Cell Biology, 37*(5), 977–990.

64. Ruff, R. M., & Parker, S. B. (1993). Gender- and age-specific changes in motor speed and eye-hand coordination in adults: Normative values for the finger tapping and grooved pegboard tests. *Perceptual and Motor Skills, 76*(3_suppl), 1219–1230.

65. Salthouse, T. A. (2010). Selective review of cognitive aging. *Journal of the International Neuropsychological Society, 16*(5), 754–760.

66. Salvioli, S., Capri, M., Bucci, L., Lanni, C., Racchi, M., Uberti, D., & Franceschi, C. (2009). Why do centenarians escape or postpone cancer? The role of IGF-1, inflammation and p53. *Cancer Immunology, Immunotherapy, 58*(12), 1909–1917.

67. Sanders, J. L., & Newman, A. B. (2013). Telomere length in epidemiology: A biomarker of aging, age-related disease, both, or neither? *Epidemiologic Reviews, 35*(1), 112–131.

68. Sarwar, N., Danesh, J., Eiriksdottir, G., Sigurdsson, G., Wareham, N., Bingham, S., & Gudnason,

V. (2007). Triglycerides and the risk of coronary heart disease: 10,158 incident cases among 262,525 participants in 29 Western prospective studies. *Circulation, 115*(4), 450–458.

69. Seeger, T., & Boon, R. A. (2015). MicroRNAs in cardiovascular aging. *Journal of Physiology, 594*(8), 2085–2094.
70. Sharma, S., Rais, A., Sandhu, R., Nel, W., & Ebadi, M. (2013). Clinical significance of metallothioneins in cell therapy and nanomedicine. *International Journal of Nanomedicine, 8*, 1477–1488.
71. Simm, A., Muller, B., Nass, N., Hofmann, B., Bushnaq, H., Silber, R. E., & Bartling, B. (2015). Protein glycation—Between tissue aging and protection. *Experimental Gerontology, 68*, 71–75.
72. Slijepcevic, P. (2008). DNA damage response, telomere maintenance and aging in light of the integrative model. *Mechanisms of Ageing and Development, 129*(1–2), 11–16.
73. Stewart, J. A., Chaiken, M. F., Wang, F., & Price, C. M. (2012). Maintaining the end: Roles of telomere proteins in end-protection, telomere replication and length regulation. *Mutatation Research, 730*(1–2), 12–19.
74. Studenski, S., Perera, S., Patel, K., Rosano, C., Faulkner, K., Inzitari, M., & Guralnik, J. M. (2011). Gait speed and survival in older adults. *JAMA, 305*(1), 50–58.
75. Su, Y. P., Chang, C. K., Hayes, R. D., Perera, G., Broadbent, M., To, D., & Stewart, R. (2014). Mini-Mental State Examination as a predictor of mortality among older people referred to secondary mental healthcare. *PLoS ONE, 9*(8), e105312.
76. Tedone, E., Arosio, B., Gussago, C., Casati, M., Ferri, E., Ogliari, G., & Mari, D. (2014). Leukocyte telomere length and prevalence of age-related diseases in semisupercentenarians, centenarians, and centenarians' offspring. *Experimental Gerontology, 58*, 90–95.
77. Van den Beld, A. W., Visser, T. J., Feelders, R. A., Grobbee, D. E., & Lamberts, S. W. (2005). Thyroid hormone concentrations, disease, physical function, and mortality in elderly men. *The Journal of Clinical Endocrinology & Metabolism, 90*(12), 6403–6409.
78. Vermeulen, J., Neyens, J. C., van Rossum, E., Spreeuwenberg, M. D., & de Witte, L. P. (2011). Predicting ADL disability in community-dwelling elderly people using physical frailty indicators: A systematic review. *BMC Geriatrics, 11*(1), 33.
79. Visser, M., Pahor, M., Taaffe, D. R., Goodpaster, B. H., Simonsick, E. M., Newman, A. B., & Harris, T. B. (2002). Relationship of interleukin-6 and tumor necrosis factor-α with muscle mass and muscle strength in elderly men and women: The Health ABC Study. *The Journals of Gerontology Series A: Biological Sciences and Medical Sciences, 57*(5), M326–M332.
80. Visser, M., Pahor, M., Tylavsky, F., Kritchevsky, S. B., Cauley, J. A., Newman, A. B., & Harris, T. B. (2003). One- and two-year change in body composition as measured by DXA in a population-based cohort of older men and women. *Journal of Applied Physiology, 94*(6), 2368–2374.
81. Vlachopoulos, C., Xaplanteris, P., Aboyans, V., Brodmann, M., Cifkova, R., Cosentino, F., & Laurent, S. (2015). The role of vascular biomarkers for primary and secondary prevention. A position paper from the European Society of Cardiology Working Group on peripheral circulation: Endorsed by the Association for Research into Arterial Structure and Physiology (ARTERY) Society. *Atherosclerosis, 241*(2), 507–532.
82. Von Zglinicki, T., Burkle, A., & Kirkwood, T. B. (2001). Stress, DNA damage and aging—An integrative approach. *Experimental Gerontology, 36*(7), 1049–1062.

83. Wagner, K. H., Wallner, M., Molzer, C., Gazzin, S., Bulmer, A. C., Tiribelli, C., & Vitek, L. (2015). Looking to the horizon: The role of bilirubin in the development and prevention of age-related chronic diseases. *Clinical Science, 129*(1), 1–25.

84. Wallner, M., Blassnigg, S. M., Marisch, K., Pappenheim, M. T., Mullner, E., Molzer, C., & Wagner, K. H. (2012). Effects of unconjugated bilirubin on chromosomal damage in individuals with Gilbert's syndrome measured with the micronucleus cytome assay. *Mutagenesis, 27*(6), 731–735.

85. Wallner, M., Marculescu, R., Doberer, D., Wolzt, M., Wagner, O., Vitek, L., & Wagner, K. H. (2013). Protection from age-related increase in lipid biomarkers and inflammation contributes to cardiovascular protection in Gilbert's syndrome. *Clinical Science, 125*(6), 257–264.

86. Weinert, B. T., & Timiras, P. S. (2003). Invited review: Theories of aging. *Journal of Applied Physiology, 95*(4), 1706–1716.

87. Wessner, B., Gryadunov-Masutti, L., Tschan, H., Bachl, N., & Roth, E. (2010). Is there a role for microRNAs in exercise immunology? A synopsis of current literature and future developments. *Exercise Immunology Review, 16*, 22–39.

Chapter 6

THE IMPACT OF THE ENVIRONMENT ON AGE-RELATED DISEASES AND ORGAN FUNCTION CHANGES

Contents

Introduction

It is reasonable to expect that as we age, the biological changes that occur in our bodies will also lead to changes in our susceptibility to disease. For certain diseases, like those in which early exposure to antigens leads to lifelong immunity, the likelihood of resistance typically rises, and the occurrence of the disease decreases as individuals grow older. For certain illnesses, such as those resulting from long-term, repeated exposures, the likelihood of occurrence may rise as a person gets older.

The disease susceptibility varies throughout the human life cycle and is thought to be influenced by multiple factors, such as alterations in the immune system and the rate of cellular proliferation. Exposure to substances that cause cancer or damage to the nervous system during infancy and childhood (or in old age) may result in more intense reactions compared to those that happen during the middle stages of life. While there are logical theoretical reasons to believe that certain disease patterns may be a natural part of the aging process, further research is required to better understand the potential mechanisms involved. Conducting controlled studies on animal populations is necessary to ascertain the natural prevalence of diseases during the aging process, as well as the alterations in immune response, metabolic functions, and reactions to foreign substances (xenobiotics) throughout the entire lifespan.

This chapter examines various animal and human studies that investigate the connections between the environment and age-related diseases in specific organ systems. The chapter also examines evidence of age-related alterations in typical physiological processes, such as visual perception, bone remodeling, and immune response. Table 6.1 displays several illustrations.

Table 6.1. Main Characteristics of the Blood Biochemistry-Based and Psychological Status-Based Calculators

Study	Sample	Validation Strategy and Model Characteristics	Model Parameters	Comments
Putin et al., 2016	62,419 samples from the Eastern European population (90% of Russia)	1. Highly biased markers excluded. 2. The dataset divided into training and test sets of 56,177 and 6242 samples, respectively. 3. 40 deep neural networks (DNNs) trained on 56,177 blood test samples. 4. Modular ensemble comprising 21 DNNs of varying depth, structure and optimization to predict human chronological age using a basic blood test. The full version is based on 41 blood chemistry parameters.	Best performance (DNN): 81.5% epsilon-accuracy r = 0.90, $R^2 = 0.80$, MAE = 6.07 years within a 10-year frame. Overall performance (ensemble): 83.5% epsilon-accuracy r = 0.91, $R^2 = 0.82$, MAE = 5.55 years.	5 most important markers for chronological age estimation identified: albumin, glucose, alkaline phosphatase, urea, and erythrocytes An algorithm developed based on a single source of clinical data.

Mamoshina et al., 2018	20,699 samples for the Canadian population, 65,760 samples for the South Korean population, and 55,920 samples for the Eastern European population	55,751 samples from the NHANES with blood test values used to measure the predictive power of the models	The best-performing predictor trained on the Eastern European population-specific dataset demonstrated an MAE of 6.25, an R^2 of 0.69 Best performing predictors: Canadian population: MAE = 6.36 years, R^2 = 0.52 South Korean population: MAE = 5.59, R^2 = 0.49 Eastern European population: MAE = 6.25, R^2 = 0.69	Population type identified as a major feature for age estimation in all 3 populations
Zhavoronkov et al., 2020	The final dataset contained 6071 participants (U.S. residents)	(1) Series of DNNs were trained based on data from anonymized questionnaire responses from MIDUS 1, MIDUS 2 and MIDUS Refresher longitudinal surveys (2) 50 most important features were selected to build the final models (modifiable factors) (3) Final models were trained with five-fold cross-validation (CV) using all MIDUS 1 samples. MIDUS 2 and MIDUS Refresher were used for model validation purposes	Best performance (DNN): MAE = 6.70 years and epsilon accuracy = 0.78 for PsychoAge; MAE = 7.32 years and epsilon accuracy = 0.74 for SubjAge Model validation (using other datasets): MAE = 7.18/7.73 years and epsilon accuracy = 0.73/0.70 for PsychoAge; MAE = 8.53/8.56 years and epsilon accuracy = 0.66/0.65 for SubjAge	Additionally, variables that remain highly important (top-25) across all age groups were defined. These variables form the psychological aging core.

Source: *Erema, V. V., Yakovchik, A. Y., Kashtanova, D. A., Bochkaeva, Z. V., Ivanov, M. V., Sosin, D. V., Matkava, L. R., Yudin, V. S., Makarov, V. V., Keskinov, A. A., et al. Biological age predictors: The status quo and future trends. International Journal of Molecular Sciences. 2022; 23(23), 15103. https://doi.org/10.3390/ijms232315103.*

Orientation and Directional Terms:

Term	Definition	Illustration
Age-related diseases	Diseases that typically occur as individuals age, such as Alzheimer's disease, arthritis, heart disease, and osteoporosis. These conditions are often influenced by genetic, environmental, and lifestyle factors.	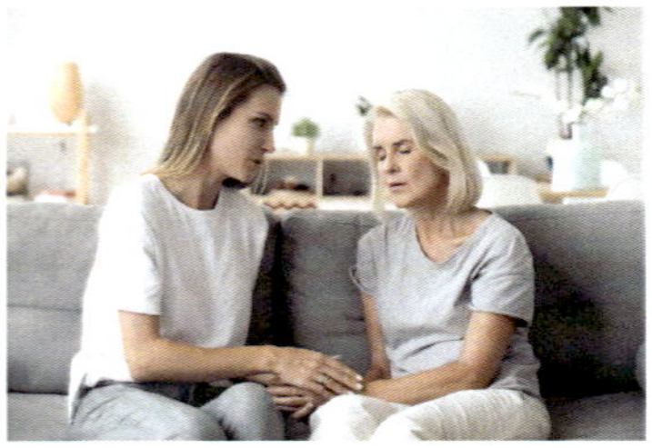
Heart disease mortality	The death rate due to heart diseases, which includes conditions such as coronary artery disease, heart attacks, and heart failure. It is often used as a key indicator of public health.	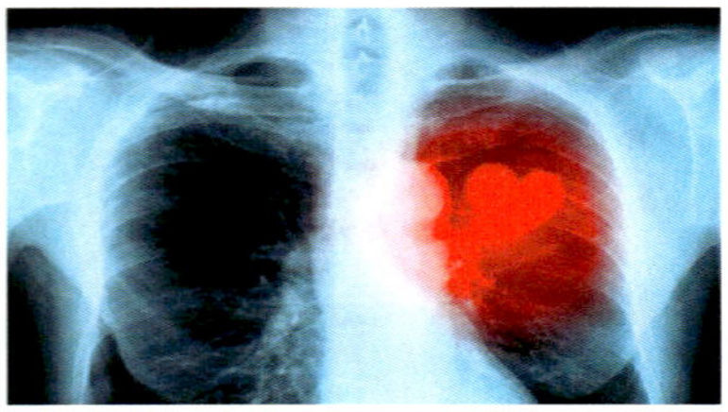
Cerebrovascular disease	A group of conditions that affect the blood vessels and blood supply to the brain, including stroke, transient ischemic attack (TIA), and aneurysms.	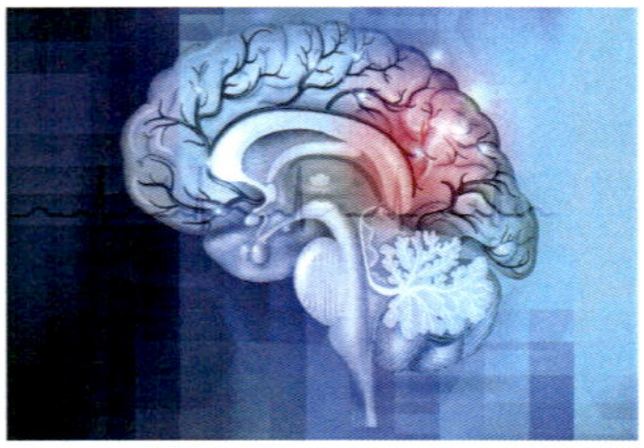
Arteriosclerosis	The thickening, hardening, and loss of elasticity of the walls of arteries, often leading to restricted blood flow and increased blood pressure.	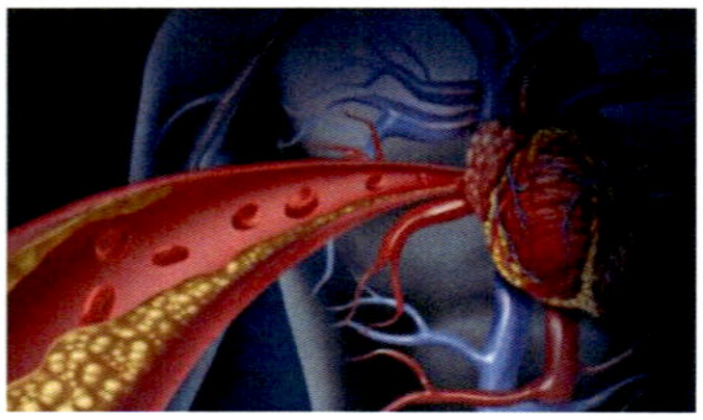
Noise-induced hearing loss	Hearing loss caused by exposure to loud noises, which can damage the hair cells in the inner ear. It can be temporary or permanent, depending on the intensity and duration of noise exposure.	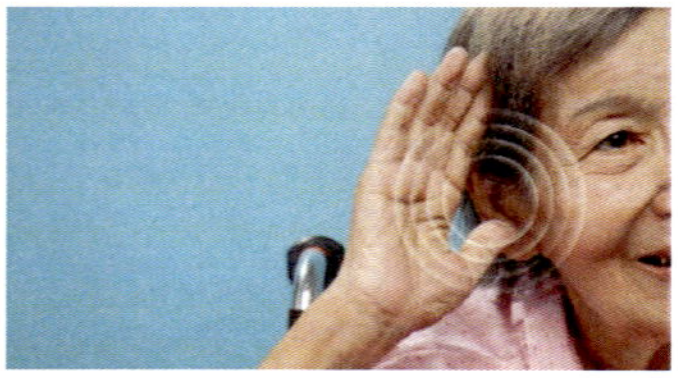
Biological toxins	Toxic substances produced by living organisms, including bacteria, plants, and animals. These toxins can cause various diseases and health issues in humans and other organisms.	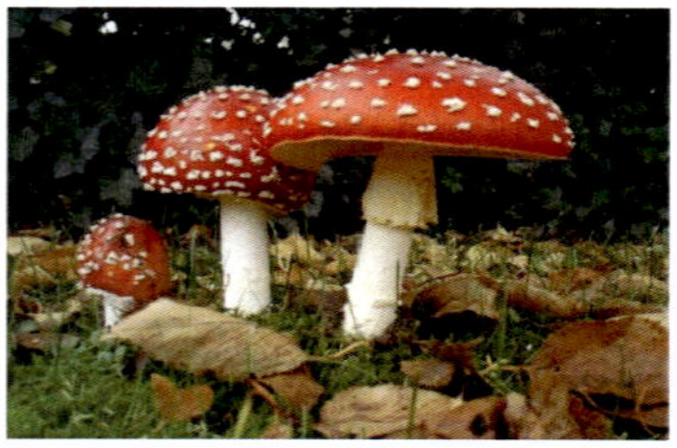

6.1. Demographics of Age-associated Diseases

The incidence of most human diseases appears to be primarily determined by age. Distinct age patterns of risk have been identified for all diseases, and many of these patterns have served as the foundation for significant etiological theories. For instance, the highest occurrence of a specific type of Hodgkin's disease during the third decade of life indicated a potential infectious cause (MacMahon, 1971). Similarly, the stable occurrence of breast cancer between the ages of 45–55 indicated a possible influence of the cessation of ovarian function on the disease's development (Petrakis et al., 1982). The incidence curves for breast cancer in premenopausal and postmenopausal women in various countries indicate that environmental factors have a greater impact on the development of postmenopausal breast cancer. On the other hand, genetic, endocrinologic, and other internal factors have a stronger influence on premenopausal breast cancer (Figure 6.1).

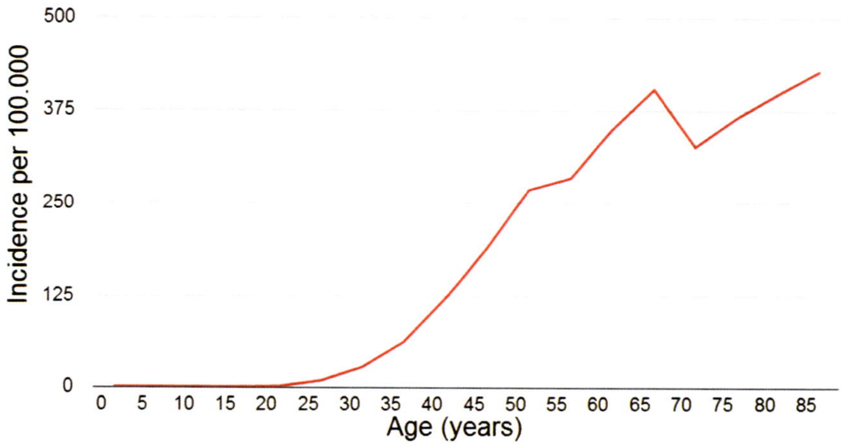

Figure 6.1. *Age-specific incidence rates for female breast.*

Source: By Mikael Häggström. When using this image in external works, it may be cited as:Häggström, Mikael (2014). "Medical gallery of Mikael Häggström 2014." WikiJournal of Medicine 1 (2). DOI:10.15347/wjm/2014.008. ISSN 2002-4436. Public Domain.orBy Mikael Häggström, used with permission. – Own work, CC0, https://commons.wikimedia.org/w/index.php?curid=16543428.

The role of age as an independent factor associated with increasing incidence appears to be direct in some diseases. In some cases, factors such as obesity and duration of exposure are the direct causes of time and age-related effects, rather than age itself. It is necessary to evaluate the correlation between disease susceptibility and age, which could be influenced by intrinsic factors, extrinsic factors, or a combination of both, for each specific disease. For instance, researchers have extensively studied the impact of certain internal and external factors on adult-onset diabetes mellitus. However, additional studies are necessary to fully comprehend the relative significance and interplay between natural and external factors in the disease.

Both morbidity and mortality data can be utilized to assess the correlation between disease and age in the elderly population (aged 65 and above). Morbidity data can be used to measure either the number of new cases of a disease that occur during a specific time period (incidence) or the total number of cases of the disease at a particular point in time (prevalence). The choice between these two measures depends on the study design or the method used to collect the data. Incidence and prevalence are two distinct measures of disease frequency that offer valuable insights. Incidence provides information about the risk of a disease in a population, while prevalence indicates the overall burden of the disease. Both measures are crucial for a comprehensive understanding of a specific disease. Mortality data, which are more easily accessible than morbidity data for the entire population, correspond to incidence data for conditions that are highly dangerous and brief in duration, such as certain types of cancer and cardiovascular disease. However, they are less valuable for assessing other diseases, such as diabetes and chronic obstructive pulmonary disease.

The majority of deaths in the United States, specifically two-thirds, happen to individuals who are 65 years old or older. Additionally, 30% of deaths occur in individuals who are over the age of 80. In both 1979 and 1950, heart disease, cancer, and stroke were responsible for 75% of deaths in the elderly population (NCHS, 1981b). Two notable aspects of the recent cause-specific mortality patterns in the elderly are worth mentioning—the decrease in mortality rates for cardiovascular and cerebrovascular diseases among the elderly, and the consistent rates for cancer (Figure 6.2). Between 1950 and 1979, there was a 17% decline in the mortality rate for individuals aged 65 and older. When mortality rates are adjusted for age (to account for the significant increase in the population aged 85 and over), there was a decrease of over 27% in mortality. Additionally, the decline in mortality for females was twice as much as that for males, as shown in Figure 6.2.

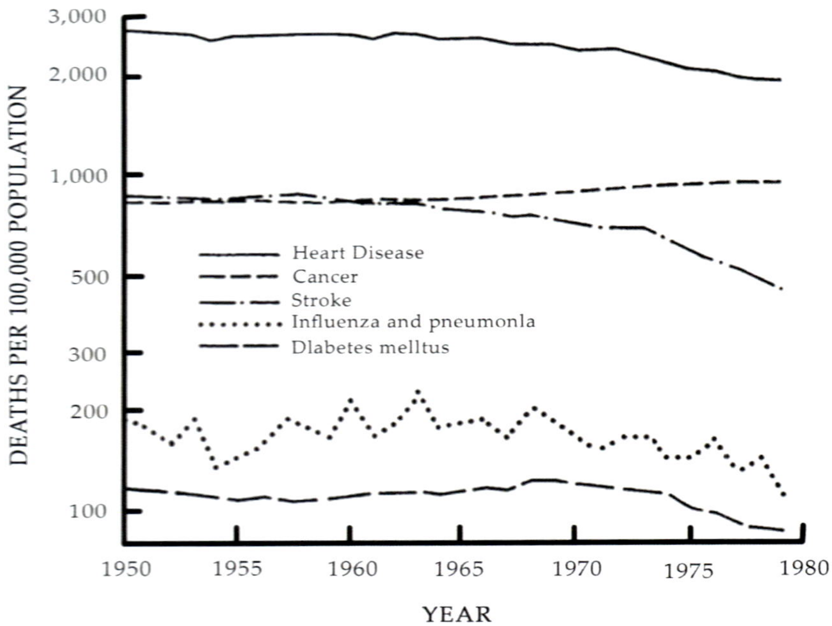

Figure 6.2. *Age-adjusted death rates for persons 65 years of age and over, according to leading causes of death: United States, 1950–1979.*

Source: National Center for Health Statistics (1982).

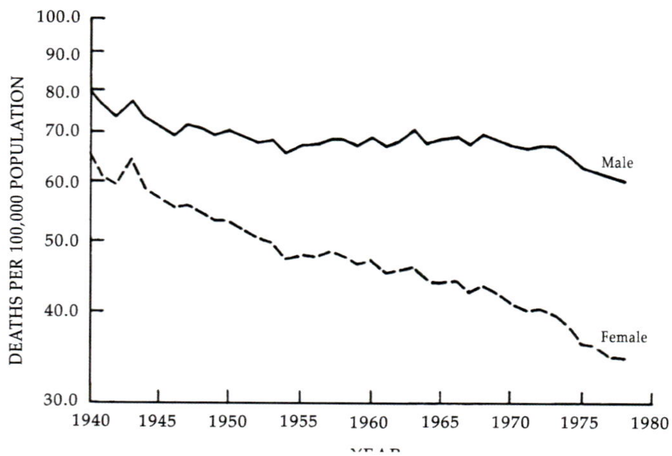

Figure 6.3. *Age-adjusted death rates for persons 65 years of age and over, according to sex: United States, 1940–1978.*

Source: National Center for Health Statistics (1981b).

Heart disease mortality contributed to approximately 50% of the overall decrease, while cerebrovascular disease mortality accounted for an additional 25% of the overall decrease. In this age group, heart diseases have the highest mortality rate, while cerebrovascular diseases have the third highest mortality rate. The mortality rate due to cancer, which is the second most significant factor and the only major one that demonstrated a rise, experienced a 13% increase. The majority of cancer-related deaths in the elderly population are attributed to lung, colon, genital, and breast (in females) cancers. Among males, the mortality trends for cancer show a slight decrease in the significant yearly rise in lung cancer mortality. Additionally, there is a gradual increase in mortality rates for colon and prostate cancers. While cancer mortality rates in males have increased, there has been a slight decrease in overall cancer mortality rates in women aged 65 and over from 1950 to 1978, as shown in Figures 6.4 and 6.5. Female individuals experience a significant rise in lung cancer mortality and a decline in mortality rates for stomach and uterine cervix cancers.

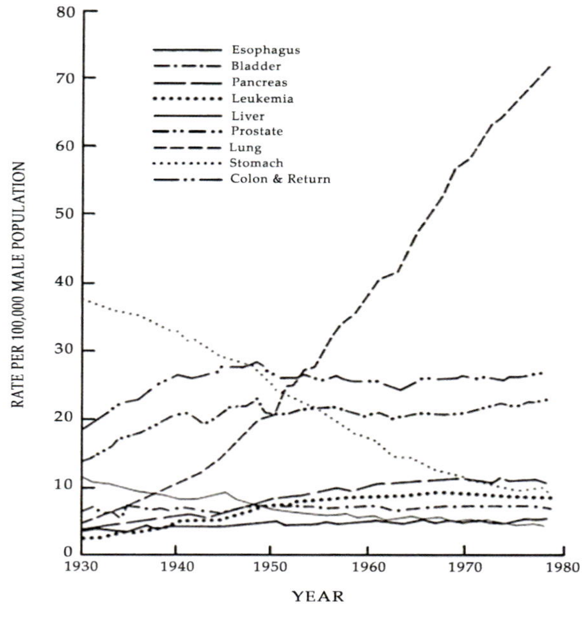

Figure 6.4. *Age-adjusted cancer death rates for selected sites, males: United States, 1930–1978.*

Source: U.S. OTA (1985).

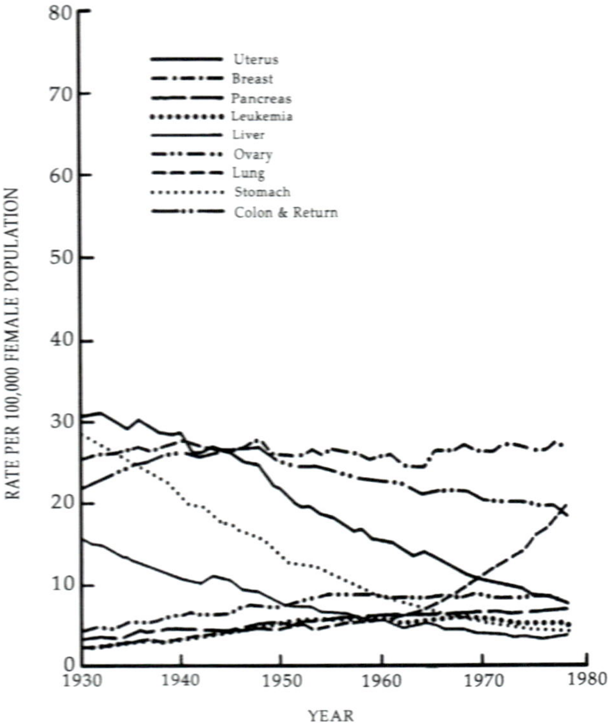

Figure 6.5. *Age-adjusted cancer death rates for selected sites, females: United States, 1930–1978.*

Source: U.S. OTA (1985).

Figure 6.6 demonstrates a significant rise in mortality as age increases for cardiovascular disease, while Figure 6.7 shows no such increase for all types of cancer combined. Cancer mortality rates, encompassing all sites, experience a sharp rise during middle age and then exhibit a more gradual increase until the age of 65. Between the ages of 65 and 69, cancer is responsible for around 30% of all deaths. However, by the time individuals reach the age of 80, cancer only accounts for 12% of deaths. Conversely, the percentage of deaths attributed to cardiovascular disease rises from 50% among individuals aged 65–69 to 65% among those aged 80. According to Brody (1983, 1987), the slight rise in cancer mortality rates after the age of 65 may indicate that cancer development is not strongly linked to the aging process and vulnerability of the host. Brody also predicts that by the year 2000, cancer will cause less than 10% of deaths in individuals aged 85 and above, which is the age group where half of all deaths will occur.

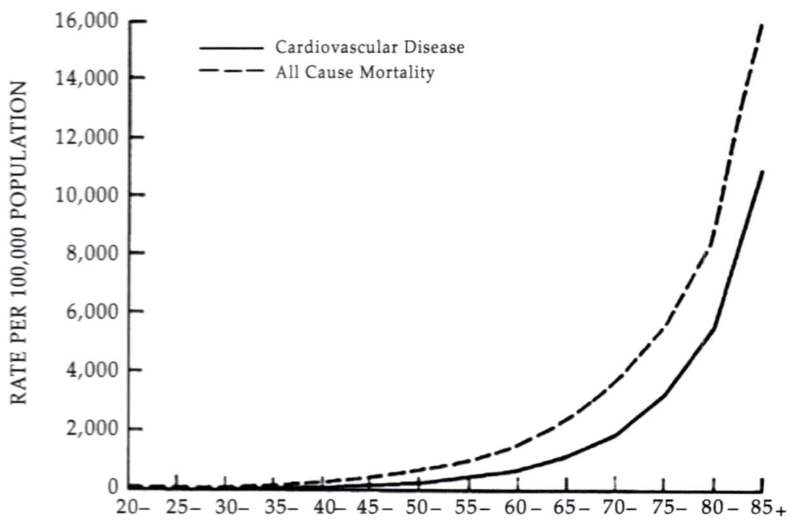

Figure 6.6. *Major cardiovascular diseases: age-specific mortality rates versus all causes of mortality.*

Source: National Center for Health Statistics (1985a).

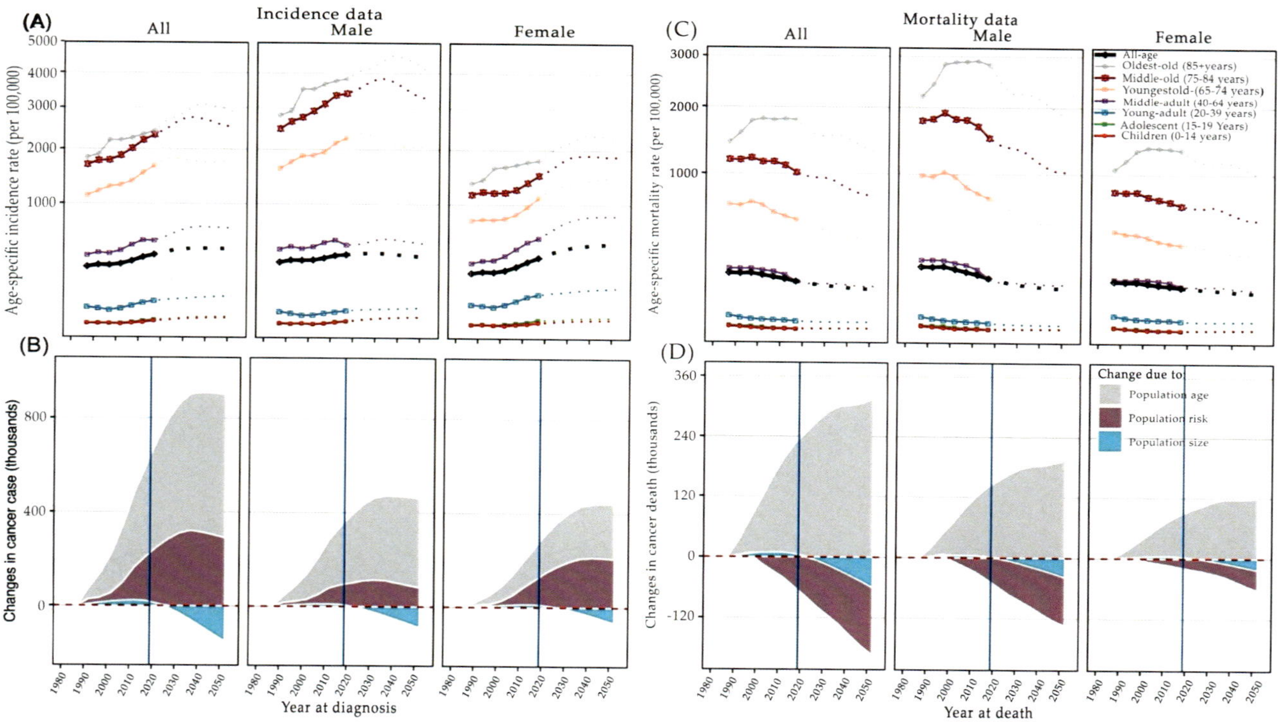

Figure 6.7. *Projections of age-specific incidence rates (Panel (A)) and mortality rates (Panel (C)), and decomposed changes in new cancer cases (Panel (B)) and deaths (Panel (D)).*

Source: Nguyen PT, Saito E, Katanoda K. Long-term projections of cancer incidence and mortality in Japan and decomposition analysis of changes in cancer burden, 2020–2054: An empirical validation approach. Cancers. 2022; 14(24):6076. https://doi.org/10.3390/cancers14246076.

Before conducting a comprehensive evaluation of epidemiologic observations linking cancer mortality to aging processes, it is crucial to consider several important factors. Smoking is the primary factor responsible for the rise in mortality rates from respiratory cancer and overall cancer among elderly individuals of both genders. While it is true that a greater percentage of older men smoke compared to women, the disparity in smoking habits between the sexes has significantly decreased in recent times. The prevalence of smoking among men aged 65 and older decreased from 28.5% in 1965 to 17.9% in 1980, while the prevalence among women increased from 9.6% to 16.8%. The disparity in smoking cessation rates between genders is particularly significant for individuals who have previously smoked and are at a higher risk for respiratory cancer. Among individuals aged 65 and above, the percentage of men who have quit smoking increased from 28.1% in 1965 to 47.4% in 1980, while the percentage of women increased from 4.5% to 14.2% during the same period.

The disparities in smoking habits between elderly men and women undoubtedly contribute to the variations in cancer mortality rates, particularly in respiratory cancer mortality. Cigarette smoking is responsible for approximately 80–85% of deaths caused by lung cancer and 30% of all deaths caused by cancer, according to estimates by Doll and Peto in 1981.

The hypothesis that the aging of the immune system is responsible for the higher occurrence of cancer in older individuals has been proposed. However, the current epidemiological evidence does not substantiate this claim, except for certain types of tumors. Due to the presence of various time-related factors, such as prolonged exposure to carcinogens, it becomes challenging to distinguish the impact of increasing age from the impact of heightened exposure to carcinogens.

Nonetheless, two pieces of evidence can elucidate the impact of age on cancer occurrence. In 1975, Peto et al. conducted a comprehensive and well-regulated study on mice of different ages. The study focused on the effects of benzo[a]pyrene on mice's skin. The occurrence of epithelial cancers was not influenced by the age at which exposure began but was directly associated with the length of exposure. A recent examination of the existing empirical data from animal studies (Hornig, in press) discovered limited evidence to support the idea that there is a universal rise in vulnerability to the impacts of all cancer-causing agents as one gets older. Furthermore, the existence of factors such as time-related cumulative damage and physiological changes linked to aging that can impact vulnerability implies that there may not be a definitive answer to the question of the connection between advancing age and susceptibility to cancer. This connection is likely to vary depending on the specific organ, type of cell, toxic exposure, and animal species involved (Birnbaum, 1987).

Epidemiological evidence substantiates the hypothesis that the rise in lung cancer susceptibility with age is not influenced by the increase in risk associated with smoking. The impact of the duration of exposure can be assessed by observing the rise in occurrence over a specific period, measured from the initiation of smoking in smokers and from birth in nonsmokers. The occurrence rates remain consistent over time. Nevertheless, the impact of age can be approximated by observing the occurrence of a particular event over a period of time, starting from birth in all individuals. In the case of smokers, the incidence of this event tends to rise at a faster rate as time progresses (Doll and Peto, 1978; Peto and Doll, 1984).

Doll (1978) observed that immune factors play a significant role in tumors such as non-Hodgkin's lymphoma and soft-tissue sarcomas, which are derived from mesenchymal tissue. These types of tumors do not show a sharp increase in incidence with age, unlike the more common epithelial cancers. The rapid increase in the occurrence of lymphomas in transplant recipients following treatment with immunosuppressive drugs is significantly different from the extended periods of time observed for the development of epithelial tumors caused by exposure to chemical carcinogens (Hoover and Fraumeni, 1973). The observations indicate that the mesenchymal tumors associated with immune factors may have a different, potentially viral, cause. There is a higher occurrence of squamous carcinoma of the skin in patients who are taking immunosuppressive agents, which indicates that this type of tumor is also influenced by the immune system (Kripke, 1974).

The mortality rates for diseases of the heart, influenza and pneumonia, cerebrovascular disease, arteriosclerosis, and accidents significantly rise with age. On the other hand, the rates for other causes such as cancer, diabetes mellitus, bronchitis, emphysema and asthma, and nephritis and nephrosis show a less significant increase (Table 6.2). There is no apparent correlation between age and mortality from cirrhosis of the liver in the elderly population.

Table 6.2. Death Rates for the Ten Primary Causes of Death Among Individuals Aged 65 and above, Categorized by Age, in the Year 1976

	Deaths per 100,000			
Cause of Death	**65 Years and Over**	**65–74 Years**	**75–84 Years**	**85 Years and Over**
All causes	5,428.9	3,127.6	7,333.6	15,486.9
Heart diseases	2,393.5	1,286.9	3,263.7	7,384.3
Malignant neoplasms	979.0	786.3	1,248.6	1,441.5
Cerebrovascular diseases	694.6	280.1	1,014.0	2,586.8
Influenza and pneumonia	211.1	70.1	289.3	959.2
Arteriosclerosis	122.2	25.8	152.5	714.3
Diabetes mellitus	108.1	70.0	155.8	219.2
Accidents	104.5	62.2	134.5	306.7
Motor vehicle	25.2	21.7	32.3	26.0
All other	79.3	40.4	102.2	280.7
Bronchitis, emphysema, and asthma	76.8	60.7	101.4	108.5
Cirrhosis of liver	36.5	42.6	29.3	18.0
Nephritis and nephrosis	25.0	15.2	34.1	64.6
All other causes	677.5	427.8	908.6	1,638.8

The National Health Interview Study found that the occurrence of every chronic condition examined is more common among individuals aged 65 and older. However, it is important to note that these estimates may not fully capture the impact of age, as they do not account for elderly individuals residing in nursing homes (Table 6.3).

Table 6.3. Prevalence of Selected Impairments by Age and Sex, United States, 1981

	Prevalence, Number of Persons Per 1,000	
Condition	**All Ages**	**65 or Older**
Visual impairment	40.4	136.6
Hearing impairment	82.9	283.6
Paralysis (complete or partial)	5.9	19.6
Heart conditions	76.4	277.0
Hypertensive disease	113.4	378.6
Cerebrovascular disease	8.3	45.4
Chronic bronchitis	35.3	46.1
Emphysema	9.3	42.9
Functional or symptomatic upper gastrointestinal tract disorders	17.4	39.9

Diverticula of intestine	6.8	38.4
Diabetes	24.3	84.8
Urinary system disease	25.9	56.6

By the 1960s, there was increasing evidence that cardiovascular risk factors could be modified to reduce the chances of illness and death. This was supported by various studies such as the Hypertension Detection and Follow-up Program Cooperative Group (1985, 1987), Langford et al. (1986), the Multiple Risk Factor Intervention Trial Research Group (MRFIT) (1982, 1986), Paffenberger (1979), Paffenberger et al. (1978), U.S. Public Health Service (1968), and Veterans' Administration Cooperative Study Group (1967, 1970), as well as Wald (1976).

The study of human aging processes and the influence of environmental factors has been increasingly limited due to a decrease in autopsy rates. Various factors have been cited for the decrease in autopsy rates (American Medical Association, Council on Scientific Affairs, 1987), one of which is the removal of the requirement by the Joint Commission on the Accreditation of Hospitals (JCAH) to have a minimum autopsy rate for accreditation. Currently, the percentage of deaths in hospitals that undergo autopsy is only 14–15%, whereas around 30–40 years ago, it was approximately 50% (Guariglia and Abrahams, 1985). The Institute of Medicine's declaration on national autopsy policy underscored the crucial significance of autopsy, as stated by Mortimer in 1985. Prior research indicated that the frequency of autopsies was lower for deaths in older individuals compared to younger individuals, and this distinction seems to have endured. The current autopsy rates for deaths among individuals over 65 may be as low as 1%.

This phenomenon leads to a deprivation of crucial pathological data for research on human aging, data that cannot be replaced by any other means (Kohn, 1982). Without postmortem examinations, epidemiological studies on age-related diseases and mortality depend on diagnoses made before death or the cause of death recorded on death certificates. Up to 50% of deaths may have inaccurate death certificate information for certain causes of death. Furthermore, the presence of a system to guarantee the gathering, examination, and preservation of pertinent tissues, cells, and bodily fluids would facilitate research on the accumulation of environmental substances in the body and the evaluation of possible cause-and-effect relationships between these substances and tissue alterations.

6.2. Skin

Environmental factors are widely believed to play a role in the effects of aging and age-related diseases, although there are limited instances to support this claim. One of the most well-documented phenomena is photoaging, which refers to the alterations in the appearance and functioning of the skin caused by regular exposure to the sun, rather than solely by the natural aging process.

Photoaging, also known as premature aging and dermatoheliosis, is commonly associated with "true" chronological aging and has only recently been distinguished, even by dermatologists (Gilchrest, 1984). Photoaging is clinically defined by the presence of various skin conditions such as coarseness, wrinkling, mottling, laxity, telangiectasia (enlarged blood vessels), atrophy, fibrotic depigmentation (scar-like patches), and ultimately the development of malignant tumors on the face, neck, hands, and other frequently exposed areas of the body. Individuals with fair skin who reside in regions with high solar intensity and engage in frequent occupational or recreational sun exposure experience the earliest and most severe effects. However, most white Americans exhibit these changes to some extent by their fifth decade, and many by their third decade. The clinical changes typically exhibit a gradual and continuous progression over the course of an individual's lifetime.

Cigarette smoking is a known environmental factor that has been consistently observed to cause premature aging of the skin. This has been demonstrated in a recent study that was carefully designed to control variables such as age, social class, sun exposure, and recent weight change (Model, 1985). Out of the 116 patients between the ages of 35 and 69, individuals who had smoked a minimum of 10 cigarettes per day for at least 10 years were significantly more prone to having severely wrinkled, thin, and tough skin compared to those who did not smoke. Regrettably, the potential negative impact of smoking on the aging of the skin has not been investigated in experiments involving animals or cell cultures.

The significant body of epidemiological and experimental animal evidence has linked the ultraviolet (UV) component of sunlight, specifically UVB (290–320 nm), to both photoaging (Kligman, 1969; Kligman et al., 1982; Smith et al., 1962) and photocarcinogenesis (Blum, 1959; Urbach et al., 1974). Additionally, longer ultraviolet (UV) wavelengths and even infrared (heat) energy may also play a role in this phenomenon (Kligman et al., 1985; Strickland, 1986). There is currently no data available that either confirms or rules out the possibility of interactions between UV radiation and other environmental exposures, such as chemical or dietary factors, in those processes. According to Gilchrest (1984), photoaging is responsible for over 90% of cosmetic skin issues related to aging. These issues can have a negative impact on people's self-esteem (Graham and Kligman, 1985) and how society perceives them (Dion et al., 1972). Abundant epidemiologic evidence indicates that photoaging plays a causal role in a comparable proportion of basal cell and squamous cell carcinomas (Urbach et al., 1974), which collectively make up over 50% of all malignancies in the United States. The sun is also believed to be a contributing factor in a smaller, yet undetermined, number of cases of malignant melanoma. This is a significant public health issue due to the rising number of cases and high mortality rate associated with it. In addition to its widespread negative impact on appearance and its significant contribution to the development of skin cancer, regular exposure to the sun has now been acknowledged as worsening various age-related functional declines in human skin. An instance of potential medical significance is immune responsiveness. The elderly population exhibits impaired establishment and expression of delayed hypersensitivity in the skin, as documented by Smith et al. (1962) and Waldorf et al. (1968). The impairment is partially caused by the well-documented age-related declines in T-lymphocyte function (Mackay, 1977).

Furthermore, studies have observed a decline in the quantity of epidermal Langerhans cells, which are immune cells derived from bone marrow and responsible for immune response in the skin (Gilchrest et al., 1982b; Thiers et al., 1984). Two separate studies, utilizing different methods of examining tissue samples, have found that skin regularly exposed to the sun experiences a decrease of 20–50% in Langerhans cells (Gilchrest et al., 1983; Thiers et al., 1984). Additionally, a third study has shown a comparable reduction in the susceptibility to allergic reactions to dinitrochlorobenzene in elderly volunteers, with sun-exposed skin areas exhibiting a decrease in sensitivity compared to sun-protected areas (O'Dell et al., 1980). According to the immune-surveillance theory of carcinogenesis, which is one of several theories that are debated, this aspect of photoaging may play a role in the high occurrence of skin cancer that is strongly linked to aging.

The cellular and clinical effects of environmental factors on skin aging have been studied using the in vitro model developed by Hayflick 25 years ago (Hayflick, 1965; Hayflick and Moorhead, 1961). It is widely acknowledged that human fibroblasts have a limited and consistent lifespan when grown in a controlled environment (Hayflick, 1979). This lifespan is found to decrease as the age of the donor increases (Martin et al., 1970; Schneider and Mitsui, 1976). Additionally, fibroblasts derived from individuals with certain disorders associated with premature aging have a shorter lifespan compared to fibroblasts from age-matched healthy donors (Martin et al., 1970).

In order to investigate the impact of regular sun exposure on the aging process of skin cells, dermal fibroblasts (Schneider and Mitsui, 1976) and epidermal keratinocytes (Gilchrest, 1980) were cultured from biopsy sites on both the sun-protected inner and sun-exposed outer areas of the upper arms of nine healthy, fair-skinned, male volunteers aged 28–86. The volunteers had similar levels of annual exposure throughout their lives and did not have any significant exposure within 4 months prior to the biopsy. The paired cultures were kept in the same standardized conditions and continuously transferred until they reached a state of senescence.

The cultures originating from sites protected from the sun experienced a greater number of population doublings compared to the cultures originating from sun-exposed sites. This difference became more pronounced as the age of the donor and the severity of photoaging changed increased. Comparable findings were achieved when examining fibroblast cultures obtained from distinct paired locations, specifically sun-exposed and sun-protected skin areas adjacent to the ears of older women who underwent face-lift procedures (Gilchrest et al., 1983). The data indicate that regular sun exposure does expedite cellular aging, as determined by at least one measure.

Photoaging and chronologic or intrinsic aging in the skin exhibit notable similarities, but they can be differentiated at the electron microscopic level (Braverman and Fonferko, 1982a,b; Lavker, 1979). The capacity to differentiate between these factors provides the potential for distinguishing the impact of environmental elements, apart from sun exposure, on aging. This can be achieved even without control tissue that has not been environmentally exposed, which is particularly advantageous in the context of skin. Sufficient understanding of typical morphological and physiological changes associated with aging is necessary to accomplish this. Nevertheless, it will not be readily achieved. When comparing habitually exposed areas like the face or hand to protected areas like the buttock or breast in middle-aged or elderly individuals, it becomes evident that there are different rates of aging. These differences are seen along the lines where clothing is typically worn, rather than being determined by specific anatomical regions.

However, the significant impact of the environment on skin aging has only recently been acknowledged. Convincing scientists and the public of other negative environmental effects on the perceived aging process will necessitate substantial and compelling evidence.

6.3. Vision

Several alterations occur in the eye tissues because of the aging process. A significant proportion of older individuals experience blindness and visual impairment due to certain factors. The understanding of the influence of environmental factors on these "biologic markers" of aging is still in its early stages. Approximately 6% of individuals aged 65 and above experience significant visual impairment, while this number increases to 46% for individuals aged 85 and above. Aging-related macular degeneration, which is linked to alterations in the retinal epithelium, is responsible for a portion of these cases. The remaining cases are attributed to nonneuronal changes, such as cataracts and glaucoma.

6.3.1. Cataracts

- Cataracts, which are the clouding of the lenses of the eyes, are strongly associated with the natural aging process. In fact, it has been proposed that cataracts would develop in every individual if they lived for a sufficiently long period of time. Approximately 17 million individuals (about the population of New York) worldwide have impaired vision due to cataracts, with cataracts being the primary cause of treatable blindness in developing nations. Cataract affects approximately one million individuals in the United States and is a leading cause of blindness in the country. Approximately 60% of individuals in the United States aged 65 to 74 exhibit indications of cataract.
- Epidemiological data reveal significant regional disparities in the occurrence of cataracts and indicate that environmental factors contribute to its cause (to restore vision). For instance, the occurrence of cataracts is exceptionally high in Tibet and Nepal, and there is a significant three-fold variation in the occurrence of cataracts among various climatic zones in northern India. Population studies have revealed a significant contrast in the occurrence of cataracts among different age groups in the United States and India. Specifically, for individuals aged 52–64, 65–74, and 75–85, the prevalence rates were 5%, 18%, and 46% respectively in the United States, whereas in India, the rates were 29%, 43%, and 82% respectively.
- The etiology of age-related cataracts is influenced by several significant risk factors, which include:
    - **Intercourse:** Women have a higher likelihood of experiencing negative outcomes, indicating that hormonal factors may play a significant role. Additional investigation is required on this topic.
    - **Exposure to Ultraviolet Radiation:** Geographical research has indicated that there is a higher likelihood of developing cataracts in regions with abundant sunlight or at elevated altitudes. The elevated incidences of cataracts in Tibet and Nepal indicate a correlation between prolonged exposure to sunlight and higher levels of UV irradiation, which are more prevalent at higher altitudes. According to a current hypothesis, the initial reactions involve oxidative mechanisms that can affect proteins in the lens, including membrane Na+-K+ ATPase. This protein plays a crucial role in regulating the distribution of salt and water in tissues. Overhydration of the lens leads to swelling and disruption of the cellular membranes, resulting in cellular destruction and ultimately

obstructing the transmission of light through the lens. Various types of ionizing radiation have been proven to cause experimental cataracts, making them acknowledged occupational hazards associated with cataract development.

- · **Diabetes:** Metabolic alterations in glucose occur in the lens due to biochemical changes in both the lens itself and the surrounding fluid. In the case of experimental "sugar" cataracts, glucose metabolism occurs through an alternative oxidative metabolic pathway instead of the usual anaerobic series of energy-producing reactions. This leads to the buildup of sorbitol, a type of sugar alcohol, in the lens fibers (McLean et al., 1985). The elevated sorbitol concentration creates a difference in osmotic pressure, leading to the movement of water from the aqueous humor into the lens fibers. This causes the lens fibers to expand and eventually break down, resulting in the clouding of the lens. Aldose reductase is responsible for the production of sorbitol, and the use of inhibitors has successfully prevented experimental cataracts (Kador et al., 1985).

6.3.2. Glaucoma

Glaucoma, specifically primary open-angle glaucoma, is linked to the process of getting older. Glaucoma is defined by the reduction of visual field, alterations in the optic nerve's appearance, and elevated intraocular pressure (pressure exceeding the eye's capacity to withstand). The regulation of intraocular pressure involves a delicate equilibrium between the production of aqueous humor and its drainage through the trabecular meshwork. Glaucoma is characterized by the presence of ultrastructural factors in the meshwork that impede the filtration process and result in elevated intraocular pressure.

Empirical studies have demonstrated a significant rise in the occurrence of glaucoma as individuals grow older. Based on the information gathered, the prevalence rates for glaucoma in predominantly white populations range from 2% to 6%. The prevalence of a certain condition at the age of 70 is significantly higher than at the age of 40, according to the U.S. National Advisory Eye Council in 1983. Nevertheless, the data are obtained from studies carried out under diverse circumstances and in populations of varying magnitudes, and they indicate the identification of glaucoma in relatively limited numbers of patients. Empirical evidence has indicated that the incidence of glaucoma is higher among individuals of African descent compared to individuals of European descent. A recent comprehensive survey conducted in Baltimore has revealed that the overall occurrence of glaucoma among individuals of African descent is 5.8%. This prevalence is distributed as follows: 1.9% among individuals aged 40–49, 4.7% among individuals aged 50–59, 7.4% among individuals aged 60–69, and 12% among individuals aged 70 and above. The data from a white population that can be compared are currently being analyzed (Tielsch et al., 1986).

An investigation into the size and shape of trabecular meshwork samples taken from healthy eyes revealed a gradual decline in the number of cells as individuals age (Alvarado et al., 1981). Measurements of tissues from eyes with glaucoma showed that the process sped up in glaucoma, indicating that the meshwork in glaucoma ages prematurely (Alvarado et al., 1984a,b).

6.3.3. Diabetic Retinopathy

Diabetic retinopathy has a more pronounced impact on the central macular area of the retina, which is the part responsible for the highest level of visual clarity, compared to the peripheral areas. The primary clinical manifestations of retinopathy include vasoconstriction, vascular leakage, and neovascularization, which is characterized by the development of fragile and permeable blood vessels. The resultant hemorrhages frequently result in the formation of scar tissue, causing tension on the retina, leading to its detachment and subsequent blindness.

Approximately 90% of individuals with insulin-dependent diabetes that have persisted for 15 years exhibit some level of retinopathy; after 30 years, around 50% develop proliferative retinal vascular changes. If diabetes can be ascribed to environmental factors like diet, then it is possible to prevent diabetic retinopathy.

6.3.4. Aging-Related Macular Degeneration

Aging-related macular degeneration, previously referred to as senile macular degeneration, specifically impacts the central region of the retina responsible for high-quality vision, resulting in significant visual impairment. This disease is a significant factor in causing vision loss among individuals who are 60 years of age or older. Approximately 90% of the elderly population experience some type of retinal degeneration. Most individuals experience the mild "dry" or nonexudative form, which typically advances at a slow pace. In the more severe form of the disease known as exudative maculopathy, neovascularization takes place. This refers to the abnormal growth of new blood vessels that extend from the choroid, penetrate Bruch's membrane, and reside beneath the retinal pigment epithelium. Hemorrhaging from the newly formed blood vessels triggers mechanisms that degrade the retinal pigment epithelium, raise the position of the retina, and impair visual function. In cases of nonexudative maculopathy, the blood vessels have not breached Bruch's membrane. However, it is important to note that this type of maculopathy has the potential to develop into exudative maculopathy. Laser photocoagulation is effective in reducing maculopathy.

A recent analysis of the causes of aging-related macular degeneration reveals that the risk factors include the presence of drusen, choroidal vascular disease, and a deficiency in vitamin C (Feeney-Burns and Ellerseick, 1985). Drusen, which are small yellowish structures that can be seen under the macula in Bruch's membrane using an ophthalmoscope, typically become more common as a person gets older. Maculopathy is characterized by distinct alterations in both the quantity and visual characteristics of certain elements. A recent study using electron microscopy examined the alterations in Bruch's membrane that occur as a person gets older (Tso, 1985). The macular region underwent progressive morphologic changes starting in the second decade.

6.4. Hearing

Hearing loss is a prevalent condition among older adults, impacting over 25% of individuals aged 65 and above (Katzman and Terry, 1983). Most cases are idiopathic, meaning that their cause is often genetic. These cases occur when there is a loss of sensory hair cells in the inner ear and the auditory nerve is affected. However, it is also well known that drug ingestion can lead to ototoxicity. The potential impact of chronic environmental noise pollution throughout one's lifetime remains uncertain, although it is well-established that prolonged exposure to excessively loud noises can result in permanent hearing impairment (World Health Organization, 1980). Noise-induced hearing loss (NIHL) occurs because of prolonged and regular exposure to loud sounds over an extended period, typically spanning months or years. Over time, small insults accumulate and eventually result in permanent hearing loss. Most hearing losses observed in the workplace are of this type.

Presbycusis refers to the progressive decline in auditory function that occurs because of the natural aging process. It is yet to be established if there is a connection between presbycusis and NIHL and if an individual's susceptibility to NIHL is influenced by their age. Previous research by Helmkamp et al. (1984) and Spoor (1967) has proposed that the relationship between presbycusis and NIHL is not solely additive.

6.5. Nervous System

6.5.1. Changes Associated with Aging

The process of aging is linked to significant alterations in the nervous system (Katzman and Terry, 1983). As individuals age, there is a decline in neural function, which may enable previously dormant neurotoxic disorders to manifest clinically (Calne et al., 1986). Observations from clinical practice have shown that older individuals, particularly those with metabolic abnormalities or with impaired liver or kidney function, are more vulnerable to the harmful effects of foreign substances (Silverstein, 1982). Nevertheless, comprehensive investigations into the impacts of chemical neurotoxicants on laboratory animals of different age groups have not been conducted.

The aspects of normal human aging that have been extensively studied and well-documented are the changes in intellect and memory. Intellectual performance, as assessed through tests evaluating vocabulary, information retention, and comprehension, reaches its highest point between the ages of 20 and 30. In the absence of any illnesses, this level of performance is sustained throughout adulthood, at least until the mid-70s. Perceptual processing and choice reaction times are diminished as individuals age. Elderly individuals consistently experience impairment in the acquisition, retention, and recall of information related to short-term memory.

Motor tasks, such as locomotion, handwriting, and other purposeful movements, are executed with reduced speed, strength, or coordination. Muscle atrophy is a frequent occurrence, resulting in decreased strength and making it challenging to elicit tendon reflexes (Katzman and Terry, 1983). As individuals age, their ability to sense vibrations gradually declines. They also experience a decrease in touch sensitivity, impaired ability to distinguish between different temperatures, and a slight increase in the threshold for feeling pain. Age-related changes include impaired thermoregulation and reduced tear production. There is a change in sleeping patterns.

The process of aging in humans is accompanied by neurobehavioral changes, which are linked to modifications in the structure or function of the central and peripheral nervous systems. According to Katzman and Terry (1983), alterations in vascular and cardiac reflexes, galvanic skin response, potency, micturition, and pupillary response are likely caused by changes in the autonomic nervous system. The elderly often experience sympathetic hyperactivity, which can negatively impact cognitive functioning, particularly during psychological testing conducted under stressful conditions. Individuals with sympathetic hyperactivity are likely to have an increased vulnerability to chemical toxicants that possess sympathomimetic properties. Alterations in cerebral blood flow, which are crucial for the preservation of optimal brain function, may manifest after the age of 80. Normally aging individuals have been found to exhibit cerebral cortical atrophy and ventricular enlargement. Certain areas of the brain are more prone to losing neurons. These include the locus ceruleus and substantia nigra, which experience the greatest reduction in cell count during the third and fourth decades of life and continue to decline gradually afterward. Other affected cells include Purkinje's cells and putamen neurons, which linearly decrease in number. However, multiple cranial nuclei and the olivary nucleus exhibit consistent and unchanging populations. The number of neurons in the cerebral cortex can decrease by as much as 50% between the ages of 20 and 80. Additionally, there are further reductions and changes in the branching patterns of their dendrites and the connections they make with other neurons. The amount of lipofuscin, a yellow pigment that cannot be dissolved, increases in a linear manner in most neurons as age increases. However, there is no proof that this substance is harmful to cells.

Additional neuronal abnormalities observed in aged brains consist of neurofibrillary tangles, neuritic plaques, and granulovacuolar bodies. Neuronal changes and cell loss lead to significant changes in the levels of neurotransmitters, such as dopamine, norepinephrine, serotonin, gamma-aminobutyric acid, and choline acetyltransferase, an enzyme necessary to produce the neurotransmitter acetylcholine (Katzman and Terry, 1983).

The peripheral nervous system undergoes morphologic age-related changes, which likely involve a decrease in sensory neurons, an elevated occurrence of demyelination in spinal roots and peripheral nerves, an increase in connective tissue, and a slight loss of myelinated fibers (Spencer and Ochoa, 1981). Dorsal root ganglion cells commonly experience distal dystrophic and degenerative changes in their central processes. Motor neuron count decreases slightly with age (Tomlinson and Irving, 1977), and there are observed degenerative changes in the endings of motor axons. Characteristic features include alterations in sensory and motor nerve conduction, accompanied by a gradual deceleration of nerve action potentials.

6.5.2. Induced Disorders and Diseases

There is a significant overlap between the neurological effects of aging and those caused by chemical substances. This overlap may suggest that the nervous system has a restricted range of biological expression or that the processes involved in neural aging can be attributed to the harmful effects of circulating metabolites originating from both internal and external sources.

It is widely accepted that the symptoms of neural dysfunction caused by aging become apparent only after the extensive redundancy in the structure and function of the nervous system has been overcome. For instance, a persistent state of Parkinson's disease only manifests after a significant depletion of neurons in the substantia nigra, and it can arise because of the aging process. Certain individuals may have an increased susceptibility to neurotoxic disorders due to genetic factors, such as being slow acetylators which can lead to isoniazid toxicity. Other factors that can contribute to this risk include abnormal metabolic states, such as malnutrition, compromised blood-brain regulatory interfaces, such as liver dysfunction, or the natural process of aging, which can result in poor renal clearance. Older individuals are typically more vulnerable than younger individuals to the potential neurotoxic side effects of therapeutic drugs and other chemical substances.

Calne et al. (1986) have suggested that the aging process and the development of degenerative diseases in the elderly, which impact cognitive and motor abilities, may be attributed to environmental factors, such as exposure to chemical toxicants and environmental toxins. Presenile dementia of the Alzheimer's, Parkinson's disease, and amyotrophic lateral sclerosis are believed to result from subclinical environmental damage to specific regions of the central nervous system that are especially susceptible to age-related neuronal loss. The hypothesis regarding parkinsonism is being investigated in individuals who have experienced subclinical damage to the substantia nigra following exposure to MPTP (Langston, 1985). Due to the age-related decline of nigral neurons, distinct characteristics of the disease will probably develop later in life.

The indigenous population of Guam is particularly vulnerable to amyotrophic lateral sclerosis, presenile dementia, and parkinsonism (Spencer et al., 1987). Researchers in the field of epidemiology have discovered that being exposed to the environment of Guam during the first 20 years of life is enough to create the necessary conditions for the development of amyotrophic lateral sclerosis or parkinsonism-dementia many years later (Garruto et al., 1980). The potential causes of the condition are the cycad plant (*Cycas circinalis*) (Spencer et al., 1987) and aluminum (Perl et al., 1982).

6.5.3. Neurotoxicants

Lead and mercury are prominent environmental pollutants that have the potential to cause neurotoxicity. However, the number of people in North America who have clear neurotoxic disorders directly caused by these pollutants is likely to be small. Moreover, a wide range of plants and animals produce or possess powerful toxins, some of which disrupt the transmission of nerve signals. One particular toxin, known as ciguatoxin, is a significant contributor to sudden neurotoxicity in the Pacific region, particularly among individuals who consume fish that have been contaminated with it (Kaplan, 1980). Additional neurotoxins, such as α-bungarotoxin and α-latrotoxin, have an impact on synaptic transmission. Both categories can generate severe, potentially fatal situations. Certain agents infiltrate the food and water that humans consume. Certain chemicals that have been scientifically demonstrated to have neurotoxic effects on animals are utilized as food additives (such as monosodium glutamate), flavors and fragrances (such as 2,6-dinitro-3-methoxy-4-tert-butyl toluene), and anti-seborrheic agents (such as zinc pyridinethione). However, there have been no reported instances of neurotoxic diseases in humans resulting from these sources.

Biological toxins such as *Clostridium botulinum*, *C. tetani*, and Corynebacterium diphtheriae, as well as neurotoxic agents found naturally in food like cassava, cycad, and Lathyrus spp., or as contaminants like ergot and aflatoxin, along with pesticides, are likely responsible for a significant number of neurotoxic disorders in developing countries. Pesticide poisoning is a global issue. Cholinergic crises that are not controlled can frequently occur among agricultural and pesticide workers in certain regions, and in some cases, can result in death (Bull, 1982). Additionally, surviving individuals have been observed to experience enduring alterations in their electroencephalograms and behavior (Duffy et al., 1979). Some pesticides contain organochlorines or synthetic pyrethroids that can cause tremors and seizures by disrupting neurotransmission (Taylor et al., 1979; Narahashi, 1984). The global issue of substance abuse, specifically involving ethanol, hallucinogens, narcotics, central nervous system stimulants, solvents, and nitrous oxide, results in different forms of temporary or prolonged neurological impairment.

Various substances commonly found in the workplace, such as solvents, monomers, and catalysts, have been linked to a range of neurological disorders, including polyneuropathy and organic brain syndrome. Workers who were exposed to the industrial neurotoxicant Lucel-7 (2-tert-butylazo-2-hydroxy-5-methylhexane) for a short period of a few weeks developed a range of disorders, as observed in a study conducted by Spencer et al. in 1985.

Exposure to pharmaceuticals can lead to the development of dementia, delirium, and depression. In the study by Learoyd (1972), it was discovered that 16% of the 236 elderly patients who were admitted to the hospital for behavioral disturbances had disorders that were directly caused by the effects of psychoactive drugs. In a recent study of 107 unselected outpatients who were referred for evaluation of global mental impairment, which includes symptoms such as memory loss, confusion, slow thought, inability to care for oneself, and self-neglect, Larson et al. (1984) discovered that 15 patients exhibited potentially reversible dementias. These dementias are characterized by a chronic and progressive decline in higher intellectual function. Medication was the primary cause.

The potential causes of dementia included amantadine-induced confusion, insulin-induced hypoglycemia, and haloperidol-induced oversedation and parkinsonism. Several drug combinations were involved: clorazepate and lorazepam; meprobamate, protriptyline, and thioridazine; and reserpine, diazepam, and meprobamate.

Reversible dementia can occur, especially when triggered by medications, toxic metals, or industrial chemicals (Cummings et al., 1980). Drugs associated with dementia can be classified into four primary categories: psychotropic medications (including phenothiazines, butyrophenones, benzodiazepines, tricyclic antidepressants, and lithium carbonate), anticonvulsants (such as phenytoin, mephenytoin, and carbamazepine), antihypertensive agents (including clonidine, methyldopa, and propranolol), and anticholinergic compounds (such as atropine and antihistamines). Heavy metals, such as lead, mercury, thallium, and arsenic, can result in intellectual impairments. However, these impairments can be reversed through the process of chelation or by reducing exposure to these metals.

Despite the decreased availability of proprietary bromide preparations compared to the past, it is important to consider bromide intoxication as a potential hidden cause of dementia (Raskind et al., 1978). According to a report by Crapper et al. (1976), the level of aluminum in the brains of patients who died of senile dementia of Alzheimer's type is 10–30 times higher than the usual concentration. Subsequent research has identified the presence of aluminum in cells containing neurofibrillary tangles (Perl and Brody, 1980). However, the exact contribution of aluminum to the development of the disease is still a subject of debate (Glenner, 1982). Prolonged exposure to industrial substances such as trichloroethylene, toluene, carbon disulfide, organophosphates, and carbon monoxide has been found to cause changes in mental state. However, these changes can be reversed by removing the substances responsible for them (Cummings et al., 1980).

Delirium refers to organic brain syndromes that exhibit a sudden onset of cognitive dysfunction, which includes fluctuating impairments in attention, memory, and orientation. Typical symptoms of this condition include difficulty sleeping or decreased alertness, perceptual disturbances such as false perceptions and seeing things that are not there, and changes in physical activity, especially restlessness. Older individuals, especially those who already have dementia, are at a higher risk of experiencing drug-induced delirium (Barnes and Raskind, 1980). Levodopa, amantadine, corticosteroids, and various drugs with anticholinergic properties are frequently the cause. Barbiturates and other sedative hypnotic agents have the potential to induce paradoxic agitated delirium in susceptible patients.

Drug therapy can lead to the development of depression as a complication. Antihypertensive medications, including reserpine, methyldopa, and clonidine, have been found to induce depressive symptoms. However, beta-blockers appear to have a higher occurrence of these symptoms compared to centrally acting agents. There is abundant anecdotal evidence indicating that patients without any previous psychiatric conditions may experience feelings of unease, unhappiness, or severe clinical depression when they begin treatment with beta-adrenergic antagonists. Additionally, the occurrence of central nervous system side effects from propranolol varies in frequency, ranging from 1% to more than 70% (Paykel et al., 1982). The reported symptoms encompass depression, somnolence, insomnia, and hallucinations.

Moreover, there is a notable increase in the utilization of tricyclic antidepressants among patients who are prescribed beta-blockers, with a rate of 23% over 2 years. This percentage is significantly higher compared to patients who are taking hydralazine or hypoglycemics (both at 15%) or methyldopa or reserpine (both at 10%). Nevertheless, the strength of the correlation between beta-blockers and depression treatment was observed to decrease as individuals grew older (Avorn, 1986). The suggested reasons were a decrease in receptor sensitivity due to aging and the physicians' failure to recognize dysphoria or other abnormal side effects in an older patient as significant. Beta-blockers may exert their central effect by interfering with the function of nonadrenergic neurotransmitters in the brain, which is believed to be involved in the development of depression in certain cases.

Typically, the signs and symptoms of drug-induced neurologic disorders are nearly identical to those observed in disorders not caused by drugs. However, these symptoms can usually be reversed if detected early enough (Lane and Routledge, 1983). Prolonged therapeutic treatment with anticonvulsants, anticholinergics, neuroleptics, antineoplastics, and antiparkinsonian drugs often leads to neurotoxicity. Furthermore, a newly identified iatrogenic neurotoxicity is the sensory neuropathy syndrome linked to pyridoxine megavitamin therapy, which is commonly prescribed to treat premenstrual tension (Schaumburg et al., 1983).

The prevalence of subclinical neurologic and behavioral disorders linked to chemical substances remains uncertain, although it is speculated by certain individuals to be substantial. Instances encompass the ongoing disputes regarding childhood cognitive impairment caused by environmental lead contamination and the neurobehavioral consequences linked to long-term occupational exposure to various industrial solvents.

6.6. Respiratory System

The growth and development of the lungs persist until the second decade of life, after which pulmonary function starts to deteriorate. The decrease can be most readily assessed using tests that measure forced expiration. Several epidemiological studies suggest that the forced expiratory volume in 1 second (FEV1) consistently decreases with age, even among individuals who do not smoke and are in good health. The rate of loss is higher in older individuals compared to younger individuals (Fletcher, 1976; Higgins et al., 1982; Beaty et al., 1984; Burrows et al., 1986). Smokers experience a more rapid decline in pulmonary function compared to nonsmokers. However, if smokers quit smoking, their rate of decline returns to the level observed in nonsmokers (Fletcher,

1976). Despite limited knowledge about the connection between aging and environmental damage to the lungs, two notable features have significant pathophysiologic correlations. Age and smoking have significant effects on the measurement of the structure and function of small airways. Even in young smokers who are assumed to be in good health, there is clear evidence of inflammatory reactions in the outer airways (Niewoehner et al., 1974).

The prevalence of small-airway dysfunction tends to rise as individuals age and is evident in smokers across all age groups (Enjeti et al., 1978).

The recognition of the significance of peripheral lung structure and function in the progression of lung aging or disease, as well as the emphasis on studying peripheral lung function in assessing environmental exposures, has been driven by these observations (Macklem, 1972).

Airway reactivity is the second crucial aspect of lung function. The airway responses are usually heightened in individuals with asthma, but they may also be heightened in non-asthmatic individuals who smoke (Gerrard et al., 1980; Mullen et al., 1986), after viral infections, and following exposure to oxidants, such as ozone (Boushey et al., 1980). Airway reactivity can be assessed in a controlled laboratory setting by administering bronchoconstricting agents. Several studies indicate that heightened airway reactivity may be a significant risk factor for accelerated decline in function associated with aging (Orie, 1960; Barter and Campbell, 1976; Vollmer, 1985).

The connection between the levels of air pollutants in the environment and the decrease in lung function, as people get older, is a subject of debate and disagreement (U.S. EPA, 1986). Nevertheless, the genuine possibility of environmental exposures, whether they occur outdoors or indoors, affecting vulnerable individuals cannot be denied.

There is strong epidemiological evidence that both age and environmental factors, specifically smoking, are linked to a decline in lung function. Additionally, there is a significant correlation between lung dysfunction and mortality from all causes, including both pulmonary and nonpulmonary causes. Consistent and robust associations between lung function and mortality have been consistently observed in epidemiological studies conducted in Tecumseh (Higgins and Keller, 1970), Framingham (Ashley et al., 1975), and Baltimore (Beaty et al., 1982; Menkes et al., 1985). It cannot be attributed to smoking habits and partially represents deaths caused by chronic lung disease or lung cancer (Skillrud, 1986).

While the exact foundation of this fascinating connection remains unknown, two explanations are particularly appealing. Increased exposure to environmental toxins or heightened susceptibility of the host can disrupt the lungs, as well as other bodily systems since the lungs typically serve as a barrier between the body and the environment. Furthermore, dysfunctions in organ systems other than the lungs can potentially result in abnormalities in lungs that are otherwise functioning normally. Both explanations emphasize the significance of lung function in determining environmental exposure and evaluating an individual's vulnerability to both nonpulmonary and pulmonary aging and disease.

6.7. Cardiovascular System

Age-related changes in the cardiovascular system include stenotic coronary vascular disease caused by atherosclerosis, stiffening of the large arteries, an increase in systolic blood pressure, and mild cardiac hypertrophy. These changes also result in a reduced cardiac filling rate, while the cardiac filling volume and resting cardiac output remain unchanged (Lakatta, 1985a, b, 1986).

Exercise can reveal more subtle signs of aging. As people age, their response to intense exercise changes. This includes a decrease in the increase of heart rate, an increase in heart size (which is normal when resting) both at the end of the filling period and at the end of the contraction period, and a decrease in the increase of ejection fraction (the proportion of the filling volume pumped with each contraction of the heart) (Rodeheffer et al., 1984).

The observed changes can be attributed to a decline in the cardiovascular system's responsiveness to catecholamines, which are produced when the sympathetic nervous system is activated during exercise, and this decline is associated with aging. Extensive evidence from studies on both animals and humans has shown that the autonomic modulation of cardiac and vascular tissue in response to β-adrenergic agonists becomes less sensitive with age. This has been demonstrated in various experiments conducted by Bertel et al. (1980), Conway et al. (1971), Fleisch (1981), Kuramoto et al. (1978), Vestal et al. (1979), Yin et al. (1979, 1981).

Although there is a significant amount of information available on how aging affects cardiovascular physiology, there has been little focus on how the elderly population might be more susceptible to the harmful effects of drugs, chemicals, and other environmental substances. A study conducted by Algeo et al. (1983) examined whether there is a variation in the reaction of the older heart muscle to cardiac glycosides, such as ouabain and digoxin, in both animals and humans. The tension and rate of tension development in isometric trabeculae carneae were approximately four times higher in young Wistar rat myocardium compared to aged myocardium (Gerstenblith et al., 1979). There was no variation in the inhibition of Na+-K+-ATPase induced by ouabain based on age, which is a proposed mechanism of action for ouabain and other digitalis preparations. On the other hand, the activity of the Na+-K+ ATPase was 50% lower in aged Fischer 344 rats compared to younger rats. Additionally, the toxicity of ouabain was inversely correlated with the enzyme activity (Baskin et al., 1977).

Ouabain exhibited a greater inhibition of enzyme activity in older rats compared to younger rats. According to a study by Wollenberger et al. in 1953, the amount of ouabain that caused death in adult and aged guinea pigs was the same, regardless of their age (up to approximately 5–6.5 years old).

No age difference in the inotropic response to digitalis was found in elderly humans (Cokkinos et al., 1980). The inotropic response, as assessed by systolic intervals, to the intravenous administration of deslanoside (1.2 mg) was found to be comparable between a group of 20 healthy males and females (with a mean age of 34.3 years) and a group of 20 healthy older individuals (with a mean age of 65.3 years). The clinical outcomes of acetyldigoxin in congestive heart failure and digoxin in atrial fibrillation are not influenced by age, as demonstrated by Aravanis (1969) and Chamberlain et al. (1970). Therefore, besides the rise in plasma digoxin caused by reduced kidney excretion in older individuals, there is limited proof to substantiate the commonly held belief that the inherent responsiveness of the heart muscle to digitalis is heightened in old age.

Age-related data on antiarrhythmic agents are more limited compared to the available data on cardiac glycosides. However, these data generally suggest that there is no significant increase in sensitivity or toxicity in older individuals, if there is no abnormal conduction. A recent clinical study revealed that there was a change in the responsiveness to verapamil, which is a type of medication that blocks calcium channels. Elderly patients exhibited higher plasma concentrations compared to young patients due to age-related variations in pharmacokinetics (Abernethy et al., 1986).

Doxorubicin (Adriamycin), a chemotherapeutic drug belonging to the anthracycline class, exhibits significant cardiac toxicity that is associated with aging. An inherent issue in the administration of doxorubicin for therapeutic intentions is the occurrence of frequently irreversible and potentially lethal congestive heart failure. The impact appears to be dependent on the dosage, and when cumulative doses exceed 550 mg/m2, there is a significant rise in the occurrence of heart failure (Lefrak et al., 1973). When more precise methods are employed to assess heart function, such as systolic intervals, around 15% of patients show signs of cardiac damage following doxorubicin therapy at doses exceeding 400 mg/m2 (Dresdale et al., 1983). Cardiac histology undergoes degenerative changes in almost all cases when the dosage exceeds 240 mg/m2 (Bristow et al., 1978). In a retrospective survey of 4,000 patients conducted by Von Hoff et al., (1979), it was found that in addition to cumulative dose, old age was identified as the primary risk factor.

It has been observed by others that aging increases the risk of developing cardiotoxicity (Bristow et al., 1978; Dresdale et al., 1983). However, this is not due to a higher occurrence of coronary heart disease in older patients (Von Hoff et al., 1979). The precise mechanism underlying the cardiotoxicity of doxorubicin remains unknown; however, it is hypothesized that the generation of free radicals may play a role (Olson et al., 1981; Unverferth et al., 1982). The detoxification pathways for free radicals are less active in certain tissues of aging laboratory animals (Stohs et al., 1982), which suggests that the ability to remove free radicals in the heart might be compromised in elderly patients.

The clinical observations regarding doxorubicin indicate that other substances and environmental factors that generate free radicals could potentially be linked to myocardial damage, with the possibility of the effects being more pronounced in older individuals. Regrettably, there is a lack of available data on that specific aspect. In fact, it seems that the influence of age on cardiovascular toxicity has been largely disregarded by professionals in the fields of toxicology and epidemiology.

6.8. Renal System

Chronic nephropathy, characterized by glomerular sclerosis, mesangial cell injury, and excessive production of mesangial matrix, is frequently observed in aged rats (Durand et al., 1964; Coleman et al., 1977). Young rats exhibit comparable progressive lesions following surgical reduction of kidney mass (Chanutin and Ferris, 1932; Shimamura and Morrison, 1975; Purkerson et al., 1976). Similarly, in humans, these lesions typically occur at advanced ages after kidney damage caused by disease, once the initial disease process has ceased (Brenner et al., 1982). A study conducted by Maeda et al. in 1985 found that reducing the protein intake in rat diets slows down the progression of nephropathy, which is a kidney disease that commonly occurs with aging. This effect was also observed in rats that underwent surgery to reduce kidney mass, as reported by Hostetter et al. in 1981, Laouari et al. in 1983, and Moise and Smith in 1927.

Furthermore, there is empirical evidence indicating that decreasing the amount of protein consumed by individuals can decelerate the advancement of chronic renal failure toward end-stage disease (Mitch, 1984). Brenner et al. (1982) proposed that a reduction in dietary protein inhibits glomerular hyperperfusion and hyperfiltration, which they believed to be the cause of lesion progression and subsequent decline in renal function.

Iwasaki et al. (1986) recently discovered that the progression of kidney lesions in male Fischer 344 rats during the natural aging process can be slowed down by incorporating soy protein into their diet as the primary source of protein, without decreasing their overall protein consumption. This discovery holds significance in two regards: as a means to study aging using animal models, and as a potential treatment for chronic renal failure in humans. The male Fischer 344 rat has been extensively used as a prominent animal model (National Research Council, 1981b) for studying aging. This is due to its genetic uniformity and its resistance to age-related obesity, which is commonly observed in other rat strains. Nevertheless, a significant issue with this strain, like other rat strains, is the occurrence of renal failure as the rat age. This hinders the investigation of normal aging processes in some rats by the time they reach 18 months (about 1 and a half years), and in many rats after they reach 24 months (about 2 years) of age. Diets that exclusively use soy protein as the only source of protein can largely overcome the issue and therefore make it easier to conduct comprehensive studies on the lifespan of Fischer 344 rats.

Restricting dietary protein in patients with chronic renal failure has been shown to delay the progression of renal function loss and extend the time before dialysis or transplantation is required, according to available data. However, this treatment carries the risk of protein malnutrition, as well as depletion of minerals and vitamins (Mitch, 1984). Choosing the appropriate dietary protein source could potentially provide a treatment for chronic renal failure that is equally effective as protein restriction but without the associated risks.

6.9. Immune System

The immune system is a crucial defense mechanism of the body. Environmental factors that can affect the immune system include the impact of psychological stress (such as bereavement), dietary intake, ambient temperature, living conditions, light exposure, noise levels, and exposure to chemicals. Certain environmental factors that impact immune function can influence life expectancy, and consequently, can affect vulnerability to diseases or the aging process itself.

Nutrition has the most profound impact on both immunity and life span in rodents among all environmental factors. Restricting the amount of calories consumed by mice and rats to about half of what they would normally eat prevents the decline in immune function that occurs with age, decreases the occurrence of various diseases (including cancer), and increases lifespan. Research has demonstrated that undernutrition can extend the lifespan of various short-lived strains of mice, as discussed in the review by Good et al. (1980). The impact of a comparable dietary regimen on the lifespan of higher organisms, including humans, remains uncertain.

There is undeniable evidence that the boundary between an organism and its surroundings changes as it ages (refer to Weksler, 1986 for a comprehensive review). The immune function of the skin and the mucosal lining of the respiratory and gastrointestinal tracts undergo alterations as a person ages. However, these changes do not always occur in sync with the changes in overall immunity.

Considerably more information is available regarding the alterations in systemic immunity that occur with age in both rodents and humans. One notable anatomical change is the gradual shrinking of the thymus gland, which starts at sexual maturity and is fully completed by middle age (around 45–50 years in humans). This process leads to the loss of two important functions of the thymus. Age-related decline in thymic function primarily affects the ability to facilitate the development of T-cell precursors that travel from the bone marrow to the thymus gland. The second factor is the decline in the concentration of thymic hormone in the bloodstream, which starts shortly after reaching sexual maturity. Thymic hormone activity becomes untraceable in the bloodstream of humans after reaching middle age.

The thymus, which produces fully developed T lymphocytes, has a crucial function in cell-mediated immune responses and the control of the immune response. As expected, immune senescence is marked by a decline in thymus-dependent functions that are necessary for both cellular immunity and the control of humoral immunity. The susceptibility of elderly individuals to diseases caused by various pathogens, such as viruses, fungi, neoplastic cells, and certain environmental agents, is heightened due to the reliance on cell-mediated immunity for the response against these agents. The significant rise in illness and death related to influenza in older individuals is a frequent clinical outcome of weakened immune function due to aging.

Furthermore, the decline in cell-mediated immunity that occurs with aging is accompanied by the impairment of thymic function, which disrupts the regulation of immune responses. The notable rise in the occurrence of autoantibodies and the production of monoclonal immunoglobulins as individuals age is a clear indication of this phenomenon. The decline in suppressor-cell function in elderly individuals is believed to be a contributing factor to the age-related rise in autoantibodies and monoclonal proteins. The autoimmune reactions in elderly individuals may be intensified when they are prescribed drugs such as procainamide, α-methyldopa, or estrogens, as these medications themselves promote the production of autoantibodies. Autoantibodies and autoantigens combine to create immune complexes. The presence of circulating immune complexes can contribute to vascular damage, leading to the progression of atherosclerosis in older individuals.

Advancements have been achieved in comprehending the cellular foundation of lymphocyte activity, which can be attributed to the inability of T lymphocytes to undergo cell division. The evidence indicates that the cellular mechanism underlying immune senescence is comparable to what Hayflick proposed two decades ago (Hayflick, 1965) in cultured fibroblasts, which is the decline in replicative capacity. Therefore, any environmental factor that impairs the ability of cells to divide would likely reduce immune function and hasten the aging of the immune system.

6.10. Sexuality

The apprehension of experiencing a decline in sexual prowess or physical allure can cause significant distress among individuals as they age. Men commonly experience anxiety regarding sexual impotence, while women often worry about the decline in their physical attractiveness and desirability. Several gradual and predictable physiological changes do happen as a person ages, but these changes do not prevent active and fulfilling sexual functioning in old age.

The majority of the sexual changes experienced by older women are a direct consequence of the decline in female hormones, particularly estrogen, during menopause. Various environmental factors, including ionizing radiation, pharmaceuticals, and cigarette smoking, have been proven to affect the timing of menopause, also known as ovarian failure (Chapman, 1983; Mattison and Ross, 1983; Mattison, 1985). Nevertheless, a significant majority of women, approximately 60%, do not encounter significant physical or emotional symptoms related to menopause. Among those who do experience symptoms, the majority only have mild to moderate physical issues such as headaches, neckaches, hot flashes, fatigue, and emotional instability.

As men age, they do not experience a loss of their ability to have erections and ejaculations if they are physically healthy. However, certain changes may occur. As men age, they typically experience an increase in the time it takes to achieve an erection and reach orgasm compared to when they were younger.

Medications, whether taken as prescribed or not, can exacerbate these effects and induce additional sexual complications. Certain substances disrupt the functioning of the autonomic nervous system, which plays a role in regulating sexual response. External factors can influence one's mood and level of alertness, as well as modify the production or functioning of sex hormones. According to a study published in 1983, medications were found to be the cause or a contributing factor in 25% of sexual problems experienced by men (Butler and Lewis, 1986). While there is limited information on the relationship between drugs and female sexuality, it can be inferred that drugs that impact men are likely to have similar effects on women (Butler and Lewis, 1986).

Tranquilizers, antidepressants, and certain antihypertensive medications have all been linked to erectile dysfunction in men. The impact of these medications on women is not as comprehensively understood. Arthritis medications known as corticosteroids can cause a temporary condition of erectile dysfunction. Analgesics can decrease sensitivity, which can consequently impact male sexual function. Prolonged use of aspirin decreases fertility. Cimetidine, a commonly sold medication in the United States used to treat ulcers, has the potential to cause erectile dysfunction. Excessive alcohol consumption diminishes male potency and impairs female orgasmic ability. Nicotine itself can contribute to the occurrence of impotence. While aging leads to certain expected and gradual changes in sexual function, these changes are often complicated by the influence of environmental factors.

6.11. Role of Environment in Bone Metabolism and Vitamin D Nutrition

One significant issue linked to the process of aging is the reduction in bone density. Approximately 10 million elderly individuals in the United States are estimated to experience a significant decrease in bone density, which weakens the structure of their skeleton and greatly increases their vulnerability to fractures. The extent of this public-health issue is apparent in the approximately 200,000 hip fractures that happen annually. According to estimates from Cummings et al. (1985), the annual expenditure for the acute care of individuals with age-related fractures amounts to $6 billion.

The elderly experience bone loss due to various factors, including insufficient absorption of vitamin D and calcium, which are influenced by estrogen levels. There is extensive documentation in Great Britain, a country that does not regularly fortify foods with vitamin D, indicating that over 40% of males and 30% of females with hip fractures have a deficiency in vitamin D (Chalmers et al., 1967; Aaron et al., 1974), it has been presumed that vitamin D deficiency is not a significant health issue in the United States due to the fortification of foods with vitamin D. A study conducted in the Southwest found that more than 60% of the elderly individuals living independently were consuming less than 25% of the recommended daily allowance (RDA) of vitamin D through their diets (Omdahl et al., 1982). Two additional studies found that approximately 30% of elderly patients with hip fractures exhibited indications of vitamin D deficiency (Sokoloff, 1978; Doppelt et al., 1983).

A significant factor contributing to inadequate vitamin D levels among older individuals in the United States is a reduction or complete avoidance of milk and dairy product intake. The decline is associated with the prevalent misconception among older individuals that they no longer require milk consumption, as milk is solely crucial for maintaining a strong skeletal system in developing children. Additionally, gastrointestinal discomfort arises due to insufficient lactase, the enzyme responsible for breaking down lactose in milk. Only a small number of foods contain vitamin D naturally, such as fish liver oil, eggs, liver, and milk. Additionally, some foods like milk, certain cereals, and margarine are fortified with vitamin D in certain countries. A quart of milk contains 400 international units (10 g) of vitamin D, which meets the Recommended Daily Allowance (RDA) (Holick, 1986).

For an elderly individual who does not consume milk or other vitamin D-rich foods, or take a vitamin D supplement, it is crucial to expose themselves to sunlight to produce sufficient vitamin D3 for maintaining a healthy skeletal system. Nevertheless, due to the heightened understanding that being exposed to sunlight can lead to skin cancer and parched and creased skin, it is frequently recommended that older individuals shield their skin by wearing protective clothing or applying sunscreen before venturing outside. These measures serve to prevent both the harmful impact of solar radiation and the advantageous impact – the synthesis of vitamin D3 in the skin (MacLaughlin and Holick, 1985).

A Closer Look

Biological toxins

Biological toxins play a significant role in the aging process, and recent advances have shed light on their complex interactions within the body. These toxins, ranging from environmental pollutants to metabolic byproducts, can accelerate aging by inducing oxidative stress, inflammation, and cellular damage. Oxidative stress, in particular, arises when toxins generate an imbalance between free radicals and antioxidants, leading to cellular dysfunction and contributing to age-related diseases such as cardiovascular conditions and neurodegenerative disorders.

Advances in research have highlighted the diverse sources and mechanisms through which biological toxins impact aging. Environmental toxins like heavy metals and air pollutants accumulate in tissues over time, exacerbating oxidative damage and impairing cellular repair mechanisms. Similarly, metabolic byproducts such as advanced glycation end-products (AGEs) form through reactions between sugars and proteins, accumulating in tissues and promoting inflammation and tissue stiffening associated with aging.

Moreover, the microbiome has emerged as a critical player in toxin metabolism and aging. Gut bacteria produce metabolites that can either mitigate or exacerbate toxin-induced damage, influencing overall health and longevity. Research into the gut-brain axis has shown how toxins and their metabolites can affect cognitive function and neurodegenerative processes, linking intestinal health to brain aging.

Advances in understanding biological toxins in aging have spurred research into preventive strategies and interventions. These include dietary modifications to reduce toxin intake, antioxidant therapies to combat oxidative stress, and microbiome-targeted treatments to optimize toxin metabolism. Integrative approaches that consider both environmental exposure and metabolic processes hold promise for mitigating the impact of biological toxins on aging, potentially extending healthspan and improving quality of life in aging populations.

Continued research into the intricate relationships between biological toxins and aging promises to uncover new therapeutic targets and strategies for promoting healthy aging and preventing age-related diseases.

Summary

- Age-associated diseases and changes in organ function are influenced by a variety of environmental factors. This chapter explores the impact of environmental elements such as pollution, diet, lifestyle, and social determinants on aging processes and related health outcomes.
- Pollution, including air, water, and soil contaminants, plays a significant role in the development and progression of age-related diseases. Fine particulate matter and other pollutants can exacerbate respiratory conditions, cardiovascular diseases, and neurodegenerative disorders, contributing to the overall burden of age-associated illnesses.
- Dietary habits are crucial determinants of health in aging populations. A diet rich in fruits, vegetables, whole grains, and lean proteins can mitigate the risk of age-related diseases such as diabetes, cardiovascular diseases, and certain cancers. Conversely, a diet high in processed foods, sugar, and unhealthy fats can accelerate the aging process and increase susceptibility to disease.
- Lifestyle factors such as physical activity, smoking, and alcohol consumption also play a pivotal role in aging and disease development. Regular exercise can improve cardiovascular health, maintain muscle mass, and enhance cognitive function, while smoking and excessive alcohol intake can accelerate aging processes and increase the risk of chronic diseases.
- Social determinants, including socioeconomic status, education, and access to healthcare, profoundly impact health outcomes in aging populations. Individuals with lower socioeconomic status are more likely to experience poor health outcomes due to limited access to healthcare, unhealthy living conditions, and higher levels of stress.

References

1. Agostini, M., Traldi, P., & Hamdan, M. (2023). Mass spectrometry-based proteomics: Analyses related to drug-resistance and disease biomarkers. *Medicina, 59*(1), 1722. https://doi.org/10.3390/medicina590101722.
2. Alfano, R., Herceg, Z., Nawrot, T. S., Chadeau-Hyam, M., Ghantous, A., & Plusquin, M. (2018). The impact of air pollution on our epigenome: How far is the evidence? (A systematic review). *Current Environmental Health Reports, 5*(4), 544–578. https://doi.org/10.1007/s40572-018-0223-0.
3. Arneson, A., Haghani, A., Thompson, M. J., Pellegrini, M., Kwon, S. B., Vu, H., Maciejewski, E., Yao, M., Li, C. Z., Lu, A. T., et al. (2022). A mammalian methylation array for profiling methylation levels at conserved sequences. *Nature Communications, 13*(1), 783. https://doi.org/10.1038/s41467-022-28444-4.
4. Baker, G. T., 3rd, & Sprott, R. L. (1988). Biomarkers of aging. *Experimental Gerontology, 23*(3), 223–239. https://doi.org/10.1016/0531-5565(88)90025-3.
5. Baranyi, G., Deary, I. J., McCartney, D. L., Harris, S. E., Shortt, N., Reis, S., Russ, T. C., Thompson, C. W., Vieno, M., & Cox, S. R., et al. (2022). Life-course exposure to air pollution and biological ageing in the Lothian Birth Cohort 1936. *Environment International, 169*, 107501. https://doi.org/10.1016/j.envint.2022.107501.
6. Bell, C. G., Lowe, R., Adams, P. D., Baccarelli, A. A., Beck, S., Bell, J. T., Christensen, B. C., Gladyshev, V. N., Heijmans, B. T., & Horvath, S., et al. (2019). DNA methylation aging clocks: Challenges and recommendations. *Genome Biology, 20*(1), 249. https://doi.org/10.1186/s13059-019-1824-y.
7. Bell, J. T., Tsai, P. C., Yang, T. P., Pidsley, R., Nisbet, J., Glass, D., Mangino, M., Zhai, G., Zhang, F., & Valdes, A., et al. (2012). Epigenome-wide scans identify differentially methylated regions for age and age-related phenotypes in a healthy ageing population. *PLoS Genetics, 8*(4), e1002629. https://doi.org/10.1371/journal.pgen.1002629.
8. Bell, M. L., Dominici, F., Ebisu, K., Zeger, S. L., & Samet, J. M. (2007). Spatial and temporal variation in PM(2.5) chemical composition in the United States for health effects studies. *Environmental Health Perspectives, 115*(7), 989–995. https://doi.org/10.1289/ehp.9621.
9. Belsky, D. W., Caspi, A., Arseneault, L., Baccarelli, A., Corcoran, D. L., Gao, X., Hannon, E., Harrington, H. L., Rasmussen, L. J., & Houts, R., et al. (2020). Quantification of the pace of biological aging in humans through a blood test, the DunedinPoAm DNA methylation algorithm. *eLife, 9*, e54870. https://doi.org/10.7554/eLife.54870.
10. Belsky, D. W., Caspi, A., Corcoran, D. L., Sugden, K., Poulton, R., Arseneault, L., Baccarelli, A., Chamarti, K., Gao, X., & Hannon, E., et al. (2022). DunedinPACE, a DNA methylation biomarker of the pace of aging. *eLife, 11*, e73420. https://doi.org/10.7554/eLife.73420.
11. Bocklandt, S., Lin, W., Sehl, M. E., Sanchez, F. J., Sinsheimer, J. S., Horvath, S., & Vilain, E. (2011). Epigenetic predictor of age. *PLoS ONE, 6*(6), e14821. https://doi.org/10.1371/journal.pone.0014821.
12. Bogdan, A. R., Miyazawa, M., Hashimoto, K., & Tsuji, Y. (2016). Regulators of iron homeostasis: New players in metabolism, cell death, and disease. *Trends in Biochemical Sciences, 41*(3), 274–286. https://doi.org/10.1016/j.tibs.2015.11.012.

13. Bohlin, J., Haberg, S. E., Magnus, P., Reese, S. E., Gjessing, H. K., Magnus, M. C., Parr, C. L., Page, C. M., London, S. J., & Nystad, W. (2016). Prediction of gestational age based on genome-wide differentially methylated regions. *Genome Biology, 17*, 207. https://doi.org/10.1186/s13059-016-1063-0.

14. Borkan, G. A., & Norris, A. H. (1980). Assessment of biological age using a profile of physical parameters. *Journal of Gerontology, 35*(2), 177–184. https://doi.org/10.1093/geronj/35.2.177.

15. Boyer, K., Domingo-Relloso, A., Jiang, E., Haack, K., Goessler, W., Zhang, Y., Umans, J. G., Belsky, D. W., Cole, S. A., & Navas-Acien, A., et al. (2023). Metal mixtures and DNA methylation measures of biological aging in American Indian populations. *Environment International, 178*, 108064. https://doi.org/10.1016/j.envint.2023.108064.

16. Butler, R. N., Sprott, R., Warner, H., Bland, J., Feuers, R., Forster, M., Fillit, H., Harman, S. M., Hewitt, M., & Hyman, M., et al. (2004). Biomarkers of aging: From primitive organisms to humans. *The Journals of Gerontology: Series A, 59*(6), B560–B567. https://doi.org/10.1093/gerona/59.6.B560.

17. Cantone, L., Tobaldini, E., Favero, C., Albetti, B., Sacco, R. M., Torgano, G., Ferrari, L., Montano, N., & Bollati, V. (2020). Particulate air pollution, clock gene methylation, and stroke: Effects on stroke severity and disability. *International Journal of Molecular Sciences, 21*(9), 3090. https://doi.org/10.3390/ijms21093090.

18. Caulton, A., Dodds, K. G., McRae, K. M., Couldrey, C., Horvath, S., & Clarke, S. M. (2021). Development of epigenetic clocks for key ruminant species. *Genes, 13*(1), 96. https://doi.org/10.3390/genes13010096.

19. Chen, B. H., Marioni, R. E., Colicino, E., Peters, M. J., Ward-Caviness, C. K., Tsai, P. C., Roetker, N. S., Just, A. C., Demerath, E. W., & Guan, W., et al. (2016). DNA methylation-based measures of biological age: Meta-analysis predicting time to death. *Aging, 8*(9), 1844–1865. https://doi.org/10.18632/aging.101020.

20. Chen, M., Fu, Y., Wang, X., Wu, R., Su, D., Zhou, N., & Qi, Y. (2022). Metformin protects lens epithelial cells against senescence in a naturally aged mouse model. *Cell Death Discovery, 8*, 8. https://doi.org/10.1038/s41420-022-00934-0.

21. Chen, M., Wong, E. M., Nguyen, T. L., Dite, G. S., Stone, J., Dugue, P. A., Giles, G. G., Southey, M. C., Milne, R. L., Hopper, J. L., et al. (2019). DNA methylation-based biological age, genome-wide average DNA methylation, and conventional breast cancer risk factors. *Scientific Reports, 9*, 15055. https://doi.org/10.1038/s41598-019-51369-0.

22. Chen, Q., Thompson, J., Hu, Y., & Lesnefsky, E. J. (2021). Chronic metformin treatment decreases cardiac injury during ischemia-reperfusion by attenuating endoplasmic reticulum stress with improved mitochondrial function. *Aging, 13*(6), 7828–7845. https://doi.org/10.18632/aging.202875.

23. Christensen, B. C., Houseman, E. A., Marsit, C. J., Zheng, S., Wrensch, M. R., Wiemels, J. L., Nelson, H. H., Karagas, M. R., Padbury, J. F., Bueno, R., et al. (2009). Aging and environmental exposures alter tissue-specific DNA methylation dependent upon CpG island context. *PLoS Genetics, 5*(8), e1000602. https://doi.org/10.1371/journal.pgen.1000602.

24. Clark, J., Bulka, C. M., Martin, C. L., Roell, K., Santos, H. P., O'Shea, T. M., Smeester, L., Fry, R., & Dhingra, R. (2022). Placental epigenetic gestational aging in relation to maternal sociodemographic factors and smoking among infants born extremely preterm: A descriptive

study. *Epigenetics, 17*(24), 2389–2403. https://doi.org/10.1080/15592294.2022.2108796.

25. Dammering, F., Martins, J., Dittrich, K., Czamara, D., Rex-Haffner, M., Overfeld, J., de Punder, K., Buss, C., Entringer, S., Winter, S. M., et al. (2021). The pediatric buccal epigenetic clock identifies significant aging acceleration in children with internalizing disorder and maltreatment exposure. *Neurobiology of Stress, 15*, 100394. https://doi.org/10.1016/j.ynstr.2021.100394.
26. Danial, C., Sarin, K. Y., Oro, A. E., & Chang, A. L. (2016). An investigator-initiated open-label trial of sonidegib in advanced basal cell carcinoma patients resistant to vismodegib. *Clinical Cancer Research, 22*(6), 1325–1329. https://doi.org/10.1158/1078-0432.CCR-15-1856.
27. Darrow, S. M., Verhoeven, J. E., Revesz, D., Lindqvist, D., Penninx, B. W., Delucchi, K. L., Wolkowitz, O. M., & Mathews, C. A. (2016). The association between psychiatric disorders and telomere length: A meta-analysis involving 14,827 persons. *Psychosomatic Medicine, 78*(7), 776–787. https://doi.org/10.1097/PSY.0000000000000356.
28. Dato, S., Bellizzi, D., Rose, G., & Passarino, G. (2016). The impact of nutrients on the aging rate: A complex interaction of demographic, environmental and genetic factors. *Mechanisms of Ageing and Development, 154*, 49–61. https://doi.org/10.1016/j.mad.2016.02.005.
29. Davinelli, S., Trichopoulou, A., Corbi, G., De Vivo, I., & Scapagnini, G. (2019). The potential nutrigeroprotective role of Mediterranean diet and its functional components on telomere length dynamics. *Ageing Research Reviews, 49*, 1–10. https://doi.org/10.1016/j.arr.2018.11.003.
30. De Magalhaes, J. P., Curado, J., & Church, G. M. (2009). Meta-analysis of age-related gene expression profiles identifies common signatures of aging. *Bioinformatics, 25*(7), 875–881. https://doi.org/10.1093/bioinformatics/btp073.
31. De Prado-Bert, P., Ruiz-Arenas, C., Vives-Usano, M., Andrusaityte, S., Cadiou, S., Carracedo, A., Casas, M., Chatzi, L., Dadvand, P., & Gonzalez, J. R., et al. (2021). The early-life exposome and epigenetic age acceleration in children. *Environment International, 155*, 106683. https://doi.org/10.1016/j.envint.2021.106683.
32. Dugue, P. A., Bassett, J. K., Joo, J. E., Baglietto, L., Jung, C. H., Wong, E. M., Fiorito, G., Schmidt, D., Makalic, E., & Li, S., et al. (2018). Association of DNA methylation-based biological age with health risk factors and overall and cause-specific mortality. *American Journal of Epidemiology, 187*(3), 529–538. https://doi.org/10.1093/aje/kwx291.
33. Dupras, C., Beck, S., Rothstein, M. A., Berner, A., Saulnier, K. M., Pinkesz, M., Prince, A. E. R., Liosi, S., Song, L., & Joly, Y. (2019). Potential (mis)use of epigenetic age estimators by private companies and public agencies: Human rights law should provide ethical guidance. *Environmental Epigenetics, 5*(3), dvz018. https://doi.org/10.1093/eep/dvz018.
34. Dutta, S., Haggerty, D. K., Rappolee, D. A., & Ruden, D. M. (2020). Phthalate exposure and long-term epigenomic consequences: A review. *Frontiers in Genetics, 11*, 405. https://doi.org/10.3389/fgene.2020.00405.
35. Epel, E. S., Blackburn, E. H., Lin, J., Dhabhar, F. S., Adler, N. E., Morrow, J. D., & Cawthon, R. M. (2004). Accelerated telomere shortening in response to life stress. *Proceedings of the National Academy of Sciences, 101*(49), 17312–17315. https://doi.org/10.1073/pnas.0407162101.
36. Evich, M. G., Davis, M. J. B., McCord, J. P., Acrey, B., Awkerman, J. A., Knappe, D. R. U., Lindstrom, A. B., Speth, T. F., Tebes-Stevens, C., & Strynar, M. J., et al. (2022). Per- and polyfluoroalkyl substances in the environment. *Science, 375*(6577), eabg9065. https://doi.org/10.1126/science.abg9065.

37. Fang, F., Zhou, L., Perng, W., Marsit, C. J., Knight, A. K., Cardenas, A., Aung, M. T., Hivert, M. F., Aris, I. M., & Goodrich, J. M., et al. (2023). Evaluation of pediatric epigenetic clocks across multiple tissues. *Clinical Epigenetics, 15*(1), 142. https://doi.org/10.1186/s13148-023-01583-4.

38. Field, A. E., Robertson, N. A., Wang, T., Havas, A., Ideker, T., & Adams, P. D. (2018). DNA methylation clocks in aging: Categories, causes, and consequences. *Molecular Cell, 71*(6), 882–895. https://doi.org/10.1016/j.molcel.2018.08.008.

39. Fiorito, G., Caini, S., Palli, D., Bendinelli, B., Saieva, C., Ermini, I., Valentini, V., Assedi, M., Rizzolo, P., & Ambrogetti, D., et al. (2021). DNA methylation-based biomarkers of aging were slowed down in a two-year diet and physical activity intervention trial: The DAMA study. *Aging Cell, 20*(10), e13439. https://doi.org/10.1111/acel.13439.

40. Fleischer, J. G., Schulte, R., Tsai, H. H., Tyagi, S., Ibarra, A., Shokhirev, M. N., Huang, L., Hetzer, M. W., & Navlakha, S. (2018). Predicting age from the transcriptome of human dermal fibroblasts. *Genome Biology, 19*, 221. https://doi.org/10.1186/s13059-018-1599-6.

41. Florath, I., Butterbach, K., Muller, H., Bewerunge-Hudler, M., & Brenner, H. (2014). Cross-sectional and longitudinal changes in DNA methylation with age: An epigenome-wide analysis revealing over 60 novel age-associated CpG sites. *Human Molecular Genetics, 23*(5), 1186–1201. https://doi.org/10.1093/hmg/ddt531.

42. Fox, B. C., Mobley, H. L., & Wade, J. C. (1989). The use of a DNA probe for epidemiological studies of candidiasis in immunocompromised hosts. *Journal of Infectious Diseases, 159*(3), 488–494. https://doi.org/10.1093/infdis/159.3.488.

43. Franzago, M., Pilenzi, L., Di Rado, S., Vitacolonna, E., & Stuppia, L. (2022). The epigenetic aging, obesity, and lifestyle. *Frontiers in Cell and Developmental Biology, 10*, 985274. https://doi.org/10.3389/fcell.2022.985274.

44. Fraszczyk, E., Luijten, M., Spijkerman, A. M. W., Snieder, H., Wackers, P. F. K., Bloks, V. W., Nicoletti, C. F., Nonino, C. B., Crujeiras, A. B., & Buurman, W. A., et al. (2020). The effects of bariatric surgery on clinical profile, DNA methylation, and ageing in severely obese patients. *Clinical Epigenetics, 12*, 14. https://doi.org/10.1186/s13148-020-0808-x.

45. Fries, G. R., Bauer, I. E., Scaini, G., Wu, M. J., Kazimi, I. F., Valvassori, S. S., Zunta-Soares, G., Walss-Bass, C., Soares, J. C., & Quevedo, J. (2017). Accelerated epigenetic aging and mitochondrial DNA copy number in bipolar disorder. *Translational Psychiatry, 7*, 1283. https://doi.org/10.1038/s41398-017-0048-8.

46. Galkin, F., Kovalchuk, O., Koldasbayeva, D., Zhavoronkov, A., & Bischof, E. (2023). Stress; diet, exercise: Common environmental factors and their impact on epigenetic age. *Ageing Research Reviews, 88*, 101956. https://doi.org/10.1016/j.arr.2023.101956.

47. Galvez-Fernandez, M., Powers, M., Grau-Perez, M., Domingo-Relloso, A., Lolacono, N., Goessler, W., Zhang, Y., Fretts, A., Umans, J. G., & Maruthur, N., et al. (2022). Urinary Zinc and Incident Type 2 Diabetes: Prospective Evidence from the Strong Heart Study. *Diabetes Care, 45*(11), 2561–2569. https://doi.org/10.2337/dc22-0664.

48. Garagnani, P., Bacalini, M. G., Pirazzini, C., Gori, D., Giuliani, C., Mari, D., Di Blasio, A. M., Gentilini, D., Vitale, G., & Collino, S., et al. (2012). Methylation of ELOVL2 gene as a new epigenetic marker of age. *Aging Cell, 11*(6), 1132–1134. https://doi.org/10.1111/acel.12005.

49. Garcia, D. N., Saccon, T. D., Pradiee, J., Rincon, J. A. A., Andrade, K. R. S., Rovani, M. T., Mondadori, R. G., Cruz, L. A. X., Barros, C. C., & Masternak, M. M., et al. (2019). Effect of caloric restriction and rapamycin on ovarian aging in mice. *Geroscience, 41*(4), 395–408. https://doi.org/10.1007/s11357-019-00074-3.

50. Gensous, N., Garagnani, P., Santoro, A., Giuliani, C., Ostan, R., Fabbri, C., Milazzo, M., Gentilini, D., Di Blasio, A. M., & Pietruszka, B., et al. (2020). One-year Mediterranean diet promotes epigenetic rejuvenation with country- and sex-specific effects: A pilot study from the NU-AGE project. *Geroscience, 42*(3), 687–701. https://doi.org/10.1007/s11357-020-00184-0.

51. Glass, D., Vinuela, A., Davies, M. N., Ramasamy, A., Parts, L., Knowles, D., Brown, A. A., Hedman, A. K., Small, K. S., & Buil, A., et al. (2013). Gene expression changes with age in skin, adipose tissue, blood and brain. *Genome Biology, 14*(7), R75. https://doi.org/10.1186/gb-2013-14-7-r75.

52. Goodrich, J. M., Calkins, M. M., Caban-Martinez, A. J., Stueckle, T., Grant, C., Calafat, A. M., Nematollahi, A., Jung, A. M., Graber, J. M., & Jenkins, T., et al. (2021). Per- and polyfluoroalkyl substances, epigenetic age and DNA methylation: A cross-sectional study of firefighters. *Epigenomics, 13*(20), 1619–1636. https://doi.org/10.2217/epi-2021-0180.

53. Gravina, S., Dong, X., Yu, B., & Vijg, J. (2016). Single-cell genome-wide bisulfite sequencing uncovers extensive heterogeneity in the mouse liver methylome. *Genome Biology, 17*, 150. https://doi.org/10.1186/s13059-016-1005-1.

54. Graw, S., Camerota, M., Carter, B. S., Helderman, J., Hofheimer, J. A., McGowan, E. C., Neal, C. R., Pastyrnak, S. L., Smith, L. M., & DellaGrotta, S. A., et al. (2021). NEOage clocks—Epigenetic clocks to estimate post-menstrual and postnatal age in preterm infants. *Aging, 13*(19), 23527–23544. https://doi.org/10.18632/aging.203744.

55. GTEx Consortium, The Genotype-Tissue Expression (GTEx) project. (2013). *Nature Genetics, 45*(6), 580–585. https://doi.org/10.1038/ng.2653.

56. Guo, Y., Li, D., & Hu, Y. (2023). Appraising the Associations Between Systemic Iron Status and Epigenetic Clocks: A Genetic Correlation and Bidirectional Mendelian Randomization Study. *American Journal of Clinical Nutrition, 118*(1), 41–49. https://doi.org/10.1093/ajcn/nqad005.

57. Haftorn, K. L., Lee, Y., Denault, W. R. P., Page, C. M., Nustad, H. E., Lyle, R., Gjessing, H. K., Malmberg, A., Magnus, M. C., & Naess, O., et al. (2021). An EPIC predictor of gestational age and its application to newborns conceived by assisted reproductive technologies. *Clinical Epigenetics, 13*, 82. https://doi.org/10.1186/s13148-021-01073-9.

58. Hamlat, E. J., Prather, A. A., Horvath, S., Belsky, J., & Epel, E. S. (2021). Early life adversity; pubertal timing, and epigenetic age acceleration in adulthood. *Developmental Psychobiology, 63*(6), 890–902. https://doi.org/10.1002/dev.22185.

59. Han, Q., Gao, X., Wang, S., Wei, Z., Wang, Y., Xu, K., & Chen, M. (2023). Co-exposure to polystyrene microplastics and di-(2-ethylhexyl) phthalate aggravates allergic asthma through the TRPA1-p38 MAPK pathway. *Toxicology Letters, 384*, 73–85. https://doi.org/10.1016/j.toxlet.2023.02.012.

60. Hannum, G., Guinney, J., Zhao, L., Zhang, L., Hughes, G., Sadda, S., Klotzle, B., Bibikova, M., Fan, J. B., Gao, Y., et al. (2013). Genome-wide methylation profiles reveal quantitative views of human aging rates. Molecular Cell, 49(2), 359–367.

61. Hansen, J., Meretzky, D., Woldesenbet, S., Stolovitzky, G., & Iyengar, R. (2017). A flexible ontology for inference of emergent whole cell function from relationships between subcellular processes. Scientific Reports, 7, 17689.

62. Harper, S. (2014). Economic and social implications of aging societies. Science, 346(6209), 587–591.

63. Harvanek, Z. M., Fogelman, N., Xu, K., & Sinha, R. (2021). Psychological and biological resilience modulates the effects of stress on epigenetic aging. Translational Psychiatry, 11(1), 601.

64. Heiss, C., Spyridopoulos, I., & Haendeler, J. (2018). Interventions to slow cardiovascular aging: Dietary restriction, drugs and novel molecules. Experimental Gerontology, 109, 108–118.

65. Hershey, H. P., Barker, R. F., Idler, K. B., Murray, M. G., & Quail, P. H. (1987). Nucleotide sequence and characterization of a gene encoding the phytochrome polypeptide from Avena. Gene, 61(3), 339–348.

66. Horvath, S. (2013). DNA methylation age of human tissues and cell types. *Genome Biology, 14*, R115. https://doi.org/10.1186/gb-2013-14-10-r115.

67. Horvath, S., & Raj, K. (2018). DNA methylation-based biomarkers and the epigenetic clock theory of ageing. *Nature Reviews Genetics, 19*(6), 371–384.

68. Horvath, S., Haghani, A., Macoretta, N., Ablaeva, J., Zoller, J. A., Li, C. Z., Zhang, J., Takasugi, M., Zhao, Y., Rydkina, E., et al. (2022). DNA methylation clocks tick in naked mole rats but queens age more slowly than nonbreeders. *Nature Aging, 2*(1), 46–59.

69. Horvath, S., Haghani, A., Peng, S., Hales, E. N., Zoller, J. A., Raj, K., & Bellone, R. R. (2022). DNA methylation aging and transcriptomic studies in horses. *Nature Communications, 13*, 40.

70. Horvath, S., Haghani, A., Zoller, J. A., Raj, K., Sinha, I., Robeck, T. R., & Manoyan, M. (2022). Epigenetic clock and methylation studies in marsupials: Opossums, Tasmanian devils, kangaroos, and wallabies. *Geroscience, 44*, 1825–1845.

71. Horvath, S., Mah, V., Lu, A. T., Woo, J. S., Choi, O. W., Jasinska, A. J., & Braun, J. (2015). The cerebellum ages slowly according to the epigenetic clock. *Aging, 7*(5), 294–306.

72. Ignjatovic, V., Lai, C., Summerhayes, R., Mathesius, U., Tawfilis, S., Perugini, M. A., & Monagle, P. (2011). Age-related differences in plasma proteins: How plasma proteins change from neonates to adults. *PLoS ONE, 6*(2), e17213.

73. Jenkins, T. G., Aston, K. I., Cairns, B., Smith, A., & Carrell, D. T. (2018). Paternal germline aging: DNA methylation age prediction from human sperm. *BMC Genomics, 19*, 763.

74. Ji, X., Zhang, Y., Li, G., & Sang, N. (2018). Potential Role of Inflammation in Associations between Particulate Matter and Heart Failure. *Current Pharmaceutical Design, 24*(3), 341–358.

75. Johansson, A., Enroth, S., & Gyllensten, U. (2013). Continuous aging of the human DNA methylome throughout the human lifespan. *PLoS ONE, 8*(6), e67378.

76. Johnson, A. A., Akman, K., Calimport, S. R., Wuttke, D., Stolzing, A., & de Magalhaes, J. P. (2012). The role of DNA methylation in aging, rejuvenation, and age-related disease. *Rejuvenation Research, 15*(5), 483–494.

77. Johnson, T. E. (2006). Recent results: Biomarkers of aging. *Experimental Gerontology, 41*(12), 1243–1246.

78. Jones, M. J., Goodman, S. J., & Kobor, M. S. (2015). DNA methylation and healthy human aging. *Aging Cell, 14*(6), 924–932.

79. Jung, S. E., Shin, K. J., & Lee, H. Y. (2017). DNA methylation-based age prediction from various tissues and body fluids. *BMB Reports, 50*, 546–553.

80. Jung, S., Hodar, J. A., & Del Sol, A. (2023). Measuring biological age using a functionally interpretable multi-tissue RNA clock. *Aging Cell, 22*(5), e13799.

81. Jylhävä, J., Pedersen, N. L., & Hägg, S. (2017). Biological age predictors. *EBioMedicine, 21*, 29–36.

82. Katrinli, S., Smith, A. K., Drury, S. S., Covault, J., Ford, J. D., Singh, V., Reese, B., Johnson, A., Scranton, V., Fall, P., et al. (2023). Cumulative stress, PTSD, and emotion dysregulation during pregnancy and epigenetic age acceleration in Hispanic mothers and their newborn infants. *Epigenetics, 18*, 2231722.

83. Kawakami, Y., Hambright, W. S., Takayama, K., Mu, X., Lu, A., Cummins, J. H., Matsumoto, T., Yurube, T., Kuroda, R., Kurosaka, M., et al. (2019). Rapamycin rescues age-related changes in muscle-derived stem/progenitor cells from progeroid mice. *Molecular Therapy - Methods & Clinical Development, 14*, 64–76.

84. Khan, S. S., Singer, B. D., & Vaughan, D. E. (2017). Molecular and physiological manifestations and measurement of aging in humans. *Aging Cell, 16*, 624–633.

85. Khodasevich, D., Holland, N., Hubbard, A., Harley, K., Deardorff, J., Eskenazi, B., & Cardenas, A. (2023). Associations between prenatal phthalate exposure and childhood epigenetic age acceleration. *Environmental Research, 231*, 116067.

86. Kiecolt-Glaser, J. K., Wilson, S. J., & Disorders, P. (2016). Morbidity and mortality: Tracing mechanistic pathways to accelerated aging. *Psychosomatic Medicine, 78*, 772–775.

87. Knight, A. K., Craig, J. M., Theda, C., Baekvad-Hansen, M., Bybjerg-Grauholm, J., Hansen, C. S., Hollegaard, M. V., Hougaard, D. M., Mortensen, P. B., Weinsheimer, S. M., et al. (2016). An epigenetic clock for gestational age at birth based on blood methylation data. *Genome Biology, 17*, 206.

88. Koen, N., Jones, M. J., Nhapi, R. T., Lake, M. T., Donald, K. A., Barnett, W., Hoffman, N., MacIsaac, J. L., Morin, A. M., Lin, D. T. S., et al. (2021). Maternal psychosocial risk factors and child gestational epigenetic age in a South African birth cohort study. *Translational Psychiatry, 11*, 358.

89. Lee, Y., Choufani, S., Weksberg, R., Wilson, S. L., Yuan, V., Burt, A., Marsit, C., Lu, A. T., Ritz, B., Bohlin, J., et al. (2019). Placental epigenetic clocks: Estimating gestational age using placental DNA methylation levels. *Aging, 11*, 4238–4253.

90. Levine, M. E., Lu, A. T., Quach, A., Chen, B. H., Assimes, T. L., Bandinelli, S., Hou, L., Baccarelli, A. A., Stewart, J. D., Li, Y., et al. (2018). An epigenetic biomarker of aging for lifespan and healthspan. *Aging, 10*, 573–591.

91. Liu, Y., Eliot, M. N., Papandonatos, G. D., Kelsey, K. T., Fore, R., Langevin, S., Buckley, J., Chen, A., Lanphear, B. P., Cecil, K. M., et al. (2022). Gestational perfluoroalkyl substance exposure and DNA methylation at birth and 12 years of age: A longitudinal epigenome-wide association study. *Environmental Health Perspectives, 130*, 37005.

92. Lodge, E. K., Dhingra, R., Martin, C. L., Fry, R. C., White, A. J., Ward-Caviness, C. K., Wani, A. H., Uddin, M., Wildman, D. E., Galea, S., et al. (2022). Serum lead, mercury, manganese, and copper and DNA methylation age among adults in Detroit, Michigan. *Environmental Epigenetics, 8*, dvac018.

93. Lu, A. T., Fei, Z., Haghani, A., Robeck, T. R., Zoller, J. A., Li, C. Z., Lowe, R., Yan, Q., Zhang, J., Vu, H., et al. (2023). Universal DNA methylation age across mammalian tissues. *Nature Aging, 3*, 1144–1166.

94. Lu, A. T., Quach, A., Wilson, J. G., Reiner, A. P., Aviv, A., Raj, K., Hou, L., Baccarelli, A. A., Li, Y., Stewart, J. D., et al. (2019). DNA methylation GrimAge strongly predicts lifespan and healthspan. *Aging, 11*, 303–327.

95. Lu, T., Pan, Y., Kao, S. Y., Li, C., Kohane, I., Chan, J., & Yankner, B. A. (2004). Gene regulation and DNA damage in the ageing human brain. *Nature, 429*, 883–891.

96. Mangan, D. (2021). Iron: An underrated factor in aging. *Aging, 13*, 23407–23415.

97. Marioni, R. E., Shah, S., McRae, A. F., Chen, B. H., Colicino, E., Harris, S. E., Gibson, J., Henders, A. K., Redmond, P., Cox, S. R., et al. (2015). DNA methylation age of blood predicts all-cause mortality in later life. *Genome Biology, 16*, 25.

98. Marioni, R. E., Shah, S., McRae, A. F., Ritchie, S. J., Muniz-Terrera, G., Harris, S. E., Gibson, J., Redmond, P., Cox, S. R., Pattie, A., et al. (2015). The epigenetic clock is correlated with physical and cognitive fitness in the Lothian Birth Cohort 1936. *International Journal of Epidemiology, 44*, 1388–1396.

99. Martucci, M., Ostan, R., Biondi, F., Bellavista, E., Fabbri, C., Bertarelli, C., Salvioli, S., Capri, M., Franceschi, C., & Santoro, A. (2017). Mediterranean diet and inflammaging within the hormesis paradigm. *Nutrition Reviews, 75*, 442–455.

100. Masaldan, S., Clatworthy, S. A. S., Gamell, C., Meggyesy, P. M., Rigopoulos, A. T., Haupt, S., Haupt, Y., Denoyer, D., Adlard, P. A., Bush, A. I., et al. (2018). Iron accumulation in senescent cells is coupled with impaired ferritinophagy and inhibition of ferroptosis. *Redox Biology, 14*, 100–115.

101. Mayne, B. T., Leemaqz, S. Y., Smith, A. K., Breen, J., Roberts, C. T., & Bianco-Miotto, T. (2017). Accelerated placental aging in early onset preeclampsia pregnancies identified by DNA methylation. *Epigenomics, 9*, 279–289.

102. McEwen, L. M., O'Donnell, K. J., McGill, M. G., Edgar, R. D., Jones, M. J., MacIsaac, J. L., Lin, D. T. S., Ramadori, K., Morin, A., Gladish, N., et al. (2020). The PedBE clock accurately estimates DNA methylation age in pediatric buccal cells. *Proceedings of the National Academy of Sciences of the United States of America, 117*, 23329–23335.

103. McGill, M. G., Pokhvisneva, I., Clappison, A. S., McEwen, L. M., Beijers, R., Tollenaar, M. S., Pham, H., Kee, M. Z. L., Garg, E., de Mendonca Filho, E. J., et al. (2022). Maternal prenatal anxiety and the fetal origins of epigenetic aging. *Biological Psychiatry, 91*, 303–312.

104. Mehta, D., Bruenig, D., Pierce, J., Sathyanarayanan, A., Stringfellow, R., Miller, O., Mullens, A. B., & Shakespeare-Finch, J. (2022). Recalibrating the epigenetic clock after exposure to trauma: The role of risk and protective psychosocial factors. *Journal of Psychiatric Research, 149*, 374–381.

105. Miller, M. W., & Sadeh, N. (2014). Traumatic stress, oxidative stress and post-traumatic stress disorder: Neurodegeneration and the accelerated-aging hypothesis. *Molecular Psychiatry, 19*, 1156–1162.

106. Mitnitski, A., Collerton, J., Martin-Ruiz, C., Jagger, C., von Zglinicki, T., Rockwood, K., & Kirkwood, T. B. (2015). Age-related frailty and its association with biological markers of ageing. *BMC Medicine, 13*, 161.

107. Moher, D., Shamseer, L., Clarke, M., Ghersi, D., Liberati, A., Petticrew, M., Shekelle, P., & Stewart, L. A.; Group, P. -P. (2015). Preferred reporting items for systematic review and meta-analysis protocols (PRISMA-P) 2015 statement. *Systematic Reviews, 4*, 1.

108. Monasso, G. S., Kupers, L. K., Jaddoe, V. W. V., Heil, S. G., & Felix, J. F. (2021). Associations of circulating folate, vitamin B12 and homocysteine concentrations in early pregnancy and cord blood with epigenetic gestational age: The Generation R Study. *Clinical Epigenetics, 13*, 95.

109. Nawrot, T. S., Saenen, N. D., Schenk, J., Janssen, B. G., Motta, V., Tarantini, L., Cox, B., Lefebvre, W., Vanpoucke, C., Maggioni, C., et al. (2018). Placental circadian pathway methylation and in utero exposure to fine particle air pollution. *Environment International, 114*, 231–241.

110. Nwanaji-Enwerem, J. C., Dai, L., Colicino, E., Oulhote, Y., Di, Q., Kloog, I., Just, A. C., Hou, L., Vokonas, P., Baccarelli, A. A., et al. (2017). Associations between long-term exposure to PM(2.5) component species and blood DNA methylation age in the elderly: The VA normative aging study. *Environment International, 102*, 57–65.

111. Oblak, L., van der Zaag, J., Higgins-Chen, A. T., Levine, M. E., & Boks, M. P. (2021). A systematic review of biological, social and environmental factors associated with epigenetic clock acceleration. *Ageing Research Reviews, 69*, 101348.

112. Oluwayiose, O. A., Houle, E., Wu, H., Whitcomb, B. W., Mumford, S. L., Schisterman, E. F., Suvorov, A., Balzer, L. B., & Pilsner, J. R. (2022). Urinary phthalate metabolites and their mixtures are associated with advanced sperm epigenetic aging in a general population. *Environmental Research, 214*, 114115.

113. Oluwayiose, O. A., Wu, H., Saddiki, H., Whitcomb, B. W., Balzer, L. B., Brandon, N., Suvorov, A., Tayyab, R., Sites, C. K., Hill, L., et al. (2021). Sperm DNA methylation mediates the association of male age on reproductive outcomes among couples undergoing infertility treatment. *Scientific Reports, 11*, 3216.

114. Pang, Y., Peng, R. D., Jones, M. R., Francesconi, K. A., Goessler, W., Howard, B. V., Umans, J. G., Best, L. G., Guallar, E., Post, W. S., et al. (2016). Metal mixtures in urban and rural populations in the US: The Multi-Ethnic Study of Atherosclerosis and the Strong Heart Study. *Environment Research, 147*, 356–364.

115. Perez, R. F., Tejedor, J. R., Fernandez, A. F., & Fraga, M. F. (2022). Aging and cancer epigenetics: Where do the paths fork? *Aging Cell, 21*, e13709.

116. Peters, M. J., Joehanes, R., Pilling, L. C., Schurmann, C., Conneely, K. N., Powell, J., Reinmaa, E., Sutphin, G. L., Zhernakova, A., Schramm, K., et al. (2015). The transcriptional landscape of age in human peripheral blood. *Nature Communications, 6*, 8570.

117. Pilsner, J. R., Saddiki, H., Whitcomb, B. W., Suvorov, A., Louis, G. M. B., Mumford, S. L., Schisterman, E. F., Oluwayiose, O. A., & Balzer, L. B. (2022). Sperm epigenetic clock associates with pregnancy outcomes in the general population. *Human Reproduction, 37*(6), 1581–1593.

118. Pi-Sunyer, X. (2009). The medical risks of obesity. *Postgraduate Medicine, 121*(6), 21–33.

119. Poganik, J. R., Zhang, B., Baht, G. S., Tyshkovskiy, A., Deik, A., Kerepesi, C., Yim, S. H., Lu, A. T., Haghani, A., Gong, T., et al. (2023). Biological age is increased by stress and restored upon recovery. *Cell Metabolism, 35*(5), 807–820.e5.

120. Prado, N. A., Brown, J. L., Zoller, J. A., Haghani, A., Yao, M., Bagryanova, L. R., Campana, M. G., Maldonado, J. E., Raj, K., Schmitt, D., et al. (2021). Epigenetic clock and methylation studies in elephants. *Aging Cell, 20*(1), e13414.

121. Protsenko, E., Wolkowitz, O. M., & Yaffe, K. (2023). Associations of stress and stress-related psychiatric disorders with GrimAge acceleration: Review and suggestions for future work. *Translational Psychiatry, 13*(1), 142.

122. Quarles, E., Basisty, N., Chiao, Y. A., Merrihew, G., Gu, H., Sweetwyne, M. T., Fredrickson, J., Nguyen, N. H., Razumova, M., Kooiker, K., et al. (2020). Rapamycin persistently improves cardiac function in aged, male and female mice, even following cessation of treatment. *Aging Cell, 19*(8), e13086.

123. Quinn, E. B., Hsiao, C. J., Maisha, F. M., & Mulligan, C. J. (2023). Prenatal maternal stress is associated with site-specific and age acceleration changes in maternal and newborn DNA methylation. *Epigenetics, 18*(4), 2222473.

124. Rae, M. J., Butler, R. N., Campisi, J., de Grey, A. D., Finch, C. E., Gough, M., Martin, G. M., Vijg, J., Perrott, K. M., & Logan, B. J. (2010). The demographic and biomedical case for late-life interventions in aging. *Science Translational Medicine, 2*(40), 40cm21.

125. Raj, K., Szladovits, B., Haghani, A., Zoller, J. A., Li, C. Z., Black, P., Maddox, D., Robeck, T. R., & Horvath, S. (2021). Epigenetic clock and methylation studies in cats. *Geroscience, 43*(6), 2363–2378.

126. Rakyan, V. K., Down, T. A., Maslau, S., Andrew, T., Yang, T. P., Beyan, H., Whittaker, P., McCann, O. T., Finer, S., Valdes, A. M., et al. (2010). Human aging-associated DNA hypermethylation occurs preferentially at bivalent chromatin domains. *Genome Research, 20*(4), 434–439.

127. Ravindrarajah, R., Lee, D. M., Pye, S. R., Gielen, E., Boonen, S., Vanderschueren, D., Pendleton, N., Finn, J. D., Tajar, A., O'Connell, M. D., et al. (2013). European Male Aging Study, the ability of three different models of frailty to predict all-cause mortality: Results from the European Male Aging Study (EMAS). *Archives of Gerontology and Geriatrics, 57*(3), 360–368.

128. Ren, X., & Kuan, P. F. (2020). RNAAgeCalc: A multi-tissue transcriptional age calculator. *PLoS ONE, 15*(7), e0237006.

129. Ridker, P. M., Buring, J. E., Cook, N. R., & Rifai, N. (2003). C-reactive protein, the metabolic syndrome, and risk of incident cardiovascular events: An 8-year follow-up of 14,719 initially healthy American women. *Circulation, 107*(3), 391–397.

130. Rodwell, G. E., Sonu, R., Zahn, J. M., Lund, J., Wilhelmy, J., Wang, L., Xiao, W., Mindrinos, M., Crane, E., Segal, E., et al. (2004). A transcriptional profile of aging in the human kidney. *PLoS Biology, 2*(12), e427.

131. Sae-Lee, C., Corsi, S., Barrow, T. M., Kuhnle, G. G. C., Bollati, V., Mathers, J. C., & Byun, H. M. (2018). Dietary Intervention Modifies DNA Methylation Age Assessed by the Epigenetic Clock. *Molecular Nutrition & Food Research, 62*(8), e1800092.

132. Safaee, M. M., Dwaraka, V. B., Lee, J. M., Fury, M., Mendez, T. L., Smith, R., Lin, J., Smith, D. L., Burke, J. F., Scheer, J. K., et al. (2023). Epigenetic age biomarkers and risk assessment in adult spinal deformity: A novel association of biological age with frailty and disability. *Journal of Neurosurgery: Spine, 38*(1), 1–12.

133. Schachtschneider, K. M., Schook, L. B., Meudt, J. J., Shanmuganayagam, D., Zoller, J. A., Haghani, A., Li, C. Z., Zhang, J., Yang, A., & Raj, K., et al. (2021). Epigenetic clock and DNA methylation analysis of porcine models of aging and obesity. *Geroscience, 43*(6), 2467–2483.

134. Schulz, K., Silva, M. R., & Klaper, R. (2020). Distribution and effects of branched versus linear isomers of PFOA, PFOS, and PFHxS: A review of recent literature. *Science of the Total Environment, 733*, 139186.

135. Searle, S. D., Mitnitski, A., Gahbauer, E. A., Gill, T. M., & Rockwood, K. (2008). A standard procedure for creating a frailty index. *BMC Geriatrics, 8*, 24.

136. Sen, P., Shah, P. P., Nativio, R., & Berger, S. L. (2016). Epigenetic Mechanisms of Longevity and Aging. *Cell, 166*(4), 822–839.

137. Sfera, A., Bullock, K., Price, A., Inderias, L., & Osorio, C. (2018). Ferrosenescence: The iron age of neurodegeneration? *Mechanisms of Ageing and Development, 174*, 63–75.

138. Sheng, N., Wang, J., Xing, F., Duan, X., & Xiang, Z. (2023). Associations between exposure to phthalates and rheumatoid arthritis risk among adults in NHANES, 2007–2016. *Chemosphere, 338*, 139472.

139. Shi, W., Gao, X., Cao, Y., Chen, Y., Cui, Q., Deng, F., Yang, B., Lin, E. Z., Fang, J., & Li, T., et al. (2022). Personal airborne chemical exposure and epigenetic ageing biomarkers in healthy Chinese elderly individuals: Evidence from mixture approaches. *Environment International, 170*, 107614.

140. Shi, W., Tang, S., Fang, J., Cao, Y., Chen, C., Li, T., Gao, X., & Shi, X. (2022). Epigenetic age stratifies the risk of blood pressure elevation related to short-term PM(2.5) exposure in older adults. *Environmental Research, 212*, 113507.

141. Shiau, S., Wang, L., Liu, H., Zheng, Y., Drong, A., Joyce, B. T., Wang, J., Li, W., Leng, J., & Shen, Y., et al. (2021). Prenatal gestational diabetes mellitus exposure and accelerated offspring DNA methylation age in early childhood. *Epigenetics, 16*(2), 186–195.

142. Sidler, C., Kovalchuk, O., & Kovalchuk, I. (2017). Epigenetic Regulation of Cellular Senescence and Aging. *Frontiers in Genetics, 8*, 138.

143. Simpkin, A. J., Howe, L. D., Tilling, K., Gaunt, T. R., Lyttleton, O., McArdle, W. L., Ring, S. M., Horvath, S., Smith, G. D., & Relton, C. L. (2017). The epigenetic clock and physical development during childhood and adolescence: Longitudinal analysis from a UK birth cohort. *International Journal of Epidemiology, 46*(2), 549–558.

144. Simpson, D. J., & Chandra, T. (2021). Epigenetic age prediction. *Aging Cell, 20*(10), e13452.

145. Song, A. Y., Feinberg, J. I., Bakulski, K. M., Croen, L. A., Fallin, M. D., Newschaffer, C. J., Hertz-Picciotto, I., Schmidt, R. J., Ladd-Acosta, C., & Volk, H. E. (2022). Prenatal Exposure to Ambient Air Pollution and Epigenetic Aging at Birth in Newborns. *Frontiers in Genetics, 13*, 929416.

146. Starling, A. P., Liu, C., Shen, G., Yang, I. V., Kechris, K., Borengasser, S. J., Boyle, K. E., Zhang, W., Smith, H. A., & Calafat, A. M., et al. (2020). Prenatal Exposure to Per- and Polyfluoroalkyl Substances, Umbilical Cord Blood DNA Methylation, and Cardio-Metabolic Indicators in

Newborns: The Healthy Start Study. *Environmental Health Perspectives, 128*(12), 127014.

147. Strong, R., Miller, R. A., Bogue, M., Fernandez, E., Javors, M. A., Libert, S., Marinez, P. A., Murphy, M. P., Musi, N., Nelson, J. F., et al. (2020). Rapamycin-mediated mouse lifespan extension: Late-life dosage regimes with sex-specific effects. *Aging Cell, 19*(11), e13269.
148. Sun, D., & Yi, S. V. (2015). Impacts of Chromatin States and Long-Range Genomic Segments on Aging and DNA Methylation. *PLoS ONE, 10*(6), e0128517.
149. Sunderland, E. M., Hu, X. C., Dassuncao, C., Tokranov, A. K., Wagner, C. C., & Allen, J. G. (2019). A review of the pathways of human exposure to poly- and perfluoroalkyl substances (PFASs) and present understanding of health effects. *Journal of Exposure Science & Environmental Epidemiology, 29*(2), 131–147.
150. Tam, B. T., Morais, J. A., & Santosa, S. (2020). Obesity and ageing: Two sides of the same coin. *Obesity Reviews, 21*(1), e12991.
151. Tamatea, A. J., & Psychopathy, B. (2015). Legal, and Research Implications at the Interface of Epigenetics and Chronic Antisocial Conduct. *Behavioral Sciences & the Law, 33*(5), 629–643.
152. Tang, H., Cheng, Z., Li, N., Mao, S., Ma, R., He, H., & Xiang, H. (2020). The short- and long-term associations of particulate matter with inflammation and blood coagulation markers: A meta-analysis. *Environmental Pollution, 267*, 115630.
153. Taylor, A. M., Pattie, A., & Deary, I. J. (2018). Cohort Profile Update: The Lothian Birth Cohorts of 1921 and 1936. *International Journal of Epidemiology, 47*(4), 1042–1042r.
154. Teschendorff, A. E. (2020). A comparison of epigenetic mitotic-like clocks for cancer risk prediction. *Genome Medicine, 12*(1), 56.
155. Thompson, M. J., Chwialkowska, K., Rubbi, L., Lusis, A. J., Davis, R. C., Srivastava, A., & Pellegrini, M. (2018). A multi-tissue full lifespan epigenetic clock for mice. *Aging, 10*(10), 2832–2854.
156. Tollenaar, M. S., Beijers, R., Garg, E., Nguyen, T. T. T., Lin, D. T. S., MacIsaac, J. L., & O'Donnell, K. J. (2021). Internalizing symptoms associate with the pace of epigenetic aging in childhood. *Biological Psychology, 159*, 108021.
157. Trapp, A., Kerepesi, C., & Gladyshev, V. N. (2021). Profiling epigenetic age in single cells. *Nature Aging, 1*(12), 1189–1201.
158. Vetter, V. M., Meyer, A., Karbasiyan, M., Steinhagen-Thiessen, E., Hopfenmuller, W., & Demuth, I. (2019). Epigenetic Clock and Relative Telomere Length Represent Largely Different Aspects of Aging in the Berlin Aging Study II (BASE-II). *The Journals of Gerontology. Series A, Biological Sciences and Medical Sciences, 74*(1), 27–32.
159. Wang, K., Liu, H., Hu, Q., Wang, L., Liu, J., Zheng, Z., & Liu, G. H. (2022). Epigenetic regulation of aging: Implications for interventions of aging and diseases. *Signal Transduction and Targeted Therapy, 7*, 374.
160. Wang, Y., Karlsson, R., Jylhava, J., Hedman, A. K., Almqvist, C., Karlsson, I. K., & Hagg, S. (2019). Comprehensive longitudinal study of epigenetic mutations in aging. *Clinical Epigenetics, 11*(1), 187.
161. Ward-Caviness, C. K., Nwanaji-Enwerem, J. C., Wolf, K., Wahl, S., Colicino, E., Trevisi, L., & Schwartz, J. (2016). Long-term exposure to air pollution is associated with biological aging. *Oncotarget., 7*(46), 74510–74525.

162. Warner, H. R. (2004). Current status of efforts to measure and modulate the biological rate of aging. *The Journals of Gerontology. Series A, Biological Sciences and Medical Sciences, 59*(7), 692–696.

163. Weidner, C. I., Lin, Q., Koch, C. M., Eisele, L., Beier, F., Ziegler, P., & Wagner, W. (2014). Aging of blood can be tracked by DNA methylation changes at just three CpG sites. *Genome Biology, 15*(2), R24.

164. Welle, S., Brooks, A. I., Delehanty, J. M., Needler, N., & Thornton, C. A. (2003). Gene expression profile of aging in human muscle. *Physiological Genomics, 14*(2), 149–159.

165. Wolf, E. J., Logue, M. W., Hayes, J. P., Sadeh, N., Schichman, S. A., Stone, A., & Miller, M. W. (2016). Accelerated DNA methylation age: Associations with PTSD and neural integrity. *Psychoneuroendocrinology, 63*, 155–162.

166. Wolf, E. J., Logue, M. W., Morrison, F. G., Wilcox, E. S., Stone, A., Schichman, S. A., & Miller, M. W. (2019). Posttraumatic psychopathology and the pace of the epigenetic clock: A longitudinal investigation. *Psychological Medicine, 49*(5), 791–800.

167. Wolf, E. J., Logue, M. W., Stoop, T. B., Schichman, S. A., Stone, A., Sadeh, N., & Miller, M. W. (2018). Accelerated DNA Methylation Age: Associations with Posttraumatic Stress Disorder and Mortality. *Psychosomatic Medicine, 80*(1), 42–48.

168. Wolf, E. J., Maniates, H., Nugent, N., Maihofer, A. X., Armstrong, D., Ratanatharathorn, A., & Miller, M. W. (2018). Traumatic stress and accelerated DNA methylation age: A meta-analysis. *Psychoneuroendocrinology, 92*, 123–134.

169. Wright, R. O. (2017). Environment, susceptibility windows, development, and child health. *Current Opinion in Pediatrics, 29*(2), 211–217.

170. Wu, H., Estill, M. S., Shershebnev, A., Suvorov, A., Krawetz, S. A., Whitcomb, B. W., & Pilsner, J. R. (2017). Preconception urinary phthalate concentrations and sperm DNA methylation profiles among men undergoing IVF treatment: A cross-sectional study. *Human Reproduction, 32*(10), 2159–2169.

171. Xu, Y., Jurkovic-Mlakar, S., Lindh, C. H., Scott, K., Fletcher, T., Jakobsson, K., & Engstrom, K. (2020). Associations between serum concentrations of perfluoroalkyl substances and DNA methylation in women exposed through drinking water: A pilot study in Ronneby, Sweden. *Environment International, 145*, 106148.

172. Xu, Y., Lindh, C. H., Fletcher, T., Jakobsson, K., & Engstrom, K. (2022). Perfluoroalkyl substances influence DNA methylation in school-age children highly exposed through drinking water contaminated from firefighting foam: A cohort study in Ronneby, Sweden. *Environmental Epigenetics, 8*, dvac004.

173. Yamashita, S., Kishino, T., Takahashi, T., Shimazu, T., Charvat, H., Kakugawa, Y., & Maeda, M. (2018). Genetic and epigenetic alterations in normal tissues have differential impacts on cancer risk among tissues. *Proceedings of the National Academy of Sciences of the United States of America, 115*(6), 1328–1333.

174. Yang, Z., Wong, A., Kuh, D., Paul, D. S., Rakyan, V. K., Leslie, R. D., & Teschendorff, A. E. (2016). Correlation of an epigenetic mitotic clock with cancer risk. *Genome Biology, 17*, 205.

175. Youn, A., & Wang, S. (2018). The MiAge Calculator: A DNA methylation-based mitotic age calculator of human tissue types. *Epigenetics, 13*(2), 192–206.

176. Zannas, A. S., Arloth, J., Carrillo-Roa, T., Iurato, S., Roh, S., Ressler, K. J., & Smith, A. K. (2015). Lifetime stress accelerates epigenetic aging in an urban, African American cohort: Relevance of glucocorticoid signaling. *Genome Biology, 16*, 266.

177. Zheng, S. C., Widschwendter, M., & Teschendorff, A. E. (2016). Epigenetic drift, epigenetic clocks and cancer risk. *Epigenomics, 8*(6), 705–719.

Chapter 7

THE SCIENCE OF DIETARY AND NUTRITIONAL INTERVENTIONS IN AGING

Contents

Introduction

Aging is a widespread occurrence among humans that can be interpreted and understood in various ways. Imahori (1992) defines aging as the deterioration of bodily functions that occurs in parallel with the aging process. The term refers to an individual's behavior and skill in a range of culturally established activities, acquisition of knowledge, and changes in physiological mechanisms, as well as in perceptual, intellectual, emotional, and other psychological processes. The process in question is normative and dynamic, rather than being a fixed element of the human life cycle. As people grow older, changes can be noticed in the areas of physical, cognitive, and social functioning. The process of aging is widely recognized as a biological phenomenon that is influenced by numerous factors (Bran et al., 2009). One of its fundamental features is the programmed aging of multiple cells located in various tissues and organs that control physiological systems. Ultimately, this results in a decrease in functionality. The increase in life expectancy has required the development of strategies to maintain good health and well-being in the later years of life. Active aging is the achievement of a desirable quality of life throughout an individual's lifespan. The nutritional needs of healthy senior citizens are essentially the same as those of younger individuals, as long as the amount of calories consumed matches the amount of energy expended.

The influence of nutrition on chronic diseases and age-related decline has been recognized as a substantial factor that can be modified (Brownie, 2006; Di Iorio et al., 2006; Dominguez et al., 2017; Norman et al., 2021). In addition to affecting present health conditions, changes in dietary patterns significantly influence the probability of individuals developing diseases such as cancer, cardiovascular disease, and diabetes in the future. Population aging refers to the progressive rise in the percentage of elderly individuals in a specific population. The upcoming social transformation is a significant advancement of the present century, with extensive consequences in different areas of society, including labor and capital markets, the need for goods and services like housing, transportation, and welfare, and the structure of family arrangements. The global population is expected to undergo a demographic shift, with the proportion of elderly individuals aged 60 years and above increasing from 12.3% in 2015 to 16.5% in 2030. This will result in an estimated 1.4 billion elderly people by 2030 and nearly one billion by 2050. In 2015, a substantial portion of the worldwide population aged sixty years or older was primarily located in five countries: Russia, Japan, India, China, and the USA. More precisely, these countries together represented 50% of the mentioned population. To achieve the goals outlined in the 2030 Program of Action for Sustainable Development, it is crucial to plan for the socioeconomic changes that will occur due to an increasing elderly population (Beard & Bloom, 2015). The phenomenon of population aging is especially significant in the context of achieving objectives related to reducing poverty, safeguarding life and well-being for individuals of all age groups, advancing gender equality, and fostering job creation. The 2002 Madrid International Plan of Action on Ageing (MIPAA) was ratified at the 2nd World Assembly on Ageing. The plan highlighted the significance of including elderly individuals in the development strategy and acknowledged their entitlement to engage in and benefit from development initiatives to safeguard their physical and mental welfare. In addition, the plan proposed that societies should establish a conducive environment that enables older individuals to actively engage in development activities (Seyfang & Haxeltine, 2012).

Orientation and Directional Terms:

Term	Definition	Illustration
Human Life Cycle	The series of stages through which a human being passes during their lifetime, typically including prenatal development, infancy, childhood, adolescence, adulthood, and old age.	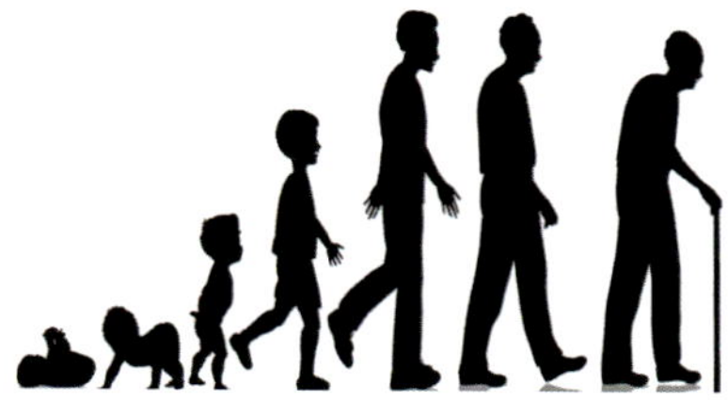
Psychological Processes	The mental functions and mechanisms that underlie human behavior and experience, including perception, cognition, emotion, motivation, learning, and memory.	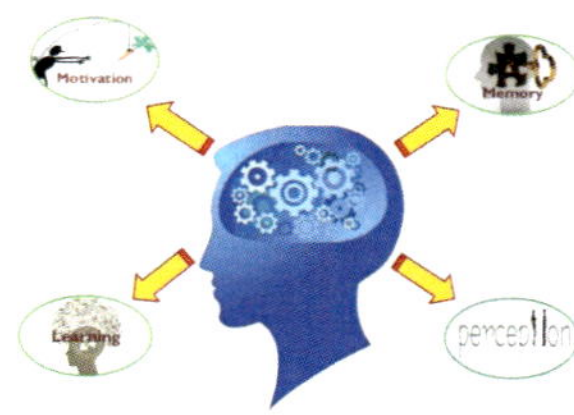
Active Aging	The process of optimizing opportunities for health, participation, and security to enhance the quality of life as people age, enabling them to continue to engage in activities and maintain independence.	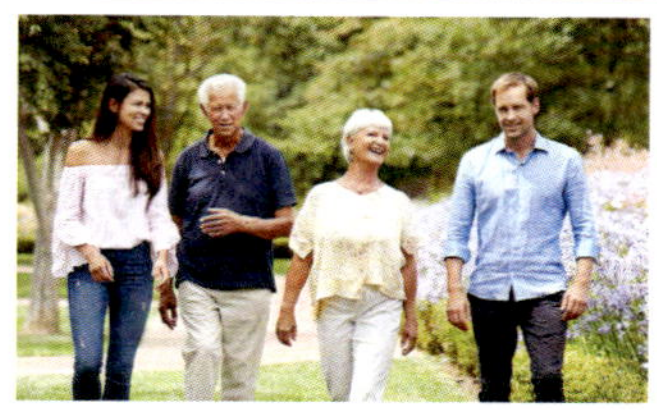
Cardiovascular Disease	A group of disorders affecting the heart and blood vessels, including coronary artery disease, hypertension, heart failure, and stroke, often caused by atherosclerosis and lifestyle factors.	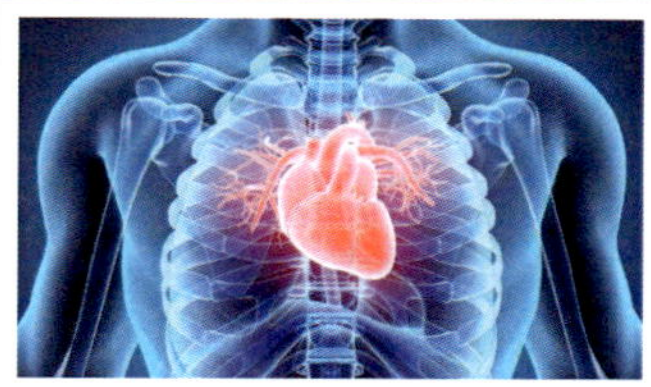
Physiological Aging	The gradual decline in physiological function and increased vulnerability to diseases and environmental stressors that occur as part of the natural aging process.	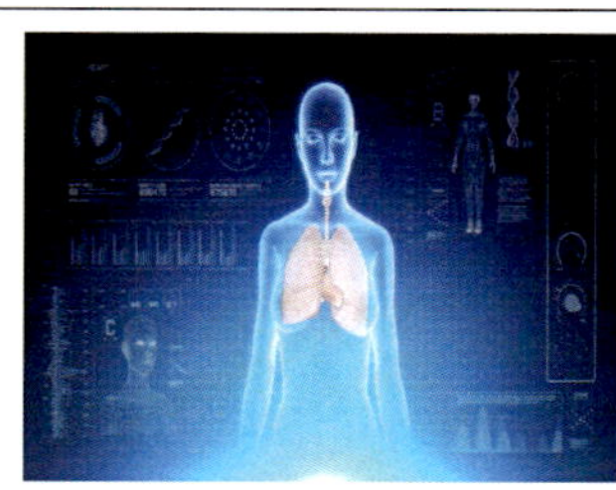
Malnutrition	A condition that occurs when a person's diet lacks the necessary nutrients or contains excessive amounts of nutrients, leading to health problems and impaired bodily functions.	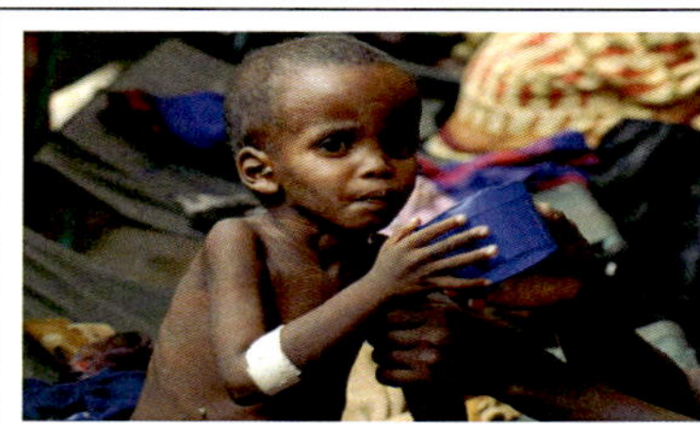

7.1. WHO Guidelines

The number of elderly individuals, specifically those aged 60 and above, is increasing in all countries. Walker & Maltby (2012) state that the World Health Organization (WHO) has developed policy guidelines to promote healthy and active aging. These guidelines consider various aspects.

- The objective is to evaluate and mitigate the consequences of disabilities, long-term illnesses, and untimely mortality.
- The objective is to reduce the risk factors associated with non-communicable diseases and decline in physical function as individuals get older, while simultaneously improving factors that promote good health.
- Providing education and training to both formal and informal caregivers.
- Ensuring the security, protection, and dignity of elderly individuals.
- As people grow older, it is crucial to support their capacity to continue participating in economic development, both in formal and informal sectors, as well as within their own households and communities.

7.1.1. Elderly Women Health

Women make up the majority of elderly individuals in all countries because they tend to live longer than men worldwide (Sohn, 2009). Asia is expected to have a population of 373 million elderly females by 2025, whereas Africa is projected to have 46 million. This concerns specific dietary needs and patterns of malnutrition, such as the high occurrence of osteoporosis in older women. Osteoporosis and its related fractures have a substantial impact on morbidity, functional impairment, healthcare expenses, and mortality. Studies have shown that there is a higher incidence of hip fractures in women, with around 80% of cases occurring in females. It is estimated that the number of fractured hips per year could reach an astonishing 6.3 million cases by 2050. Women have a minimum lifetime vulnerability of 30% for osteoporotic fractures, while men have a relatively lower risk of 13%. According to Jaspers et. al (2015), women are considered to have a greater susceptibility to bone loss because this process speeds up after menopause. Hormone therapy administered during menopause can aid in the prevention of certain conditions. Osteoporosis has been discovered to exhibit a correlation with lifestyle factors, particularly diet, physical activity, and smoking. This finding presents a chance for initial intervention to prevent a problem from occurring in the first place (Ford et al., 2008). Preventing bone fractures can be accomplished by increasing bone density during adulthood, preventing further bone loss, or restoring bone minerals. During the teenage years and early adulthood, it is important to consume enough calcium and engage in regular physical activity to ensure proper bone development (Heidrich, 1993).

7.1.2. Prevalent Health Issues in the Elderly

The elderly population experiences a decline in resistance to illnesses. Many health conditions commonly found in older individuals are degenerative in nature. These conditions include, but are not limited to, diabetes, cataracts, arthritis, bone loss, osteomalacia, heart problems, neural and mental disorders, and malignancies (Ernst, 1999). Furthermore, it is important to mention that respiratory, gastrointestinal, and urinary tract infections are commonly observed in the elderly population. Aging is commonly associated with a gradual decline in multiple bodily functions, such as heart, lung, and kidney functions, as well as muscle strength, sensory perception, nerve impulse transmission, agility, resilience, and the ability to sustain coordinated muscular effort. The changes can be ascribed to both structural and functional modifications (Van Rensburg, 2012). The aging process is linked to a reduced ability to maintain homeostasis, which is caused by the influence of external stressors. The thermoregulatory efficiency is somewhat compromised as a result of the influence of aging on the various factors that control heat dissipation and heat production from metabolism (Chappell, 1989). The process of aging is frequently linked to a decrease in psycho-physiological functions, leading to diminished capacities to carry out physical and mental tasks. The older population demonstrates a greater prevalence of cardiovascular, respiratory, musculoskeletal, and psychiatric disorders. A commonly observed phenomenon involves a substantial decrease in aerobic power, hindered thermoregulation, a slower response rate, and diminished acuity of one's special senses (Ford & Taylor, 1985).

7.2. The Impact of Food Factors on the Aging Process

The correlation between nutrition and aging can be examined from two different angles:

As people get older, there are significant physiological and structural changes that happen in the body, which can affect food preferences, dietary intake, and calorie requirements. This concerns the impact of aging on individuals, specifically regarding their eating habits and the consequent results (Axelson, 1986).

An alternative approach involves studying the possible effects of specific food items and their individual nutrients on slowing down or speeding up the aging process.

Most polyphenolic compounds consumed through food are extensively metabolized in the digestive system. Phloroglucinol is a polyphenolic compound present in plants. It undergoes microbial catalysis in the gut, resulting in the production of acetate, butyrate, and carbon dioxide (CO2). Furthermore, it has been noted to display antibacterial characteristics. As a result, it can alter the environmental equilibrium of the gut microbiota, which is considered a crucial aspect of human physiology. The interaction between the environmental system of microorganisms in the gut and the communication pathway between the gut and the brain is a crucial factor in changing how the central nervous system responds to various inflammatory conditions (Wang et al., 2007). Recent studies have reported that probiotics can enhance brain function and cognitive performance in rats with diabetes. The implementation of dietary changes has emerged as a potential approach for treating diabetes, specifically type 2 diabetes.

Several spice blends and herbs are rich in nutrients and commonly used as flavor enhancers in Indian cuisine. Most of the powerful and pungent bioactive compounds present in spices possess both antioxidant and mildly antimicrobial properties. Spices possess notable health advantages, such as assisting in the management of gastrointestinal problems and impeding the production of mutagens that can contribute to the formation of cancer. A recent study conducted in Japan has shown that consistent intake of capsaicin, a substance present in chili peppers and administered in the form of lozenges, can significantly improve upper respiratory reflexes in older adults. This measure has the potential to reduce the likelihood of aspiration and respiratory infections. Ginger and its derivatives are used for their carminative properties, which stimulate the gastrointestinal tract (Kunnumakkara et al., 2009; Khan et al., 2012; Selga et al., 2014). Ginger consumption has been proven to effectively alleviate chemotherapy-induced nausea in cancer patients. Concomitantly administering ginger and pepper herbal extracts has been shown to enhance the bioavailability of co-administered drugs. The curcumin compound found in turmeric is believed to possess anti-inflammatory and antimicrobial properties, which are thought to contribute to its potential for preventing cancer. Reports indicate that consuming turmeric has been shown to be effective in managing Alzheimer's disease. The use of fenugreek seeds has been proven effective in lowering blood sugar levels and managing diabetes. Both onion and garlic herbal extracts have been discovered to have properties that can prevent blood platelets from sticking together and lower cholesterol levels. Spices like celery, dill, fennel seeds, cumin seeds, parsley, and coriander contain bioactive compounds called phthalides, which have anticancer properties. Lemongrass, asafoetida, basil foliage, and poppy seeds are known to have anticancer properties. The physiological and anatomical changes that take place during the aging process affect the absorption of nutrients.

As individuals age, their metabolism tends to decrease, resulting in a decline in basic metabolic rate, physical activity, and appetite (Speakman, Selman, 2003). This decline in food consumption can lead to energy deficiencies and insufficiencies in various essential vitamins and minerals. The main factor contributing to reduced appetite is a diminished inclination toward food.

Loss of teeth and difficulties in chewing can lead to changes in eating habits, marked by a preference for soft and liquid foods (Sulmont-Rossé, 2020). Consequently, there are notable alterations in dietary intake, which can result in possible insufficiencies of crucial vitamins, minerals, and dietary fiber. The elderly population often demonstrates a proclivity to omit fruits and vegetables from their dietary consumption. Fruit juice consumption is preferred over whole fruit consumption (Joshipura et al., 1996).

Taste buds are the sensory organs that detect the five fundamental tastes, namely sweet, sour, salty, bitter, and umami. Atrophy causes a change in the threshold for certain tastes, which in turn leads to a shift in food preferences, including a greater liking for sweet and salty foods. Diabetes and hypertension are common among the elderly population, with sodium and sugar being significant contributing factors in these conditions (Johnson, 2007).

Hypochlorhydria leads to a reduction in the volume of gastric acid, resulting in alterations in meal order and gastric issues (Engstrand & Graham, 2020). Delayed gastric emptying and disrupted gastroesophageal reflux can cause a range of gastric disorders, leading to changes in eating patterns and avoidance of specific foods.

The atrophy of the muscular tissue in the gastrointestinal tract leads to reduced movement of the intestines, resulting in various digestive issues and hindering the intake of food, ultimately causing malnourishment.

Constipation and diarrhea are frequently reported symptoms caused by reduced gastrointestinal motility, which can have a substantial impact on an individual's eating patterns and nutrient consumption (Di Rosa et al., 2023).

Bifidobacteria have been associated with the production of diverse metabolites that possess the capacity to enhance health, including short-chain fatty acids, conjugated linoleic acid, and bacterial antibiotics. The microbiota, present throughout the entirety of a healthy adult lifespan, is a substantial constituent and plays a crucial role in maintaining gut homeostasis and overall health. This genus is highly abundant in the intestinal microbiota of healthy infants.

Aging is a natural process that causes changes in the gastrointestinal tract, immune system decline, and sometimes malnourishment. Changes in the microbiota and its function in older individuals are an unavoidable result of lifestyle modifications, dietary patterns, and pharmacological interventions. With increasing age and the presence of multiple diseases, there is a decline in both the quantity and diversity of Bifidobacterium microorganisms. These bacteria have the potential to be a significant biomarker for specific ailments in the future (Figure 7.1).

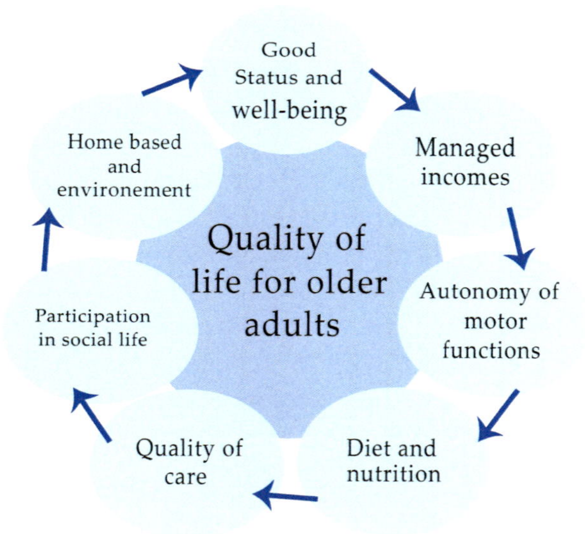

Figure 7.1. *The diagram depicts various factors that impact the well-being and quality life of elderly individuals.*

Source: Bacanoiu MV, Danoiu M. New strategies to improve the quality of life for normal aging versus pathological aging. Journal of Clinical Medicine. 2022; 11(14):4207. https://doi.org/10.3390/jcm11144207.

Physiological aging refers to the biological mechanisms that occur during the aging process, as mentioned before. Multiple physiological changes occur over several decades during this prolonged biological progression, gradually converting the normal aging process into an unhealthy one. An often mentioned example is the phenomenon of arterial wall stiffening, which is a contributing factor to the onset of hypertension and cardiovascular diseases. The acceleration of this unwelcome transition is caused by an excessive consumption of nutrients that are known to be factors contributing to degenerative diseases associated with diets, such as saturated fats, sugar, salt, and cholesterol. On the other hand, the elderly population may develop a preference for consuming liquid and soft mashed foods that do not contain important nutrients such as fruits, vegetables, and fiber. This dietary pattern may lead to a mineral and vitamin deficiency, as well as a lack of flavonoids, which are known to offer protection to older individuals.

Nutritional and dietary interventions exert a comprehensive impact on both the quality of life and the ability to withstand challenges during old age. Food restrictions, such as altering protein intake and restricting essential amino acids, are commonly practiced and have been found to positively affect lifespan. Research indicates that rodents who consume diets with lower levels of methionine or tryptophan experience beneficial results. Limiting the accessibility of these crucial molecules has the potential to delay the onset of age-related diseases and improve the quality of life in later stages of life.

7.2.1. Dietary Guidelines

Generally, older individuals tend to have lower levels of physical activity and a slower basal metabolic rate, leading to a decreased energy requirement (Freedson & Miller, 2000). Therefore, instead of consuming two large meals like lunch and dinner, it is advisable to consume 3–4 smaller meals by incorporating snacks between each meal. It is advisable to consume between 15 to 20 grams of oil per day. It is advisable to include protein-rich sources such as legumes, and dairy products like cheese and eggs, among others. Given their vulnerability to malnutrition, the elderly population necessitates a diet that is rich in calcium, micronutrients, and fiber. To ensure sufficient intake of fiber, micronutrients, and antioxidants, it is advisable to consume 200–300ml of milk and 400 grams of fruits and vegetables daily, in addition to cereals and pulses. Incorporating these items into one's diet has been proven to improve the nutritional value of eating habits and support optimal gastrointestinal function. The culinary preparations should be cooked thoroughly, have a tender texture, and contain a reduced amount of sodium and seasonings, as recommended by Ruiz et al. (2013). To prevent dehydration, hyponatremia (low sodium levels), and constipation, it is advisable to consume smaller portions of food at regular intervals and ensure sufficient hydration (Figure 7.2).

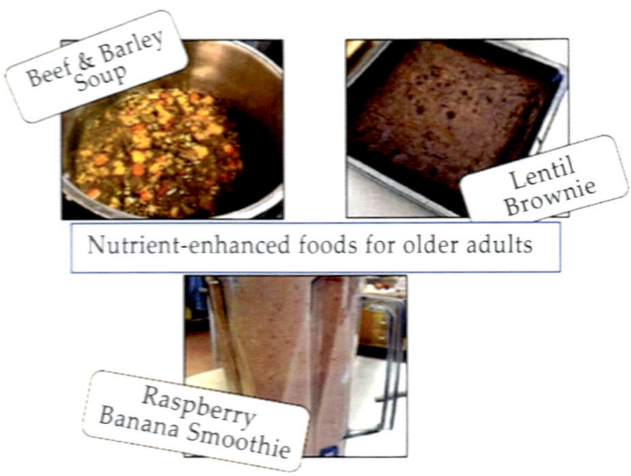

Figure 7.2. *The diagram illustrates a food planning strategy designed for the elderly population.*

Source: Romaniw OC, Rajpal R, Duncan AM, Keller HH, Duizer LM. Nutrition in disguise: Effects of food neophobia, healthy eating interests and provision of health information on liking and perceptions of nutrient-dense foods in older adults. Foods. 2021; 10(1):60. https://doi.org/10.3390/foods10010060.

7.2.2. Meal Planning

The customary dietary regimen of an older individual may consist of the following components:

At 7:00 AM. A standard portion for a modest refreshment might comprise a single glass of water, one cup of either coffee or tea and 2–3 biscuits (Roky et al., 2021).

The initial meal of the day is set for 8:30 a.m. and is commonly known as breakfast. An ideal breakfast choice is a bowl of oatmeal or wheat cereal cooked with milk, served with dried fruits like raisins and cashew nuts, cooked to the desired thickness. Dalia, a renowned Indian breakfast delicacy, can be elevated by incorporating aromatic spices such as cardamom or exclusively saffron. This dish can be enhanced by adding a single serving of fruit, such as a banana, apple, or papaya, along with a mug of milk. Sometimes, Suji upma (a dish made from semolina), poha (flattened rice), mung dal cheela (thin pancakes made from mung bean flour), and dosa (a fermented crepe made from rice batter and black lentils) can be served with a condiment like sauce or chutney.

11:00 AM. The beverage assortment comprises Bael sherbet, lime water, coconut water, and lassi. Options for dietary intake may include fruits such as oranges, grapes, custard apples, ripe guavas, watermelons, muskmelons, and pomegranates.

The allocated lunch break is planned to take place from 12:30 to 1:00 p.m. The meal comprises one cup of rice, one cup of lentils, and a maximum of two cups of vegetables such as bottle gourd, bitter squash, tori, sweet potatoes, tomato, potatoes, brinjal, legumes, ginger, onion, cloves of garlic, spinach, fennel leaves, carrots, cauliflower stalk, cabbage, and fresh peas. Furthermore, a single cup of freshly made curd is provided. At times, it may be suitable to offer dosa, idli, or chutneys. To make a salad, simply mix diced or shredded cucumber, onions, tomato, and carrots together. Season with salt and add one tablespoon of oil.

The scheduled hour for tea consumption is 4.00 p.m. One can choose to have a beverage like green herbal tea, black tea, or a glass of milk along with savory snacks or biscuits.

At 6:00 p.m. Traditional Indian snacks such as puffy rice, cooked chiwra, khandvi, and dhokla are some notable examples.

The designated time for the evening meal is 8:00 p.m. The meal comprises a pair of chapati accompanied by lentils and the option of either vegetable or paneer.

It is acceptable to occasionally offer desserts such as fruit pudding, rice kheer, and berry salad after lunch. Furthermore, one can include alternative cereals like ragi, bajra, rye, and maize in their diet, along with regular grains (Panchal, 2020).

When creating meal plans, it is crucial to consider both the culinary customs of a specific region and the personal dietary choices of individuals to improve the overall appeal of the meals. Food preferences in different regions of India vary according to their geographical location. For example, people from North India typically prefer chapatti made from atta, which is wheat flour, while those from the southern region have a greater preference for rice-based dishes such as dosa or appam.

When creating meal plans for seniors, it is crucial to take into account the significance of fully cooked foods that can be easily chewed. Legumes such as chickpeas, whole mung lentils, urad lentils, and masoor lentils can be made more easily digestible by soaking and cooking them. It is advisable to maintain the ambient temperature of food items within an optimal range, avoiding extreme levels of heat or coldness. A mixture of fennel seeds (*Foeniculum vulgare*) and ajwain (*Trachyspermum ammi*) can be lightly roasted and stored in a small container. It is recommended to consume approximately 0.25 teaspoons after meals. This practice is thought to facilitate digestion and reduce the occurrence of flatulence. Triphala is a combination of three fruits, specifically harida (*Terminalia chebula*), baheda (*Terminalia bellirica*), and amla (*Emblica officinalis*), that are dried by the sun and then ground into a fine powder. This intervention is useful in reducing the occurrence of constipation, a commonly reported ailment in the elderly population. Roughly 0.25 teaspoons in a standard cup. Plates used for serving may have a rim that makes it easier for the person to get the food. To prevent spillage, it is advisable to restrict the filling of cups and glasses to 75% capacity due to hand tremors. Reducing the physical effort needed would make it easier to lift the cup and drink from it. The objects in question have a small mass and their handles should be ergonomically designed for easy gripping.

An adequate diet is crucial for optimal physiological functioning at every stage of life (Ohlhorst et.al, 2013; Furman et al., 2019). An optimal diet should consist of a combination of protein obtained from meat, eggs, fish, and legumes, as well as five portions of vegetables and fruits per day, and carbohydrates derived from cereal grains and root vegetables. It is essential to include specific micronutrients in our diet as we age to maintain optimal health.

Malnutrition is especially prevalent among the elderly population. As people age, they experience a decrease in both muscle mass and basic metabolic rate. This leads to a decrease in the amount of energy required per kilogram of body weight. The baseline metabolic rate, also known as metabolism, is the amount of calories required to maintain the body's essential physiological functions while at rest.

Basal metabolic rate (BMR) relies on several factors, including muscle mass, lifespan, weight, and height. Gender is a significant determinant of caloric requirements, with men needing a greater caloric intake compared to women. The process of aging affects the nutritional needs for different nutrients. Individuals' dietary requirements may differ based on their age, as the suggested consumption of specific nutrients may decrease, while the need for other essential nutrients may increase in later life. The elderly population often experiences deficiencies in micronutrients, which can be caused by factors such as reduced food intake and a lack of dietary variety. Insufficient amounts of folic acid, zinc, pyridoxine, vitamins A and C (which act as antioxidants), and vitamin E have been linked to impaired immune system function and reduced antibody responses. The consumption of foods rich in small-molecule nutrients may decrease as a result of their expensive price. One contributing factor to the increasing death and illness rates among this population is the progressive deterioration of immune system functionality commonly observed in older individuals. Further changes related to the process of aging include a decrease in cognitive function and a decline in visual sharpness, both of which hinder the development of healthy eating habits and overall health during old age.

Changes in dietary patterns have been found to impact levels of risk factors throughout a person's life and may have a stronger impact on older adults. By making small adjustments to our diet and consuming less saturated fat and salt, we can lower cholesterol and blood pressure levels. This, in turn, can help reduce the occurrence of heart disease and stroke. The importance of consuming specific nutrients becomes more significant as individuals grow older. The following are the nutrients:

Calcium is a vital mineral that plays a crucial role in preserving bone health. As individuals age, there is a natural inclination for calcium to be absorbed back into the body through the bones (Cashman, 2002; Theobald, 2005; Straub, 2007). The medical condition referred to as bone loss, also known as osteoporosis, leads to the progressive degradation of bone tissue, making bones more susceptible to fractures and fragility. Calcium-rich sources include dairy products such as milk, yogurt, and cheese, as well as leafy greens and calcium-fortified cereals.

Fat: To improve cardiovascular health, it is advised that older individuals with a suitable weight limit their intake of saturated fats (Becker et al., 2004).

Fiber: As people get older, they may encounter problems with their bowels, such as constipation, which can be caused by insufficient fiber consumption (Müller-Lissner et al., 2005). It is advisable to include fiber-rich foods like wholegrain porridge, vegetables, fruits, legumes, and nuts in one's diet. Furthermore, it is recommended to encourage adequate intake of fluids in order to support optimal gastrointestinal function (Dukas et al., 2003).

As people get older, their ability to retain water decreases and their sensitivity to thirst decreases as well. This leads to a decrease in their ability to conserve fluids (Rolls & Phillips, 1990). Dehydration can lead to various negative consequences including fatigue, dizziness, irregular bowel movements, drowsiness, and cognitive decline, among other effects. Hence, it is imperative to ensure sufficient hydration levels throughout the day, regardless of thirst signals. Fluid consumption includes a range of beverages, including water, tea, coffee, fruit juices, and soups.

Iron is an essential nutrient that can be acquired from a variety of food sources.

Leafy greens, red meat, and dried fruits are effective sources of iron. Iron is used in the synthesis of hemoglobin, a protein that aids in the storage and transportation of oxygen in red blood cells, allowing for the delivery of oxygen from the lungs to other parts of the body (Terwilliger, 1998; Gupta, 2014;). Anemia occurs as a consequence of iron deficiency, leading to a diminished delivery of oxygen to cells and tissues, resulting in symptoms such as fatigue and lethargy.

Vitamin C is an essential nutrient necessary for the production of collagen, a protein that is important for wound healing and the maintenance of bone and tooth health (Ringsdorf Jr & Cheraskin, 1982; Walingo, 2005; Chambial et al., 2019). The generation of ligaments, skin, veins, and connective tissue is also considered essential. The food item in question contains a significant amount of antioxidants, which have been proven to have preventive effects against the development of coronary artery disease and malignancies. Citrus fruits, such as oranges and lemons, along with a variety of vegetables, are regarded as advantageous for their vitamin C content.

Vitamin D is essential for enhancing the absorption of calcium, which helps prevent excessive loss of calcium from bones. Exposure to direct sunlight facilitates the process of synthesizing vitamin D from ergosterol in the human body (Webb, 1988). It is crucial to enhance our diet by consuming nutrient-rich foods such as oily seafood, eggs, and fortified cereals. As people get older, their ability to produce enough vitamin D from food and sunlight may decrease. This may require them to take vitamin D supplements to ensure they get enough in their diet.

Zinc is an essential micronutrient that plays a critical role in promoting the optimal functioning of the immune system (Frassinetti et al., 2006). It is primarily found in meat, crustaceans, whole meal bread, and legumes. The combination includes supplementary nutrients, specifically vitamins C, E, B6, beta-carotene, selenium, and zinc, which are crucial for sustaining a robust immune response. Studies have shown that providing a combination of antioxidants and B vitamins can strengthen the immune system of elderly individuals.

B Vitamins: The optimal functioning of the brain necessitates the presence of B vitamins, specifically vitamins B1 and B12. Reports indicate that there is a decline in the serum levels of B12 as individuals get older (Wang, et al., 2001). There have been many cases where low levels of B12 in the blood have been associated with poor absorption due to gastric atrophy. Given the vulnerability of older individuals to frequent changes in salt and potassium levels, it is crucial to carefully monitor and control these levels following appropriate medical advice.

Vitamin E: According to Meydani et. al (2004), the administration of Vitamin E has been linked to a reduced incidence of infections in elderly individuals. Furthermore, it has been shown to have a reduced impact on the levels of influenza virus in the lungs after infection. Vitamin deficiencies are widely acknowledged to cause a range of mental symptoms, such as emotional irritability, dementia, and neurological manifestations.

Table 7.1. Anti-inflammatory and Anticancer Activities of Micronutrients Through Regulation of Specific Cell Signaling Pathways

Micronutrient	Signaling Pathway(s)	Types of Cancer	Anti-Inflammatory & Anti-Cancer Activity
Vitamin A	Activation of NF-κB, downregulation of the synthesis, and secretion of IgE through RARα	Chronic myelogenous leukemia, leukemia, cervical cancer, non-small cell lung cancer (NSCLC), head and neck cancer	Growth arrest, apoptosis, re-differentiation, halting of inflammatory cytokines
Vitamin B	Downregulation of the vascular endothelial growth factor (VEGF) signaling pathway	Lung, breast, and thyroid cancer; acute myeloid leukemia (AML); malignant lymphoma; acute lymphoblasyic leukemia; non-Hodgkin lymphoma; and melanoma	Maintenance of the VEGF levels and reduction in angiogenesis
Vitamin C	Activation of ten-eleven translocation proteins (TET) and downregulation of pluripotency factors	Primary or metastatic brain tumors, NSCLC, cervical cancer, and breast carcinoma (stage II)	Degradation of hypoxia-inducible factor (HIF-1); essential for tumor cell survival; activation of NKT cells and monocytes
Vitamin D	Activation of MAPK kinases, PI3 kinases, and phospholipase A2 and C signaling pathways (PI3K/AkT/ERK1/2/MAPK)	Skin cancer, melanoma, lymphoma, and leukemia	Inhibition of angiogenesis and metastasis; induction of apoptosis and autophagy
Vitamin E	Activation of NF-κB and downregulation of cyclooxygenase and 5-lipoxygenase-catalyzed eicosanoids	Head and neck cancer, esophageal cancer, hepatocellular cancer, AML, solid malignancies (lung, pvarian, rhinopharynx, urethral, gastric, testicular, ethmoidal, and tongue cancer), oral and uropharynx cancer.	Induction of autophagy and reduction of angiogenesis

Vitamin K	Downregulation of 12-lipoxygenase signaling pathway	solid malignancies (lung, pvarian, rhinopharynx, urethral, gastric, testicular, ethmoidal, and tongue cancer).	Differentiation and apoptosis as well as maintenance of cellular redox homeostasis
Selenium	Downregulation of Nrf2 signaling pathway	All types of cancer	Activation and proliferation of B cells and various enzyme activation
Zinc	Upregulation of NK cells	All types of cancer	Enzyme activation. Stabilization and regulation of cellular signaling
Copper	Regulation of Nrf2 signaling pathway	All types of cancer	Generation of free radicals (reactive oxygen and nitrogen species)
Magnesium	Activation of Stat3 and NF-κB signaling pathways	All types of cancer	Reduction of inflammatory biomarkers, such as C-reactive protein (CRP) and increasing nitric oxide (NO) levels
Manganese	Activation of NF-κB and hypoxia-inducible factor (HIF-1)	All types of cancer	Maintenance of superoxide dismutase (SOD) and production of reactive species

Abbreviations: NF-κB, nuclear factor kappa light-chain-enhancer of activated B cells; RARα, retinoic acid receptor alpha; NKT, natural killer T cells; MAPK, mitogen-activated protein kinase; AKT, protein kinase B; ERK, extracellular signal-regulated kinase; Nrf2, nuclear factor erythroid 2–related factor 2.

Source: Fagbohun OF, Gillies CR, Murphy KPJ, Rupasinghe HPV. Role of antioxidant vitamins and other micronutrients on regulations of specific genes and signaling pathways in the prevention and treatment of cancer. International Journal of Molecular Sciences. 2023; 24(7):6092. https://doi.org/10.3390/ijms24076092.

To improve cognitive performance in older adults, it is crucial to consume a varied diet and consider using supplements to maintain a mutually beneficial connection between nutrition, attitude, and behavior. Antioxidants have attracted considerable attention because of their potential to reduce oxidative stress, which is associated with brain aging. Consuming a significant quantity of Vitamin E in one's diet has been proposed to potentially protect against the development of Parkinson's disease. The aging process is linked to the influence of carotene and carotenoids, the antioxidant ascorbic acid, and alpha-tocopherol on cognitive function (Oliveira & Veloso, 2012).

Among elderly individuals, nutrients can influence cognitive function, mood, and behavior in diverse manners. The occurrence of stroke and related conditions significantly contributes to the overall occurrence of disability among older individuals. Consuming vitamins and minerals with protective properties, such as antioxidants, has been proven to reduce the risk of stroke and related conditions by supporting the optimal functioning of the circulatory system.

Phytochemicals, which are biologically active compounds found in plants, can have a substantial but often overlooked effect on the preservation of vascular function. Food products rich in antioxidants can help protect against the harmful effects of free radicals, which are a major cause of cognitive decline and the aging of the mind. However, older individuals often face challenges in maintaining a varied diet that can supply enough necessary micronutrients. Hence, it might be imperative to offer supplementation or fortification of food to vulnerable communities (Figure 7.3).

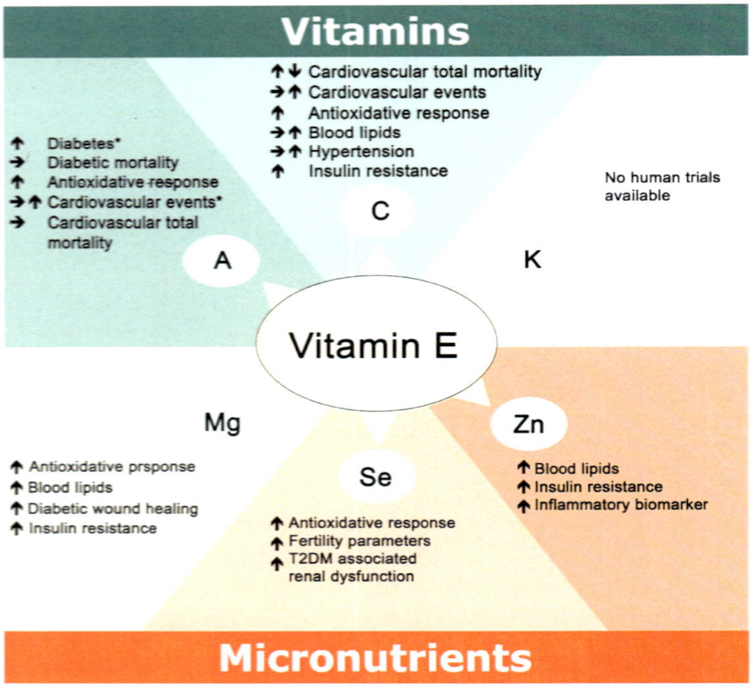

Figure 7.3. *Metabolism.*

Source: Liao S, Omage SO, Börmel L, Kluge S, Schubert M, Wallert M, Lorkowski S. Vitamin E and metabolic health: Relevance of interactions with other micronutrients. Antioxidants. 2022; 11(9):1785. https://doi.org/10.3390/antiox11091785.

The potential importance of antioxidants found in food, such as tocopherols, tocotrienols, ascorbic acid, and carotenoids, in preventing diseases is remarkable. Fruits and vegetables are abundant in antioxidants, which provide a multitude of advantages to human well-being. It has been suggested that antioxidants could have a significant effect in slowing down the progression of certain neurological disorders, as oxidative damage has been identified as a possible cause in several neurological conditions that often occur in older individuals. Phenolic acids and flavonoids are the main phytochemicals that demonstrate antioxidant properties (Khalil et al., 2011). The compounds can be obtained from a variety of food sources, such as onions, garlic cloves, ginger root, oats, soybeans, beverages, oilseeds, medicinal plants, and condiments. Berry-derived polyphenols are an essential group of micronutrients in the human diet that have been shown to improve cognitive function. The different classes of polyphenols found in berries, such as flavanols, cyan pigments, and stilbenes, particularly resveratrol, are being studied for their positive effects on human health and cognitive function as we get older, along with their impact on neurological functions. The antioxidant resveratrol is a polyphenolic compound that is frequently found in grapes and is known for its anti-aging and anti-tumor properties. It is acknowledged for its ability to provide neuroprotection against neurological inflammation and cerebral vascular disease caused by dietary factors (Leonardo & Doré, 2011).

7.3. Body Weight and Metabolism

The physical characteristics of the body's mass and shape are determined by the balance between energy intake (i.e., consumption of calories from food) and energy expenditure (i.e., burning calories through exercise and activity). Calories are essential for the optimal functioning of every organ in the human body. Calories are produced by the metabolic process of the human body when food is consumed and then used up through physical activity (Donnelly et al., 1991). Weight loss is the result of a negative energy balance, which occurs when the amount of energy consumed is less than the amount of energy expended. Excess calories that are not used for energy are stored by the body as adipose tissue. Consequently, there is a rise in body mass. Participating in physical exercise helps to regulate glucose and insulin levels, thereby promoting overall physical well-being. Various parameters are employed to assess an individual's health and physical state. The BMI appears to be the parameter that is most frequently used. Research findings suggest that maintaining a BMI of 23 is recommended for optimal health throughout one's lifespan (Martin et al., 2007).

The Body Mass Index (BMI) is a quantitative measure that evaluates an individual's body weight relative to their height. It is a universal metric that can be used to assess the physical weight of both adult males and females. The Body Mass Index (BMI) is calculated by dividing an individual's weight in kilograms by the square of their height in meters (Lissau et al., 2004) (Figure 7.4).

Example: Weight = 70 kg, Height = 170 cm (1.70 m)

Calculation: BMI = $70/(1.70 \times 1.70) = 24.22$

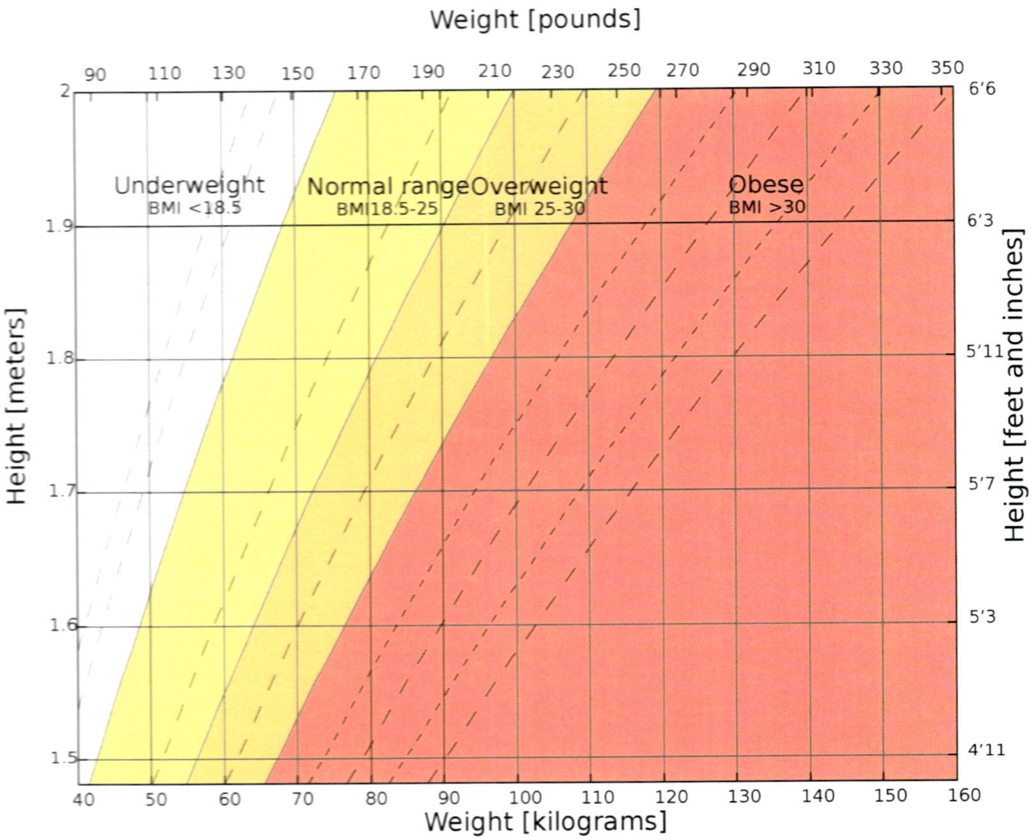

Figure 7.4. *BMI calculator.*

Source: By Invicta HOG – Own work using: Gnuplot and adobe illustrator, Public Domain, https://commons.wikimedia.org/w/index.php?curid=1208092.

There has been a noted rise in the occurrence of diseases related to one's lifestyle, which corresponds with a simultaneous increase in the percentage of adults who are overweight or obese. It is crucial to work towards achieving and maintaining an ideal body weight by following a balanced diet and regularly participating in physical activity. Participating in regular physical activity provides notable physiological and psychological benefits. Consistent physical activity not only reduces the risk of hypertension, hypercholesterolemia, hyperglycemia, adiposity, and osteopenia, but it can also help decrease the likelihood of experiencing depressive symptoms. The potential influence of immune system responses, or their lack thereof, on the aging process has been proposed. The process of aging is linked to a decline in immune system reactions, which occurs simultaneously with an increase in autoimmune disorders. Autoimmunity is the process in which the immune system produces antibodies against antigens that are produced by the same individual. Studies have shown that the manipulation of two environmental variables, specifically thermal regulation and nutrition, can influence the relationship between immune system responses and age (Kurz & Tan, 2004).

7.4. Can Nutrition Modulate the Aging Process?

Multiple studies have extensively recorded the influence of a wide range of nutrients on slowing down the aging process through different mechanisms. Implementing caloric restriction is an essential approach to facilitate the process of maintaining a healthy aging process. Empirical studies on human populations have shown that obesity presents a substantial risk to the health of older individuals and is associated with early death. Consuming this substance has the potential to cause the emergence of other non-communicable diseases that are linked to dietary habits, such as cardiovascular disease, type 2 diabetes, and cancers. Several food items, including yogurt, honey produced by bees, and other consumables, have been identified as advantageous for enhancing longevity. Furthermore, specific nutrients have been discovered to have unique functions in physiological processes that control the progression of aging.

The harmful impacts of free radicals on the aging organism can be mitigated by consuming antioxidants found in nutritional components of food, as well as non-nutrient substances present in various foods like onion, turmeric, olives, tea, and soybeans. Leafy greens, citrus fruits, and condiments are regarded as highly advantageous nutrient sources because they can scavenge free radicals and enhance the body's digestive system. These properties are recognized for their ability to enhance human well-being and offer protective benefits. The process of aging is marked by a simultaneous decrease in various enzyme systems in the body, as well as the deterioration of different tissues (Singh et al., 2019).

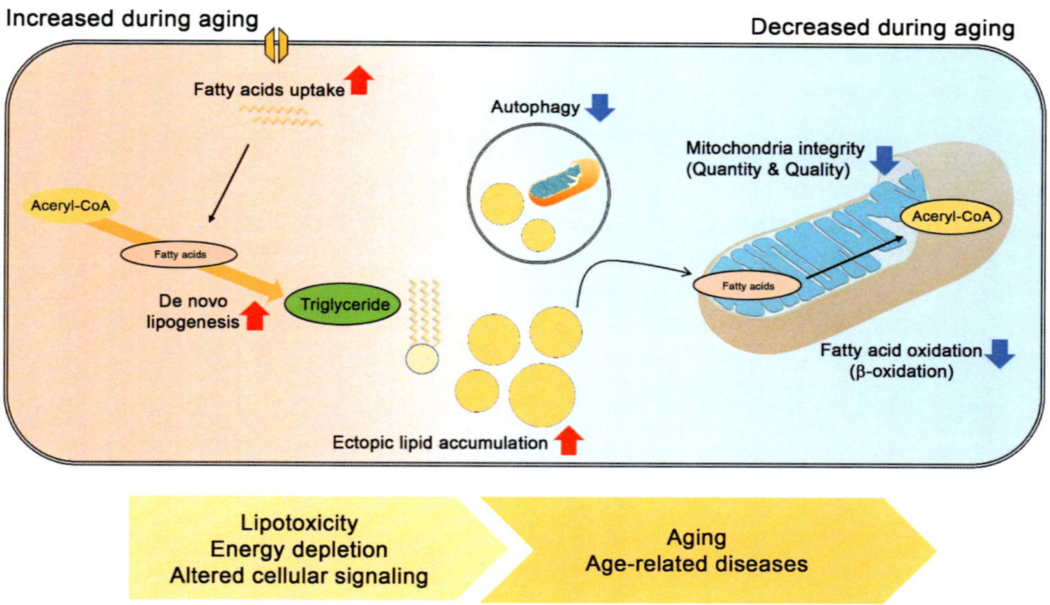

Figure 7.5. *The diagram depicts the metabolic pathways of lipids during the aging process.*

Source: Chung KW. Advances in understanding of the role of lipid metabolism in aging. Cells. 2021; 10(4):880. https://doi.org/10.3390/cells10040880.

Depressive disorders and anxiety are commonly found among the elderly population. Numerous botanical species and their derivatives have been found to have advantageous properties for managing these ailments. The use of Ashwagandha extract from a powdered root in combination with Kapikacchu dried berry powder has been recorded in literature (Kulkarni et al., 2016; Paul et al., 2021). The recommended daily calorie requirements (RDA) serve as guidelines for the optimal amount of individual nutrients to be consumed as part of a balanced diet. The table below displays the Recommended Dietary Allowances (RDA) for adult males and females. While the basic principles remain the same, individuals over the age of sixty who have sedentary jobs are also given additional amounts of certain essential nutrients. It is advisable to drink water once daily after meals (Figure 7.5).

7.5. Interventions in the Aging Process

The deceleration of the aging process is a significant issue in societies with aging populations. These societies are facing medical, interpersonal, and economic challenges due to a rising number of elderly individuals who are frail or suffering from illness. Several research studies have aimed to reduce the physical decline that occurs with aging, extend both the length and quality of life, and postpone the onset of age-related diseases (Khan et al., 2017; Tsai et al., 2021). This section focuses on specific interventions in the process of aging, specifically the use of synthetic compounds and the implementation of dietary/caloric restriction (DR/CR), along with regular exercise regimens, primarily in animal-based studies. The mechanisms and measures of aging are frequently a topic of concern, especially about age-related changes and the effects of age on energy utilization processes (FIM Craik, 2000). It suggests that procedures involving protein modifications and protein shifts, which have the potential to affect different cellular functions, may be more important.

7.5.1. Pharmacological Intervention Using Specific Chemical Compounds

A wide range of organic and synthetic compounds, as well as extracts from plants, underwent rigorous testing to assess their effectiveness in prolonging the lifespan of laboratory animals or enhancing the overall health of elderly individuals (Jackson et al., 2022). Antioxidants have been extensively studied in recent decades, especially after Denham Harman proposed the free radical hypothesis of aging in 1956. The researcher conducted experiments on rodents to explore the potential of different chemicals in prolonging lifespan. The study aimed to alleviate the adverse effects of reactive oxygen species (ROS), which are considered the most harmful free radicals in the human body. Following this, multiple studies have been conducted to extend the lifespan of test subjects or alleviate age-related diseases in humans, both of which were hypothesized to be caused by reactive oxygen species (ROS). Antioxidants, such as vitamins C and E, as well as natural compounds like polyphenols and carotenes, have been utilized. The results of the individuals' clinical trials, which were conducted to reduce the risks associated with age-related diseases, were quite disappointing. The study conducted by Mossman et. al in 2002 found that antioxidant pills were effective in animal subjects.

An extensive analysis and meta-analysis of controlled experiments conducted on more than 23,000 participants in human research revealed that the intake of antioxidant dietary supplements, specifically β-carotene, vitamins A, and E, can lead to a significant increase in overall mortality, rather than reducing it. This discovery is remarkable and justifies additional examination. The compound res, a polyphenol known for its purported "anti-aging" effects in animal studies, has not been shown to increase lifespan in different strains of mice tested in various research facilities. These strains are regarded as exemplifying the diversity of the human race. It is important to mention that the main way in which resveratrol works is not as a pure antioxidant. Consequently, the utilization of antioxidants has not yielded favorable outcomes in impeding the aging process. The hormetic effects of reactive oxygen species (ROS) have the potential to improve overall health, as evidenced by existing literature (Herrero-Zazo et al., 2013). There is a suggestion that plant polyphenols, such as catechin, may have positive effects on health not only because of their antioxidant properties, but also through indirect mechanisms. These mechanisms may involve signaling pathways or the potential induction of ROS in tissues, which can have hormetic effects. Various chemical compounds, such as rapamycin, metformin, and resveratrol, have been studied for their ability to impact the aging process in individuals. Nevertheless, this review lacks a comprehensive examination of the implications of these substances on the process of aging. Readers are advised to refer to comprehensive articles on the aforementioned topics et al. It is crucial to highlight that the improvement of health-span through a single chemical may not be all-encompassing, as older individuals often face diverse health problems that may be unrelated or have common underlying causes.

7.5.2. Dietary or Caloric Restriction Intervention

Lifelong dietary restriction or caloric restriction (DR/CR) is a well-known and easily reproducible non-genetic method to increase lifespan and reduce the occurrence of age-related diseases, such as cancer and kidney failure, in laboratory animals (Minor et al., 2010). Research indicates that implementing a calorie restriction of 30–40% during the early stages of life results in DR/CR rodents having a life span that is 30–50% longer than control animals that are provided with unlimited nourishment. The findings suggest that the schedule can influence the fundamental mechanisms of aging, as it seems to decelerate various biological and physiological changes linked to aging (Wycherley et al., 2008). Various instances can be mentioned to exemplify this assertion, including scientific articles that record the reduced activation of proteins linked to heat shock (N Gensous et al., 2019), a decline in the number of circulating dopamine receptors (Y Nagai et al., 1996), and the postponed emergence of kidney issues (Onuigbo, 2005) that accompany the progression of age (Figure 7.6).

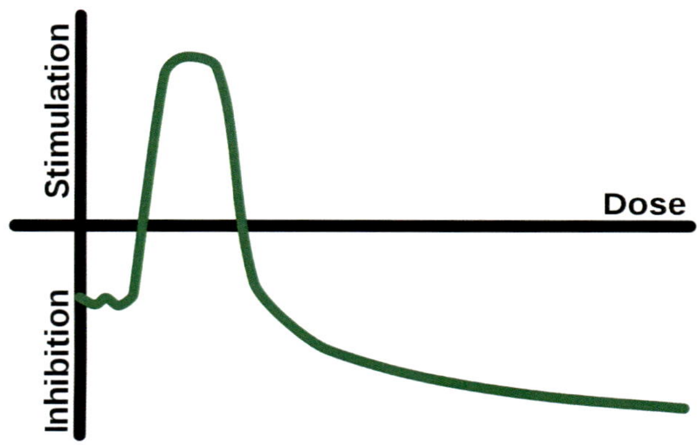

Figure 7.6. *Hormesis hypothesis.*

Source: By composed by User: Stannered – en: Image: Hormesis dose response graph.png, Public Domain, https://commons.wikimedia.org/w/index.php?curid=1831564.

It is important to mention that this intervention has been observed to enhance conditions associated with genetic abnormalities in laboratory animals, which are usually considered to be unaffected by lifestyle factors such as dietary restriction or caloric restriction. Research indicates that implementing caloric restriction (CR) can extend the lifespan of Unplanned hypertensive rats (SHR), which typically have an average lifespan of eighteen months (Brändle et al., 1997). Indeed, the lifespan of these rats can be prolonged to nearly thirty months, a duration that is similar to that of wild-type organisms. Furthermore, the application of CR has demonstrated a reduction in the frequency of heart and kidney lesions in these rats. Previous research conducted by RA Miller et. al (2005) found that caloric restriction (CR) can delay the age-related decline of the immune system in SAM rodents with defective genes. Recent reports indicate that implementing DR intervention at the early stages of life has been observed to significantly increase the life expectancy of a rodent model for Cockayne progeroid disorder. This disorder typically has a life expectancy of four to six months and is characterized by a deficiency in nucleotide excision DNA-repair enzymes. The life expectancy of the rodent model was increased by 200%. The number 52 is enclosed in square brackets. Studies have demonstrated that the administration of DR/CR can increase the lifespan of animals, irrespective of genetic abnormalities, by enhancing the factors that contribute to their reduced lifespan. Several studies, including those mentioned earlier, have utilized DR/CR during early stages of development, such as right after weaning or at the beginning of growth. Conversely, it was noted that mice who were put on a restricted diet starting at one year old experienced a 10 to 20% increase in their lifespan, as well as a reduction in the occurrence of cancer. Nevertheless, the extent of the increase in lifespans was relatively lower (around 35%) compared to the observed effects in animals that underwent lifelong calorie restriction (Valdez et al., 2010). A study reports that mice who were subjected to caloric restriction between the ages of fourteen and twenty-five months exhibited enhanced cognitive abilities. On the other hand, a different study found that rats who were subjected to caloric restriction (CR) from eighteen to twenty-six months of age until the end of their lives did not show any significant changes in their average lifespan, the occurrence of cancer, or other diseases when compared to untreated animals who were allowed to eat freely. A study found that implementing caloric restriction for 8 weeks, starting at nineteen months of age, resulted in a reduction in tumor occurrence and a significant increase in both average and maximum lifespan of the rodents (Speakman et al., 2011). According to the reports, starting DR/CR in the later stages of life has the potential to extend lifespan and postpone the onset of age-related diseases and physical limitations.

The preference for this approach stems from the potential limitations of early-onset research studies in generalizing findings to humans, making it a more favorable option compared to lifelong regimens. More precisely, if food intake is limited during childhood, it is probable that it will lead to impaired growth and other negative outcomes. Therefore, such dietary restrictions are not appropriate, even if they lead to a longer lifespan and positive effects in old age. Currently, the average life expectancy of individuals, including both males and females, in developed countries is around 80 years. The laboratory rodents and rats, commonly employed for research purposes, have an average lifespan of around 30 months when kept under well-controlled SPF conditions that closely resemble the living conditions in developed countries. The study compared the aging process in animals and humans, specifically looking at physiological decline and cognitive functions (Gallagher, 1997), as well as the development of age-related diseases like cancer (Fulop et al., 2012) and tumors, and molecular markers such as protein and DNA oxidation due to changes in mitochondria, has shown that the rate of decline is inversely related to the average lifespan in both humans and laboratory animals. The data suggests that rodents and mice experience age-related changes at a significantly faster rate than humans, estimated to be approximately thirty times faster (Rubin, 1997). Individuals aged fifty to sixty who participate in dietary restriction/caloric restriction (DR/CR) can be regarded as equivalent to rodents aged twenty to twenty-four months. In our study on interference in aging, we employed rodents and mice that fell within the designated age bracket. During the DR tests, older animals were placed in separate cages and given the option of either a gradual feeding regimen that limited their food intake to 60% of what they would normally eat, or an every-other-day feeding regimen. These tests were conducted on rats and resulted in a similar decrease in weight loss as observed in the gradual dietary restriction studies conducted on mice. These methods were documented in references and, correspondingly, in other sources. This study investigates the effects of dietary restriction (DR) on protein modification and turnover. It builds upon previous research conducted on animals that had unlimited access to food. The evaluation of protein modifications was performed by analyzing the susceptibility of digestive enzymes to heat and the occurrences of oxidative changes. Proteins of this type are likely to show reduced biological activities and may develop harmful functions, which could worsen the decline of physiological functions as we age. A study conducted on mice found that there was a higher proportion of heat-resistant aminoacyl tRNA synthetases in the brain and liver as the mice aged. The percentage of these synthetases increased from 5–15% between four and six months of age to 30–40% at 25–30 months. This discovery was documented in citation 67. The study showed that the modified enzymes were replaced by new molecules through metabolic or cellular turnover within 2 months after starting dietary restriction in individuals aged 23.5 months. This resulted in a decrease in levels similar to those found in young individuals. The likelihood of cell replacement in mature rodent hepatocytes is primarily attributed to an elevation in protein turnover rather than cell turnover, which occurs infrequently (Lindsay et al., 2010).

A study conducted by Higami et al. in 1997 examined the effects of dietary restriction (DR) on protein metabolism in a culture of inactive liver cells taken from older mice. The cells were subjected to the prescribed regimen to observe the impact. Following a 2-month period of dietary restriction (DR), the half-life of external proteins that were either established or pulse-labeled within the cells decreased by 40 to 50 percent, reaching levels similar to those seen in young animals. This statement applies to proteins that have experienced oxidative modifications. Thus, it can be deduced that dietary restriction (DR) promotes the degradation of altered protein structures in older organisms. The reduced functionality of modified digestive enzymes during dietary restriction (DR) can be attributed to the diminished oxidative stress, as well as an increase in protein turnover. This is evidenced by the production of heat-labile enzymes resulting from the exposure of enzyme components to a reactive oxygen species (ROS)-generating system. The study suggests that implementing dietary restriction (DR) has a beneficial effect on diminishing oxidative damage in older individuals (Sohal et al., 1994). The research demonstrates that the liver organs of older rats, which were exposed to dietary restriction (DR) for a period of 3.5 months, experienced a reduction in protein carbonylation from mitochondria. This reduction was similar to the levels observed in infant rodents (10-month-olds) that were given unrestricted access to food (ad libitum). Therefore, it is likely that the decrease in modified proteins observed in older animals as a result of dietary restriction can be attributed, at least in part, to the increased protein turnover and reduced oxidative stress.

The degradation of soluble protein is thought to be mainly mediated by lysosomal cytokines and/or proteasomes. Lysosomal drugs, such as ammonium chloride, did not hinder the degradation of proteins in hepatocytes. Nevertheless, the implementation of a proteasome inhibitor, Z-Leu-LeuNVaH, led to a significant reduction in protein degradation. Therefore, it is reasonable to suggest that the proteasome predominantly aids in the degradation of proteins that originate from outside the cell or proteins that are temporarily marked within cellular systems. Prior research on aging rat livers has shown that the activities of both 26S and 20S proteasomes decline as the rats grow older (Bulteau et al., 2000). The reduced functionality of the proteasome can likely be attributed to the decline that occurs with age. The current study uncovers a fascinating finding that, despite a decline in activity, the amount of proteasome significantly increases with age. This was determined by using a drug that targets a specific subunit of the proteasome. There is a a decline in the enzyme activity, which is dependent on the quantity of each subunit. This observation suggests that the changes in enzyme activity that occur as a person ages are more related to the quality of the enzymes rather than just random variations. Modified proteasomes may contribute to the formation of a self-sustaining cycle of abnormal protein accumulation as an individual gets older. The finding that the enhancement of proteasome activity took place in late-life dietary restriction (DR) is consistent with the reduced buildup of altered proteins in animals that underwent this regimen, as documented in a prior investigation. Multiple studies have presented evidence indicating a decline in the functionality of proteasomes as individuals age (Tomaru et al., 2012). This discovery provides evidence that decreased proteasome activity is a factor in the buildup of altered proteins in aging tissues. It is important to mention that the 26S proteasome can undergo reversible dissociation into its 20S catalytic core and 19S regulators under conditions of oxidative stress, as documented in scientific literature. Previous studies have indicated that the 20S proteasome selectively breaks down proteins that have been altered by oxidation. This suggests that the enzyme's separation is a consequence of stress-induced modifications.

In addition to the degradation of altered proteins that can be dissolved by proteasomes, a process known as autophagy has been observed to play a role in maintaining protein homeostasis, particularly in the aging brain. In this context, the aggregation of peptides or proteins that are unable to dissolve can result in the development of dementia and Parkinson's diseases, which are caused by the accumulation of beta-amyloid and α-synuclein, respectively. Studies have shown that the DR/CR method promotes autophagy in animal models, which helps remove abnormal protein aggregates and dysfunctional organelles. Extended periods of dietary restriction or calorie restriction are likely to enhance quality assurance processes in human muscle tissue. This is achieved by facilitating the elimination of impaired proteins and amplifying proteins subjected to heat shock, along with constituents of autophagic machinery. The influence of DR/CR on proteostasis seems to be a common occurrence in both animal models and humans.

The impaired metabolism of triglycerides and lipoproteins has been recognized as a possible factor in the progression of atherosclerosis, as well as other cardiovascular conditions that are frequently linked to the aging process (Bastien et al., 2014). The storage of lipids in adipocytes as a potential source of energy and their subsequent release for utilization in other organs depend on the existence of plasma lipoproteins. A study was conducted to examine the effect of delayed onset of diabetic retinopathy (DR) on the influence of the liver on circulating lipoproteins and their messenger ribonucleic acids (mRNAs) in a group of mice that had not eaten. Recent findings indicate a substantial rise in apolipoprotein A-IV levels in the plasma, as well as its messenger RNA (mRNA) in liver cells, after a two to a three-day period of abstinence in young mice aged six months. However, this increase is insignificant in older mice at twenty-five months of age. After a period of abstaining from food, there was a corresponding increase in the expression of apo C-II mRNA, while a significant decrease in the expression of apo C-III mRNA was observed. Apo A-IV is present in both chylomicrons and high-density lipoproteins (HDL). Previous research has demonstrated that the presence of apo C-II facilitates the activation of lipoprotein lipase (LPL), which in turn stimulates the mobilization of fatty acids. Apo C-III inhibits the function of LPL. Modulating protein synthesis in response to abstinence may enhance the uptake of fatty acids to meet the energy needs when food is scarce in young mice. Apo A-IV seemed to be moderately induced in aged animals, while fasting did not lead to a significant decrease in apo C-III mRNA levels. This suggests a possible limitation in the movement of fats. When 22-month-old rodents were put on a restricted diet (DR) for 3 months, there was a significant increase in the appearance of plasma apologize A-IV and its mRNA in the livers of the DR-fasted aged animals compared to the 25-month-old animals that were fed freely, as shown in Table 7.1. When elderly DR animals fasted, there was a reduction in the expression of apo C-III mRNA. The findings suggest that dietary restriction (DR) can cause a modification in triglyceride metabolism, leading to enhanced utilization of lipids during fasting periods. Lipoprotein lipase (LPL) activity may increase, even in situations where the individual is not fasting. Therefore, it is reasonable to suggest that restricting one's diet in later life may reduce the risk of cardiovascular diseases, such as atherosclerosis, by enhancing lipid metabolism. Chromatin structure is compacted by histones, which contain a large number of basic amino acids like Lysine and Arginine residues. The mentioned residues undergo post-translational modifications such as acetylation, methylation, and other alterations that have the potential to affect transcription. The two processes being considered involve DNA replication and DNA repair. The modifications in histones have attracted considerable interest because of their epigenetic characteristics, which occur during embryogenesis, cellular differentiation, organismal aging, and different pathological conditions. Studies have shown that the protein carbonyl, which is a marker of oxidative damage, increases with age in different animal species, including humans (Baynes & Thorpe, 1999). This increase is thought to contribute to the decline in functional cells that occurs with aging. The study found that rodent liver histones, except for H4, experience different levels of carbonylation in vivo. More specifically, H1, along with H2A/2B, exhibited higher levels of carbonylation compared to H3.

The modifications of histones, specifically H3 and H4, located at the core of nucleosomes, seem to exhibit enhanced resistance. The level of carbonylation in histones was significantly higher in the hepatic tissue of juvenile rats (5 months) compared to their mature (30 months) counterparts. This discovery challenges the prevailing pattern of increased modification that occurs as individuals grow older. Protein carbonylation predominantly occurs in amino acid sequences that possess basic properties. Modifications that mask the positive charge of Lys and Arg residues of histone can reduce their interaction with DNA. Consequently, this can impact the affinity of other amino acids, such as RNA polymerase, transcription factors, and DNA repair enzymes, by reducing their interaction with DNA. Therefore, it is reasonable to suggest that the decrease in carbonylation of histone modifications, which is linked to aging, may lead to reduced functionality of chromatin. We were motivated to study the effect of DR/CR on histone carbonylation due to a fortuitous yet reasonable discovery. After a two-month period of restricting the diet of 28-month-old rats, there was a significant increase in levels of histone carbonylation, reaching levels similar to those seen in younger animals. The discovery in question is contradictory due to the assumption that histone carbonylation is caused by oxidative stress, even though DR-animals show a decrease in carbonylation of proteins in cells overall, as reported in the literature. Previous studies have suggested that DR may plausibly cause relaxation of the chromatin framework, which in turn stimulates chromatin operations such as transcription and DNA repair in aged tissue. The aforementioned findings suggest a possible alternative physiological role of protein carbonylation that may not necessarily cause oxidative stress (Nikolaidis et al., 2008). Previous research has shown that the occurrence of oxidative damage to nuclear and mitochondrial DNA tends to increase as a person gets older. Changes in DNA bases within the nuclei can initiate carcinogenesis and potentially modify gene expression. Oxidative damage to mitochondrial DNA can hinder energy metabolism, resulting in a harmful state of organelles characterized by reduced functionality and potentially hastening the aging process. This study examined the effect of dietary restriction (DR) on the levels of 8-oxodG in the nuclear DNA of aged rat livers. According to unpublished findings by Nakamoto H and Goto S, implementing dietary restriction (DR) at twenty-eight months of maturity led to a significant decrease in the amount of 8-oxodG after two months. An increase in the expression of the repair enzymes OGG1 was observed in the group of older animals (thirty months) that were fed ad libitum, compared to the younger control group (5 months). This upregulation was aimed at repairing the damage caused by oxidative stress. The radiation protection personnel reduced the dose rate. The aforementioned observations suggest that the activity of the restoration enzyme was increased in the elderly individuals as a way to reduce the damage. Nevertheless, the increased activity became unnecessary after a 2-month period of dietary restriction, during which the damage was improved. Research indicates that delaying the implementation of dietary restriction/caloric restriction (DR/CR) can have beneficial effects on different cellular processes, thus reducing the negative impacts of aging in rodents. It is important to mention that the effect of DR/CR on the lifespan of animal models can vary among different strains, with some experiencing an increase, others showing no change, and possibly even a decrease, as reported in scientific literature. Therefore, it is crucial to exercise caution when considering the effects, particularly in terms of how long something exists, as the tendency for certain diseases, which can differ among different strains, can often impact lifespan (Gluckman et al., 2011).

When administering treatment plans to humans, it is crucial to consider the possible negative effects of dose reduction/controlled release, particularly among older individuals. This is because older individuals tend to consume fewer nutrients, such as proteins and essential micronutrients, in comparison to younger people. Humans generally have more influence over their food consumption than animals in experiments, as they are often subjected to stricter feeding protocols. Nevertheless, it is conceivable that humans may still encounter certain limitations in their daily dietary intake. The National Institutes on Aging, USA conducted a study on caloric restriction (CR) and dietary restriction (DR) involving nonhuman primates. In this study, animals that were subjected to mild food restriction were used as control subjects.

The findings suggest that the groups of monkeys that were placed on a 30% dietary restriction/caloric restriction (DR/CR) diet did not show a noteworthy increase in lifespan when compared to the group that received a standard control diet. This implies that the strict limitation of food observed in studies on rodents may not be required to achieve favorable results in primates, including humans. Nevertheless, a recent study on dietary restriction/caloric restriction (DR/CR) conducted on non-human primates revealed that the diet successfully prolonged both lifespan and health span (Kaur & Lakhman, 2012). Furthermore, studies conducted on individuals who are not obese and undergo one year of dietary restriction or calorie restriction have shown negative effects, such as a reduction in bone density and skeletal muscle. The results indicate that the DR/CR method may not have a substantial effect on increasing the duration of good health in non-obese individuals, even though the potential benefits of these regimens have been observed in animal studies.

7.5.3. Regular Exercise

Regular physical activity is widely acknowledged for its beneficial effects on health, as it can reduce the risk of age-related diseases and slow down the progressive decline of bodily functions that can adversely affect the quality of life for individuals in their middle and later years. The results of a significant long-term study investigating the link between physical activity and mortality in individuals with heart disease and cancer have shown that the opposite relationship is particularly remarkable among individuals who are 60 years old or older, rather than those who are between the ages of 20 and 59. These findings indicate that maintaining physical wellness is more effective in preserving the health of older adults. When examining the influence of physical activity on health, people frequently concentrate on its effects on the body's musculature. Nevertheless, our main focus is on the extensive ramifications of exercise interventions. While it is widely recognized that regular physical activity has positive effects on health, there are some who argue that excessive physical activity could be harmful because it may lead to higher oxygen intake and the production of ROS. Studies have shown that engaging in extensive physical activities can cause oxidative damage to DNA, protein, and lipids in the cell membranes of untrained sedentary animals. The apparent contradictory outcomes observed regarding exercise suggest that ROS can have both beneficial and detrimental impacts, depending on the extent, duration, and timing of oxidative damage to cells and connective tissue. The hypothesis suggests that participating in regular and moderate physical activity may provide advantages by enhancing the production of protective amino acids that reduce oxidative stress (Witt et al., 1992).

A study examined the influence of regular physical activity on protein oxidation in the cerebral cortex and cognitive abilities of rodents, as documented in reference 104. Animals of different ages, specifically those at 4 weeks and 14 months, underwent a regular swimming exercise routine for 9 weeks. The regimen consisted of swimming sessions that occurred 5 days a week. The cognitive abilities of animals that engaged in physical activity showed improvement in both age groups. The aforementioned changes were found to be associated with a reduction in protein carbonylation in the cerebral region. The increased expression of proteasome activity in the entire brain suggests that this enzyme is responsible for breaking down proteins that have been modified by oxidation. The exercise schedule may have caused a mild increase in oxidative stress, leading to an adaptation that enhanced enzyme activity. Reports indicate that the growth of neural cells in both laboratory cultures and living organisms is enhanced by reactive oxygen species (ROS), but this can be inhibited by administering α-lipoic acid, a potent antioxidant. The aforementioned findings may relate to the beneficial effects on the brain caused by exercise, where changes in the redox state may be involved. Engaging in physical activity has been found to increase the growth of new neurons in the cerebral cortex, as reported in studies (Uberti et al., 2023).

Furthermore, there have been reports suggesting that rats placed in an enriched environment for an extended period of time experienced an increase in the size of their cerebral cortex, while maintaining a consistent number of neuronal cells. This specific parameter is a sign of increased neural plasticity and has been observed in rodents up to the age of thirty months. This enhanced the animals' capacity to stay physically active. Epidemiological studies have shown that individuals who regularly engage in physical activity, particularly habitual walking, have a lower risk of developing dementia. There is a suggestion that a small increase in ROS levels could be the reason for the positive results observed in regular physical activity. The question of whether regular physical activity has a beneficial effect on other bodily tissues in elderly animals is a thought-provoking issue. This study examined how a regular treadmill exercise routine (four sessions per week, lasting eight weeks) affected the oxidative state of hepatocytes in elderly male rodents of two age groups: eighteen months and twenty-eight months. The study revealed that the maximum oxygen absorption was increased by approximately 40% in both age groups. The hepatic concentration of ROS was observed to be markedly elevated in sedentary individuals of advanced age when compared to those in the middle-aged group. Engaging in regular physical activity reduced the increase in oxidative damage biomarker associated with aging (Sacheck et al., 2003).

The evaluation of the redox state, determined by measuring the concentrations of glutathione, revealed a noteworthy more than twofold rise in the reduced form (GSH) among the exercise groups. The results indicate that engaging in physical activity causes a change in the cellular environment, making it more resistant to oxidative stress. This suggests that physical activity may have a beneficial effect. The current study documented an increase in the activity of NF-κB, a transcription factor that controls the expression of genes encoding inflammatory proteins such as iNOS, IL-6, Cox-2, and TNF-α, with advancing age. The rise in linking activity was observed in the nuclear samples through a deoxyoligonucleotide investigation of the reaction element, which aligns with the expected impact of increased oxidative stress. The performed exercise caused a reduction in the binding strength of NF-kB to the probe, while also causing an increase in the amount of I-κB, which is known to have a negative effect on NF-kB. The study results indicate that regularly participating in physical activity can potentially reduce or even reverse age-related changes that could otherwise worsen inflammatory processes. Glucocorticoids (GC) have anti-inflammatory properties and are given to reduce inflammation in chronic conditions such as asthma and rheumatoid arthritis. GCs have been found to inhibit the expression of genes that encode cytokines, such as interleukins and TNF-α, which are involved in promoting inflammation. Furthermore, they have been discovered to impede the function of proteins and receptors that play a role in facilitating inflammatory responses, such as iNOS and Cox-2. The GC receptors (GR) act as a transcription factor that directly or indirectly regulates the production of amino acids involved in inflammation. The study showed a significant decrease in the ability of GR to bind to the adaptable DNA element in the liver cells of aged individuals (28 – 33 months). Nevertheless, this modification was undone by a period of eight weeks of consistent physical exercise.

The results suggest that there is no significant difference in the overall quantity of GR amino acids between young adults and elderly wildlife. This suggests that the changes in the overall quality of GR, rather than its quantity, are linked to the process of aging. The serum concentration of GC significantly increased in the elderly animals that underwent exercise, compared to the control group that remained inactive. These findings support the idea that regular physical activity in older rodents may have the ability to reduce inflammation through the glucocorticoid receptor pathway, due to the anti-inflammatory properties of GC. It is important to mention that GR can interact with NF-κB, thus controlling the transcriptional activity of genes associated with inflammatory processes (Hoffmann, et al., 2006). Therefore, it is likely that transcription factors such as GR and NF-κB work together to reduce the production of inflammation-related genes caused by physical activity in older rats.

Research has shown that regularly participating in physical activity is associated with a reduced risk of developing a range of age-related conditions, such as cancer, heart attacks, diabetes, and dementia. This study examined the influence of regular physical activity on oxidative damage to nuclear and mitochondrial genetic material in elderly rats, as well as the subsequent repair process. This phenomenon could be linked to the initiation and advancement of specific pathologies. Rats, aged twenty-one months, were subjected to a consistent regimen of treadmill exercise for a period of eight weeks. The hepatic nuclear and mitochondrial genomes of aged sedentary animals showed a twofold and 1.5-fold rise in 8-oxodG levels, respectively, compared to their younger (11-month-old) counterparts. As expected, cells with mitochondria experienced higher levels of oxidative stress, resulting in a tenfold increase in oxidative damage to their DNA compared to the nuclear genetic material. After the exercise, the levels of 8-oxodG in both nuclear and mitochondrial DNA were found to have decreased to levels similar to those found in young animals. Age-related nuclear downregulation of the restoration enzyme OGG1 has been observed, whereas no corresponding downregulation was observed in its mitochondria. The physical activity resulted in a notable increase in the expression of the target gene in the nucleus, while a decrease in expression was observed in mitochondria. The repair process demonstrated distinct regulation in both organelles in response to physical exercise. The elevated levels of OGG1 activity in the mitochondria suggest that the observed reduction in oxidative damage to nuclear DNA may be partly due to an increase in its repair activity. Research indicates that engaging in physical exercise results in a reduction in the levels of mitochondrial OGG1. In addition, a study conducted on rats that were consistently taught has shown a decrease in the activity of the mitochondrial enzyme known as antioxidant GSH peroxide (Ji, 2015). This discovery implies that the decrease in oxidative damage as a result of education could be the fundamental reason.

Prolonged and intense physical activity can lead to the generation of ROS) and other detrimental consequences. Nevertheless, when the human body acquires routines to counteract harm, engaging in regular and moderate physical activity can activate cells to protect against heightened oxidative stress. Hormesis, a process that can enhance overall health and reduce the risk of disease, may be beneficial. Remarkably, the process of adaptation can occur in model organisms, even at later stages of life, in a systematic manner. It remains unverified whether this assertion is applicable to the elderly demographic.

Furthermore, it is important to highlight that moderate alcohol consumption can have positive effects on health, even though it may cause oxidative stress. Reports indicate that pre-consumption of alcohol has the potential to mitigate oxidative damage caused by ischemia/reperfusion in the DNA of experimental animals. The production of reactive oxygen species (ROS) during the NADPH-oxidase-catalyzed response is responsible for this phenomenon. Chemicals, such as polyphenols, which have long been thought to have antioxidant properties, can actually function as prooxidants and cause oxidative damage (Zhang & Tsao, 2016).

There is a proposal that humans can develop a response to better withstand oxidative damage by participating in aerobic exercise. Studies have shown that consuming antioxidant vitamins C and E can enhance the beneficial effects of physical exercise in humans. This suggests that the generation of ROS during physical activity may have triggered the improvement of health-promoting factors, such as the level of insulin in the bloodstream and the rate at which sugar is infused. Our study found that middle-aged individuals who have an active lifestyle have higher levels of oxidative stress compared to those who are sedentary. The level of urinary 8-oxodG was assessed through measurement. In addition, we noticed an increase in the antibodies (IgM) against 4-hydroxy-2-nonenal, which indicates the presence of reactive stress in the phospholipids of the cell membranes. Prior research has indicated that the quantity of this antibody is linked to protection against atherosclerosis conditions. Prior research has also recorded that middle-aged individuals who participate in consistent aerobic exercise demonstrate enhanced resistance to oxidative damage. Studies have shown that engaging in regular physical exercise can enhance the lifespan of mice carrying mutator genes in their mitochondrial human genome. This suggests that physical activity may have a beneficial effect on genetic disorders. Nevertheless, the exact mechanism responsible for this phenomenon remains ambiguous. Regular physical activity promotes good health by increasing the production of ROS, which in turn activates defense mechanisms against oxidative damage in both humans and animals. This could potentially explain the beneficial results of physical activity. Further investigation and interdisciplinary research integration are needed to fully understand the complex and not fully understood mechanisms that explain the beneficial effects of regular physical activity on the body (Hostina & Miller, 2019).

A Closer Look

Malnutrition

Malnutrition in aging is a significant concern that arises from various factors affecting dietary intake and nutrient absorption in older adults. As people age, physiological changes such as reduced appetite, altered taste and smell perception, and decreased gastrointestinal function can contribute to inadequate nutrient intake. Additionally, chronic conditions like dental problems or swallowing difficulties further complicate eating patterns, leading to a higher risk of malnutrition.

The consequences of malnutrition in aging can be severe and multifaceted. Insufficient intake of essential nutrients like vitamins, minerals, and proteins can weaken the immune system, impair wound healing, and increase susceptibility to infections. Muscle wasting and loss of strength, known as sarcopenia, are common in malnourished older adults, contributing to frailty and a higher risk of falls and fractures. Cognitive decline may also be exacerbated by inadequate nutrition, affecting memory and overall cognitive function.

Addressing malnutrition in aging requires a comprehensive approach that includes nutritional assessment, personalized dietary counseling, and potentially, oral nutritional supplements. Healthcare providers play a crucial role in identifying nutritional deficiencies early through screening tools and implementing interventions tailored to individual needs. Social factors such as isolation, limited access to nutritious food, and economic constraints also influence nutritional status in older adults, necessitating community-based support systems and nutritional education programs.

By recognizing and addressing malnutrition proactively, healthcare professionals can significantly improve the quality of life for older adults, promoting better health outcomes and maintaining independence and vitality as individuals age.

Summary

The phenomenon of aging is a complex biological process that is not fully understood despite extensive scientific investigation spanning several decades. Several theories are being proposed, suggesting that there are shared processes that can be applied to both simple eukaryotic microorganisms, such as yeast, and complex multicellular organisms, such as rats and humans. From an individual standpoint, any route that seems to contribute to the aging process should be regarded as a constituent of the overall mechanisms involved in maintaining the quality of life. Hence, it is impractical to ascribe biological aging solely to individual molecules or specific pathways. It is possible that a complete understanding of the aging process cannot be achieved by studying individual mechanisms alone, as only specific aspects can be explained using this approach. Therefore, when considering interventions for aging, we have primarily focused on methods that can influence various physiological processes, specifically, dietary restriction/caloric restriction and regular physical activity. Both methods, however, may not be easily applicable for individuals who inherently seek a comfortable lifestyle, regardless of their underlying motivation. The use of DR/CR mimetics, combined with exercise mimetics, may offer potential alternatives. However, it could be difficult, if not impossible, to find a single alternative that can fully replicate the wide-ranging benefits of following DR/CR and/or regular physical activity protocols to promote a longer period of good health.

References

1. Adav, S. S., & Wang, Y. (2021). Metabolomics Signatures of Aging: Recent Advances. *Aging and Disease, 12*(3), 646–661.
2. Amorim, J. A., Coppotelli, G., Rolo, A. P., Palmeira, C. M., Ross, J. M., & Sinclair, D. A. (2022). Mitochondrial and Metabolic Dysfunction in Ageing and Age-Related Diseases. *Nature Reviews Endocrinology, 18*(4), 243–258.
3. Barr, E. L. M., Zimmet, P. Z., Welborn, T. A., Jolley, D., Magliano, D. J., Dunstan, D. W., & Tonkin, A. M. (2007). Risk of Cardiovascular and All-Cause Mortality in Individuals with Diabetes Mellitus, Impaired Fasting Glucose, and Impaired Glucose Tolerance: The Australian Diabetes, Obesity, and Lifestyle Study (AusDiab). *Circulation, 116*(2), 151–157.
4. Benjamini, Y., & Ochberg, Y. (1995). Controlling the False Discovery Rate: A Practical and Powerful Approach to Multiple Testing. *Journal of the Royal Statistical Society. Series B (Methodological), 57*(1), 289–300.
5. Box, G. E. P., & Cox, D. R. (1964). An Analysis of Transformations. *Journal of the Royal Statistical Society. Series B (Methodological), 26*(2), 211–252.
6. Bub, A., Kriebel, A., Dörr, C., Bandt, S., Rist, M., Roth, A., & Watzl, B. (2016). The Karlsruhe Metabolomics and Nutrition (KarMeN) Study: Protocol and Methods of a Cross-Sectional Study to Characterize the Metabolome of Healthy Men and Women. *JMIR Research Protocols, 5*(4), e146.
7. Candotti, C. T., Loss, J. F., de Melo, M. O., La Torre, M., Pasini, M., Dutra, L. A., & de Oliveira, L. P. (2008). Comparing the Lactate and EMG Thresholds of Recreational Cyclists during Incremental Pedaling Exercise. *Canadian Journal of Physiology and Pharmacology, 86*(4), 272–278.

8. Canfield, C. -A., & Bradshaw, P. C. (2019). Amino Acids in the Regulation of Aging and Aging-Related Diseases. *Translational Medicine of Aging, 3*, 70–89.

9. Castro, A., Duft, R. G., de Almeida Neto, A. F., Laroche, D. P., Cardozo, A. C., & Gonçalves, M. (2015). Utility of Electromyographic Fatigue Threshold during Treadmill Running. *Muscle & Nerve, 52*(6), 1030–1039.

10. Castro, A., Duft, R. G., Ferreira, M. L. V., de Andrade, A. L. L., Gáspari, A. F., de Marchi-Silva, L., & Chacon-Mikahil, M. P. T. (2019). Association of Skeletal Muscle and Serum Metabolites with Maximum Power Output Gains in Response to Continuous Endurance or High-Intensity Interval Training Programs: The TIMES Study—A Randomized Controlled Trial. *PLOS ONE, 14*(3), e0212110.

11. Castro, A., Duft, R. G., Silva, L. M., Ferreira, M. L. V., Andrade, A. L. L., Bernardes, C. F., & Chacon-Mikahil, M. P. T. (2021). Understanding the Relationship between Intrinsic Cardiorespiratory Fitness and Serum and Skeletal Muscle Metabolomics Profile. *Journal of Proteome Research, 20*(4), 2397–2409.

12. Chak, C. M., Lacruz, M. E., Adam, J., Brandmaier, S., Covic, M., Huang, J., & Adamski, J. (2019). Ageing Investigation Using Two-Time-Point Metabolomics Data from KORA and CARLA Studies. *Metabolites, 9*(3), 44.

13. Chaleckis, R., Murakami, I., Takada, J., Kondoh, H., & Yanagida, M. (2016). Individual Variability in Human Blood Metabolites Identifies Age-Related Differences. *Proceedings of the National Academy of Sciences of the United States of America, 113*(15), 4252–4259.

14. Cheng, S., Larson, M. G., McCabe, E. L., Murabito, J. M., Rhee, E. P., Ho, J. E., & Vasan, R. S. (2015). Distinct Metabolomic Signatures Are Associated with Longevity in Humans. *Nature Communications, 6*, 6791.

15. Costanzo, M., Caterino, M., Sotgiu, G., Ruoppolo, M., Franconi, F., & Campesi, I. (2022). Sex Differences in the Human Metabolome. *Biology of Sex Differences, 13*(1), 30.

16. Cruz-Jentoft, A. J., Bahat, G., Bauer, J., Boirie, Y., Bruyère, O., Cederholm, T., & Zamboni, M. (2019). Sarcopenia: Revised European Consensus on Definition and Diagnosis. *Age and Ageing, 48*(1), 16–31.

17. Darst, B. F., Koscik, R. L., Hogan, K. J., Johnson, S. C., & Engelman, C. D. (2019). Longitudinal Plasma Metabolomics of Aging and Sex. *Aging, 11*(4), 1262–1282.

18. Feng, L., Nian, S., Tong, Z., Zhu, Y., Li, Y., Zhang, C., & Yan, Z. (2020). Age-Related Trends in Lipid Levels: A Large-Scale Cross-Sectional Study of the General Chinese Population. *BMJ Open, 10*(5), e034226.

19. Fiehn, O. (2002). Metabolomics–the Link between Genotypes and Phenotypes. *Plant Molecular Biology, 48*(1–2), 155–171.

20. Fleg, J. L., Morrell, C. H., Bos, A. G., Brant, L. J., Talbot, L. A., Wright, J. G., & Lakatta, E. G. (2005). Accelerated Longitudinal Decline of Aerobic Capacity in Healthy Older Adults. *Circulation, 112*(5), 674–682.

21. Franceschi, C., Garagnani, P., Parini, P., Giuliani, C., & Santoro, A. (2018). Inflammaging: A New Immune-Metabolic Viewpoint for Age-Related Diseases. *Nature Reviews Endocrinology, 14*(10), 576–590.

22. Gaspar, R. S., Rezende, L. F. M., & Laurindo, F. R. M. (2022). Analyzing the Impact of Modifiable Risk Factors on Cardiovascular Disease Mortality in Brazil. *PLoS ONE, 17*(3), e0269549.

23. Hartmann, A., Hartmann, C., Secci, R., Hermann, A., Fuellen, G., & Walter, M. (2021). Ranking Biomarkers of Aging by Citation Profiling and Effort Scoring. *Frontiers in Genetics, 12*, 686320.

24. Hekimi, S., Lapointe, J., & Wen, Y. (2011). Taking a "good" look at free radicals in the aging Process. *Trends in Cell Biology, 21*(9), 569–576.

25. Hertel, J., Friedrich, N., Wittfeld, K., Pietzner, M., Budde, K., Van der Auwera, S., & Nauck, M. (2016). Measuring Biological Age via Metabonomics: The Metabolic Age Score. *Journal of Proteome Research, 15*(2), 400–410.

26. Hipp, M. S., Kasturi, P., & Hartl, F. U. (2019). The Proteostasis Network and Its Decline in Ageing. *Nature Reviews Molecular Cell Biology, 20*(7), 421–435.

27. Hsu, H. -Y., Tsai, M. -C., Yeh, T. -L., Hsu, L. -Y., Hwang, L. -C., & Chien, K. -L. (2021). Association of Baseline as Well as Change in Lipid Levels with the Risk of Cardiovascular Diseases and All-Cause Deaths. *Scientific Reports, 11*(1), 7381.

28. Huang, H., Vandekeere, S., Kalucka, J., Bierhansl, L., Zecchin, A., Brüning, U., & Carmeliet, P. (2017). Role of Glutamine and Interlinked Asparagine Metabolism in Vessel Formation. *EMBO Journal, 36*(16), 2334–2352.

29. Ivanovski, I., Ješić, M., Ivanovski, A., Garavelli, L., & Ivanovski, P. (2017). Metabolically Based Liver Damage Pathophysiology in Patients with Urea Cycle Disorders—A New Hypothesis. *World Journal of Gastroenterology, 23*(43), 7930–7938.

30. Jang, C., Oh, S. F., Wada, S., Rowe, G. C., Liu, L., Chan, M. C., & Evans, R. M. (2016). A Branched-Chain Amino Acid Metabolite Drives Vascular Fatty Acid Transport and Causes Insulin Resistance. *Nature Medicine, 22*(4), 421–426.

31. Johnson, L. C., Parker, K., Aguirre, B. F., Nemkov, T. G., D'Alessandro, A., Johnson, S. A., & Martens, C. R. (2019). The Plasma Metabolome as a Predictor of Biological Aging in Humans. *GeroScience, 41*(6), 895–906.

32. Kohl, S. M., Klein, M. S., Hochrein, J., Oefner, P. J., Spang, R., & Gronwald, W. (2012). State-of-the Art Data Normalization Methods Improve NMR-Based Metabolomic Analysis. *Metabolomics, 8*(1), 146–160.

33. Kondoh, H., Kameda, M., & Yanagida, M. (2021). Whole Blood Metabolomics in Aging Research. *International Journal of Molecular Sciences, 22*(1), 175.

34. Kouchiwa, T., Wada, K., Uchiyama, M., Kasezawa, N., Niisato, M., Murakami, H., & Yokogoshi, H. (2012). Age-Related Changes in Serum Amino Acids Concentrations in Healthy Individuals. *Clinical Chemistry and Laboratory Medicine, 50*(5), 861–870.

35. Krall, A. S., Xu, S., Graeber, T. G., Braas, D., & Christofk, H. R. (2016). Asparagine Promotes Cancer Cell Proliferation through Use as an Amino Acid Exchange Factor. *Nature Communications, 7*, 11457.

36. Kyle, U. G., Genton, L., Hans, D., Karsegard, L., Slosman, D. O., & Pichard, C. (2001). Age-Related Differences in Fat-Free Mass, Skeletal Muscle, Body Cell Mass and Fat Mass between 18 and 94 Years. *European Journal of Clinical Nutrition, 55*(8), 663–672.

37. Le Couteur, D. G., Ribeiro, R., Senior, A., Hsu, B., Hirani, V., Blyth, F. M., & Cumming, R. G. (2020). Branched Chain Amino Acids, Cardiometabolic Risk Factors and Outcomes in Older

Men: The Concord Health and Ageing in Men Project. *The Journals of Gerontology: Series A, 75*(9), 1805–1810.

38. Le Couteur, D. G., Solon-Biet, S. M., Cogger, V. C., Ribeiro, R., de Cabo, R., Raubenheimer, D., & Simpson, S. J. (2020). Branched Chain Amino Acids, Aging and Age-Related Health. *Ageing Research Reviews, 64*, 101198.
39. Li, H., Ren, M., & Li, Q. (2022). (1)H NMR-Based Metabolomics Reveals the Intrinsic Interaction of Age, Plasma Signature Metabolites, and Nutrient Intake in the Longevity Population in Guangxi, China. *Nutrients, 14*(8), 2539.
40. López-Otín, C., Blasco, M. A., Partridge, L., Serrano, M., & Kroemer, G. (2013). The Hallmarks of Aging Europe PMC Funders Group. *Cell, 153*(6), 1194–1217.
41. López-Otín, C., Galluzzi, L., Freije, J. M. P., Madeo, F., & Kroemer, G. (2016). Metabolic Control of Longevity. *Cell, 166*(4), 802–821.
42. Macek, P., Terek-Derszniak, M., Biskup, M., Krol, H., Smok-Kalwat, J., Gozdz, S., & Zak, M. (2020). Assessment of Age-Induced Changes in Body Fat Percentage and BMI Aided by Bayesian Modelling: A Cross-Sectional Cohort Study in Middle-Aged and Older Adults. *Clinical Interventions in Aging, 15*, 2301–2311.
43. Markovič, R., Grubelnik, V., Vošner, H. B., Kokol, P., Završnik, M., Janša, K., & Marhl, M. (2022). Age-Related Changes in Lipid and Glucose Levels Associated with Drug Use and Mortality: An Observational Study. *Journal of Personalized Medicine, 12*(3), 280.
44. Menni, C., Kastenmüller, G., Petersen, A. K., Bell, J. T., Psatha, M., Tsai, P. C., & Valdes, A. M. (2013). Metabolomic Markers Reveal Novel Pathways of Ageing and Early Development in Human Populations. *International Journal of Epidemiology, 42*(4), 1111–1119.
45. Meyer, T. W., & Hostetter, T. H. (2007). Uremia. *New England Journal of Medicine, 357*(13), 1316–1325.
46. Milan-Mattos, J. C., Anibal, F. F., Perseguini, N. M., Minatel, V., Rehder-Santos, P., Castro, C. A., & Catai, A. M. (2019). Effects of Natural Aging and Gender on Pro-Inflammatory Markers. *Brazilian Journal of Medical and Biological Research = Revista Brasileira de Pesquisas Medicas e Biologicas, 52*, e8392.
47. Montoliu, I., Scherer, M., Beguelin, F., DaSilva, L., Mari, D., Salvioli, S., & Capri, M. (2014). Serum Profiling of Healthy Aging Identifies Phospho- and Sphingolipid Species as Markers of Human Longevity. *Aging, 6*(1), 9–25.
48. Musch, W., Verfaillie, L., & Decaux, G. (2006). Age-Related Increase in Plasma Urea Level and Decrease in Fractional Urea Excretion: Clinical Application in the Syndrome of Inappropriate Secretion of Antidiuretic Hormone. *Clinical Journal of the American Society of Nephrology, 1*(5), 909–914.
49. Niccoli, T., & Partridge, L. (2012). Ageing as a Risk Factor for Disease. *Current Biology, 22*(17), R741–R752.
50. Nicholson, J. K., & Lindon, J. C. (2008). Metabonomics. *Nature, 455*(7216), 1054–1056.
51. Orkaby, A. R. (2021). Moving beyond Chronological Age: Frailty as an Important Risk Factor for Cardiovascular Disease. *European Heart Journal, 42*(40), 3866–3868.
52. Orozco-Beltran, D., Gil-Guillen, V. F., Redon, J., Martin-Moreno, J. M., Pallares-Carratala, V., Navarro-Perez, J., & Fernandez-Gimenez, A. (2017). Lipid Profile, Cardiovascular Disease

and Mortality in a Mediterranean High-Risk Population: The ESCARVAL-RISK Study. *PLOS ONE, 12*(11), e0186196.

53. Panyard, D. J., Yu, B., & Snyder, M. P. (2022). The Metabolomics of Human Aging: Advances, Challenges, and Opportunities. *Science Advances, 8*(13), eadd6155.
54. Patti, G. J., Yanes, O., & Siuzdak, G. (2012). Innovation: Metabolomics: The Apogee of the Omics Trilogy. *Nature Reviews Molecular Cell Biology, 13*(4), 263–269.
55. Pitkänen, H. T., Oja, S. S., Kemppainen, K., Seppä, J. M., & Mero, A. A. (2003). Serum Amino Acid Concentrations in Aging Men and Women. *Amino Acids, 24*(4), 413–421.
56. Ponti, F., Santoro, A., Mercatelli, D., Gasperini, C., Conte, M., Martucci, M., & Bazzocchi, A. (2020). Aging and Imaging Assessment of Body Composition: From Fat to Facts. *Frontiers in Endocrinology, 10*, 861.
57. Prosser, G. A., Larrouy-Maumus, G., & de Carvalho, L. P. S. (2014). Metabolomic Strategies for the Identification of New Enzyme Functions and Metabolic Pathways. *EMBO Reports, 15*(7), 657–669.
58. Ramos-Chávez, L. A., Roldán-Roldán, G., García-Juárez, B., González-Esquivel, D., Pérez de la Cruz, G., Pineda, B., & Ríos, C. (2018). Low Serum Tryptophan Levels as an Indicator of Global Cognitive Performance in Nondemented Women over 50 Years of Age. *Oxidative Medicine and Cellular Longevity, 2018*, 8604718.
59. Rist, M. J., Roth, A., Frommherz, L., Weinert, C. H., Krüger, R., Merz, B., & Bub, A. (2017). Metabolite Patterns Predicting Sex and Age in Participants of the Karlsruhe Metabolomics and Nutrition (KarMeN) Study. *PLOS ONE, 12*(9), e0183228.
60. Robbins, J. M., Peterson, B., Schranner, D., Tahir, U. A., Rienmüller, T., Deng, S., & Melzer, K. (2021). Human Plasma Proteomic Profiles Indicative of Cardiorespiratory Fitness. *Nature Metabolism, 3*(6), 786–797.
61. Srivastava, S. (2019). Emerging Insights into the Metabolic Alterations in Aging Using Metabolomics. *Metabolites, 9*(12), 301.
62. Victoria, B., Nunez Lopez, Y. O., & Masternak, M. M. (2017). MicroRNAs and the Metabolic Hallmarks of Aging. *Molecular and Cellular Endocrinology, 455*, 131–147.
63. Wallace, M., Hashim, Y. Z. H. -Y., Wingfield, M., Culliton, M., McAuliffe, F., Gibney, M. J., & Brennan, L. (2010). Effects of Menstrual Cycle Phase on Metabolomic Profiles in Premenopausal Women. *Human Reproduction, 25*(4), 949–956.
64. Wishart, D. S. (2019). NMR Metabolomics: A Look Ahead. *Journal of Magnetic Resonance, 306*, 155–161.
65. Xia, J., & Wishart, D. S. (2010). MSEA: A Web-Based Tool to Identify Biologically Meaningful Patterns in Quantitative Metabolomic Data. *Nucleic Acids Research, 38*, W71–W77.
66. Yaku, K., Okabe, K., & Nakagawa, T. (2018). NAD Metabolism: Implications in Aging and Longevity. *Ageing Research Reviews, 47*, 1–17.
67. Yu, Z., Zhai, G., Singmann, P., He, Y., Xu, T., Prehn, C., & Illig, T. (2012). Human Serum Metabolic Profiles Are Age Dependent. *Aging Cell, 11*(6), 960–967.
68. Zierle-Ghosh, A., & Jan, A. (2022). Physiology, Body Mass Index. In *StatPearls* [Internet]. StatPearls Publishing: Treasure Island, FL, USA.

Chapter 8

PHYSIOLOGICAL CHANGES ACROSS THE LIFESPAN

Contents

Introduction

Age-related physiological changes are inevitable aspects of the human life cycle. These changes occur across multiple organ systems and can have profound effects on overall health and well-being. Understanding these changes is crucial for healthcare professionals to provide appropriate care and interventions for older adults.

One of the most prominent age-related changes is the decline in organ function, including the cardiovascular, respiratory, musculoskeletal, and nervous systems. For example, the cardiovascular system undergoes structural and functional alterations, such as increased arterial stiffness and decreased cardiac output, leading to a higher risk of cardiovascular diseases (CVDs) in older adults (Lakatta & Levy, 2003). Similarly, the respiratory system experiences reduced lung elasticity and muscle strength, contributing to decreased respiratory function and increased susceptibility to respiratory infections (Gross et al., 1997). Musculoskeletal changes, including loss of muscle mass and bone density, are common in aging populations, leading to sarcopenia and osteoporosis, respectively (Weaver, 2009; Cruz-Jentoft et al., 2010). These changes can result in decreased strength, mobility, and increased risk of falls and fractures in older adults.

Furthermore, age-related changes in the nervous system can lead to cognitive decline and neurodegenerative diseases, such as Alzheimer's disease and Parkinson's disease (Mattson & Magnus, 2006; Schapira, 2008). These changes can significantly impact an individual's quality of life and independence.

In addition to physiological changes, aging is also associated with changes in metabolism, immune function, and endocrine system regulation (Nikolich-Zugich, 2018; Franceschi et al., 2000). These changes can affect the body's ability to maintain homeostasis and respond to stressors, increasing the risk of chronic diseases and functional decline in older adults.

Orientation and Directional Terms

Term	Definition	Illustration
Bone density	The amount of mineral matter per square centimeter of bones, indicating their strength and density.	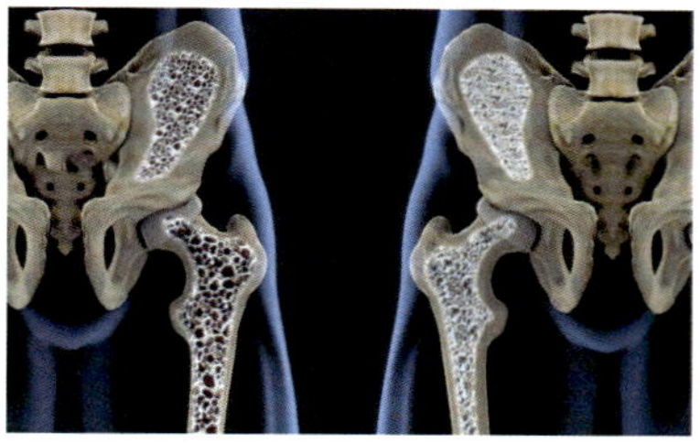
Chronic diseases	Long-lasting conditions that usually can be controlled but not cured, such as diabetes, heart disease.	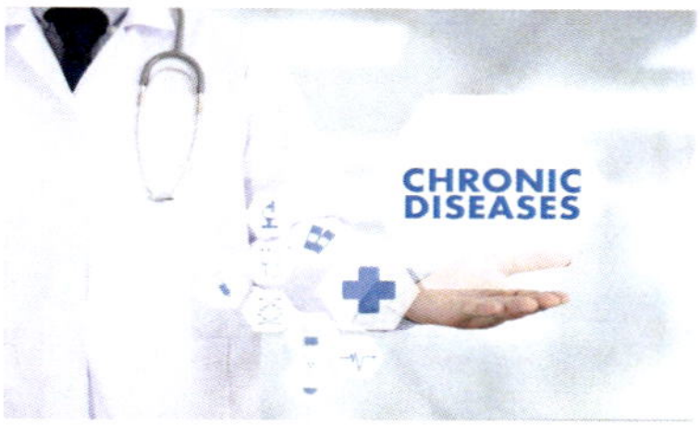
Somatosensory system	A part of the sensory system that processes sensory information from the skin, muscles, and joints.	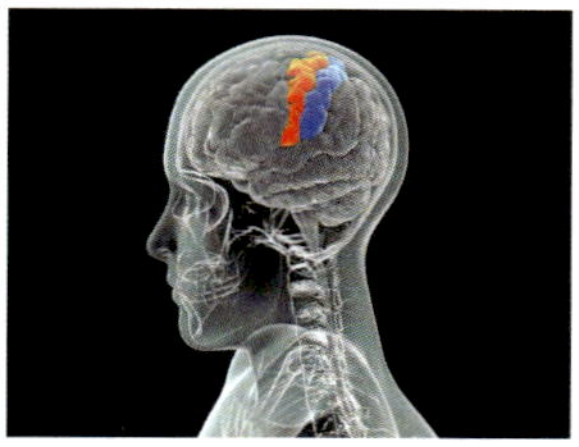
Adipose tissue	Connective tissue in which fat is stored and which has the cells distended by droplets of fat.	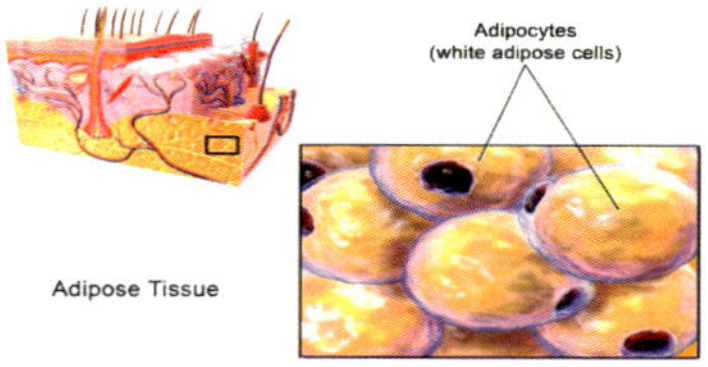
Nerve cells	Also known as neurons, these are the fundamental units of the brain and nervous system responsible for transmitting information throughout the body.	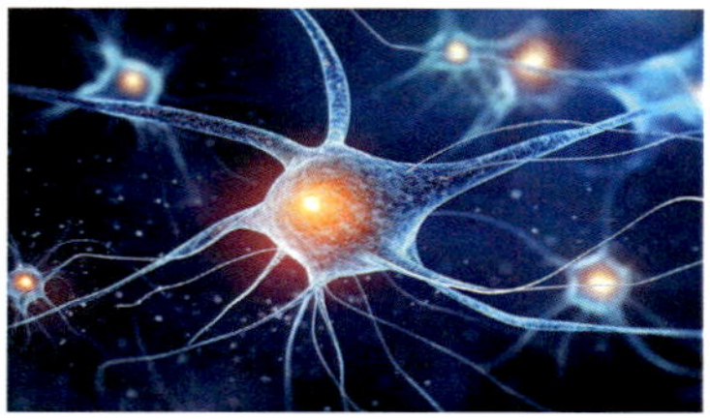
Menopause	The time in a woman's life, typically occurring between ages 45 and 55, when menstrual periods permanently cease.	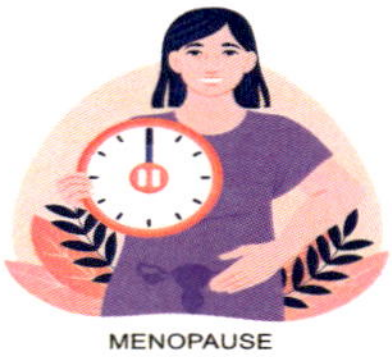

8.1. Changes in Body Composition

The process of aging is characterized by common changes, both visible and imperceptible, in physical structure such as body composition, skin, and hair, which are unavoidable with the passage of time. These changes can be quite noticeable or not noticeable at all. Individuals typically experience a decline in the proportion of their total body weight that can be attributed to water as they age. When there is a reduction in the amount of muscle tissue, there is also an increase in the proportion of adipose tissue that corresponds to this increase. After the age of fifty, there is a gradual decrease in the quantity of muscle fibers, which leads to a decline in the pliability and suppleness of muscle tissue. This, in turn, results in a decrease in the amount of muscle mass. A strenuous exercise routine, on the other hand, has the potential to prevent a significant decline in muscle tone (Rincon, Muzumdar, & Barzilai, 2005). For instance, expert athletes have demonstrated that this is possible. Individuals typically experience weight gain during their middle-aged years; however, after reaching the age of 75, there is a tendency for caloric intake to decrease, which results in weight loss. Among people in their eighties and nineties, the prevalence of obesity is uncommon, and the occurrence of older adults exhibiting exceptional muscle tone is also uncommon (Bartels, Blow, Van Citters, & Brockmann, 2006). Both phenomena are uncommon.

8.2. Changes in the Skin and Hair

Alterations in the visual and tactile qualities of the integumentary system have the potential to exert a negative influence on how elderly people perceive themselves, as well as on how others perceive them from the outside. Because of its direct exposure to environmental factors, the integumentary system of humans is distinct from that of other mammals. This is because humans do not have feathers to provide a protective covering that would mitigate the effects of solar radiation. According to Leland (2008), the primary cause of the aged appearance of skin, which is characterized by wrinkles, dryness, and increased toughness, can be attributed to the detrimental effects of ultraviolet radiation from the sun on the elastic fibers that are located beneath the surface of the skin. The production of melanin by the body, which acts as a protective mechanism, is a consequence of the exposure to the sun that was mentioned earlier. Furthermore, it causes brownish signs of aging or liver spots to appear on the face or hands. This can be a consequence of the condition. According to Ramirez and Schneider (2003), a sizeable proportion of elderly people who are members of ethnic minority groups have a skin type that is rich in melanin and displays a lower incidence of wrinkles. This contrasts with the situation among people of Caucasian descent.

As one gets older, the rate of cellular turnover that occurs within the epidermis, which is the layer of the integumentary system that is the most superficial, slows down. In addition to this, the dermis, which is the second layer of the integumentary system, experiences a decrease in thickness from the beginning of the process. The changes at the cellular level result in a reduction in the elasticity and plumpness of the skin, which in turn causes the skin to take longer to regain its original shape and causes an increase in the amount of sagging and wrinkles that appear on the skin. The elderly population can develop a sunken or emaciated appearance because of the reduction of adipose tissue in the facial region.

A decrease in the function of sweat glands and a decrease in the amount of adipose tissue and hydration in the subcutaneous layers of skin are typical symptoms of aging. According to Lane, Ingram, and Roth (2002), the blood circulation of the skin decreases as people get older. This decrease in blood circulation has the potential to compromise the effectiveness of the skin's thermoregulatory function, making older people more susceptible to extreme temperatures. We have noticed that certain elderly people tend to raise the temperature setting on the thermostat with a greater frequency than other people. To add insult to injury, the process by which they adjust to extremely high temperatures is relatively slower. Because of this, elderly people are more likely to suffer from hypothermia, which is characterized by an abnormally low body temperature, and hyperthermia, which is a condition that indicates heat stroke. According to Martin, Schoeni, and Andreski (2010), you may be familiar with instances in which elderly people have passed away during periods of extreme cold or extended heat waves (Figure 8.1).

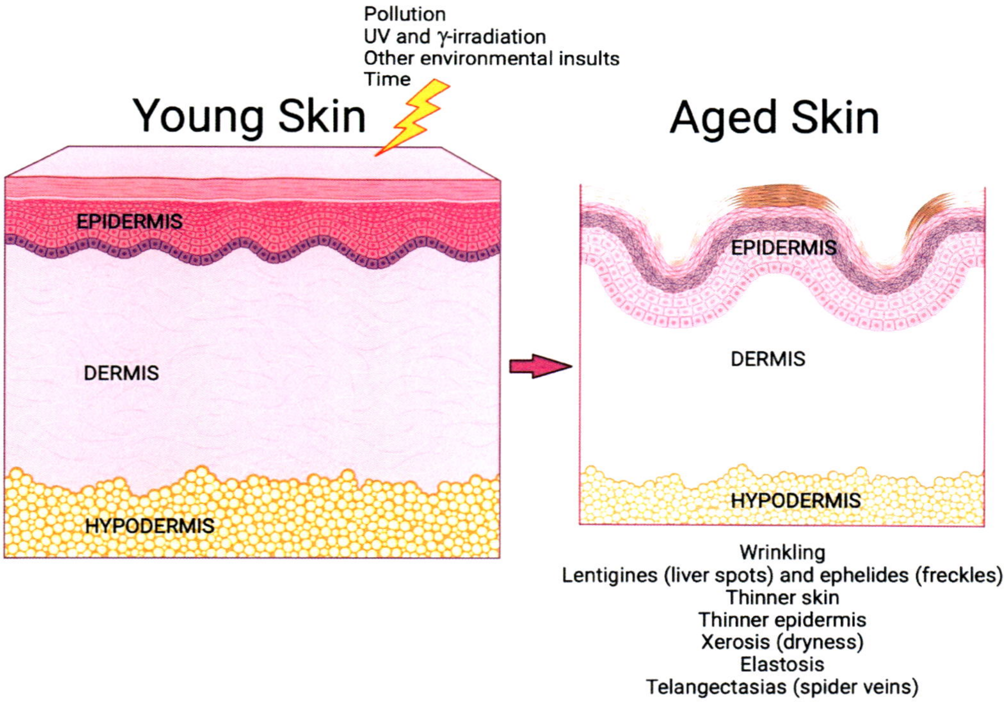

Figure 8.1. *Changes in skin and hairs during aging.*

Source: Agrawal R, Hu A, Bollag WB. The skin and inflamm.-aging. Biology. 2023; 12(11):1396. https://doi.org/10.3390/biology12111396.

The aging process causes changes to occur in the physical characteristics of our hair, including its appearance and texture. These changes occur as we progress through the process. There is a tendency for the diameter of hair to decrease, which results in the appearance of hair that is fine and limp. According to Hayflick (2000), the loss of pigmentation in the hair follicles and at the base of the hair is the phenomenon that causes graying or whitening of the hair. On the other hand, some people do not experience depigmentation throughout their lifetime and are able to achieve a significantly darker hair color even in their later years.

The study of organ systems is an essential component of both the study of anatomy and the study of health. According to Fried et al. (2001), it entails the examination and analysis of the numerous organs and tissues that are interconnected and work together to carry out specific functions within the body.

To comprehend the intricate mechanisms that regulate bodily processes and to preserve overall health and well-being, it is essential to have a solid understanding of the structure and function of organ systems. Since these changes frequently influence the elderly population's subjective state of satisfaction and their capacity to carry out routine activities, it is essential to acquire knowledge about the typical changes that occur in bodily functions (Vigil, 2015).

8.3. Musculoskeletal and Kinesthetic Systems

When it comes to height and muscular strength, some people may be experiencing a decline in their physical attributes. After approximately 25 years of age, the human body reaches its maximum size, strength, and endurance. After this point, there is a gradual decline in the number of cells and their size. After reaching the age of 30, people typically experience a reduction in height of one-sixteenth of an inch because of the passage of time.

It is interesting to note that some people in their seventies or eighties have experienced a decrease in height that is, on average, three inches. The maximum strength that an individual can demonstrate at the age of 80 is approximately 50% like the strength that a person can demonstrate at the age of twenty-five (Kanis et al., 2021). Research has shown that elderly people who maintain a regular routine of physical exercise experience significantly lower levels of decline in their cognitive abilities.

The decrease in bone mineral density and power in the trunk, arms, and legs is the cause of the curvature of the spine as well as the compression of the disks and vertebrae that make up the vertebrae spine.

Because of this, elderly people may display physical manifestations of reduced stature, such as a literal reduction in height or a stooped or hunched posture. This is the reason why elderly people may exhibit these physical manifestations. The collapse of vertebrae because of crush fractures in the spine is the defining characteristic of the medical condition known as kyphosis (Fontana & Klein, 2007).

The narrowing of the shoulder can be attributed to the deterioration of bone density, the reduction in muscular strength, and the reduction in the flexibility of the ligaments. When attempting to access high cupboards or view vehicles approaching from behind, certain elderly individuals may experience difficulties because of a decrease in their range of motion or a loss of upper body movement.

This can be a consequence of the condition. It is not unusual to come across elderly people who declare that they experience stiffness when they first get out of bed in the morning. According to Smith (2004), joint stiffness is a common occurrence that can be attributed to the thickening of cartilage within the joints as well as a reduction in the amount of fluid that lubricates the joints.

The somatosensory system is responsible for providing us with information regarding the position of our being concerning the physical environment that surrounds us. In addition to muscle weakness and decreased visual acuity, older people may exhibit a decreased capacity to accurately perceive their bodily position in physical space (Barry & Trudel, 2014). This is because age-related changes appear in the central nervous system, which is responsible for regulating the kinesthetic system.

When elderly people adopt a slow, shuffling, and purposeful gait, it is a clear indication that they are becoming more vigilant because of the changes in their strength and motor functioning. According to Fries (2002), older people who are deprived of both visual and proprioceptive cues about their spatial orientation may experience postural instability or an inability to maintain an upright stance.

This is because older people are less likely to be able to perceive their surroundings. One may have come across an elderly person who appeared to be in good health but was experiencing symptoms such as dizziness, vertigo, and a sensation of rotational movement. According to Nikolaus and Bach (2003), the elderly population is more likely to experience falls and injuries because of these falls.

This is because the confluence of age-related changes, along with decreased response speed, muscular debilitation, and diminished visual acuity, all contribute to an increased risk of falling.

8.4. Respiratory System

Around one percent of the working or reserve capacity of nearly all organ systems decreases annually after the age of thirty. This is the case for nearly all organ systems.

According to Ito and Barnes (2009), the most rapid decline occurs in fundamentally complex functions, such as vital capacity or maximum breathing capacity. These functions require the coordination of the respiratory, nervous, and muscular systems, and they are also the ones that experience the most rapid decline. Men between the ages of 25 and 70 experience a 50% decrease in the ability of their lungs to take in oxygen through the process of taking a deep breath. Imagine a reduction in volume from six quarts of air to three quarts of air. Make this mental representation.

The repercussions of the changes may become apparent in situations in which an elderly person experiences respiratory distress after climbing multiple flights of stairs on multiple occasions. Even though a decrease in vital capacity might not necessarily have a significant impact on an individual's day-to-day activities, it might cause the individual to move at a slower pace or necessitate taking breaks while climbing or descending stairs (Hornsby, 2002) (Figure 8.2).

When it comes to the physiological systems of the body, the respiratory system is the one that is most susceptible to the negative effects of environmental pollutants and infections. It is observed that the cilia, which are structures that resemble hair and are found in the airways, experience a decrease in both their quantity and their effectiveness in removing foreign particles. Because of this, there is a subsequent reduction in the amount of oxygen that is available.

According to Holloszy and Fontana (2007), the elderly population is more susceptible to chronic bronchitis, emphysema, and pneumonia because of the confluence of this change, which, in addition to compromised air quality and diminished thoracic muscle strength, makes them more susceptible to these conditions.

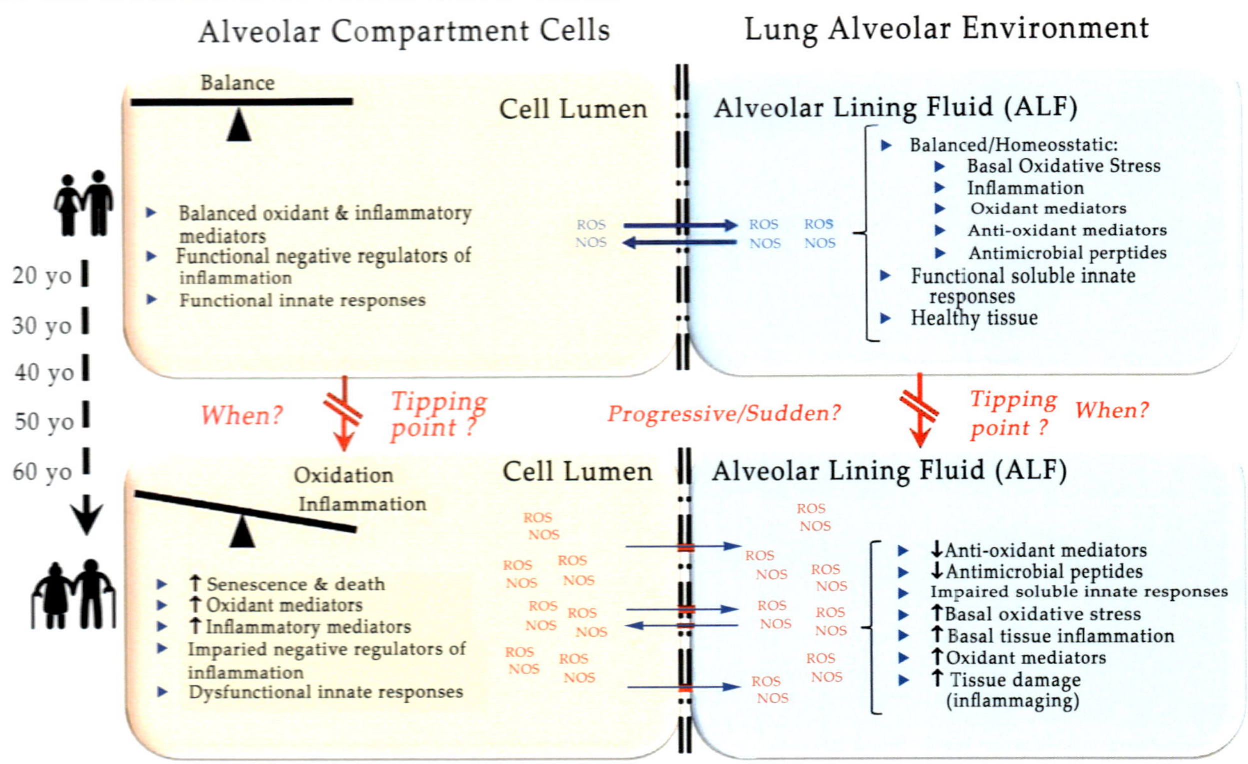

Figure 8.2. *Figure showing aging-related changes in the lungs.*

Source: Torrelles JB, Restrepo BI, Bai Y, Ross C, Schlesinger LS and Turner J (2022) The impact of aging on the lung alveolar environment, predetermining susceptibility to respiratory infections. Front. Aging 3:818700. doi: 10.3389/fragi.2022.818700.

8.5. Cardiovascular Changes

Alterations in the cardiovascular system include the replacement of myocardium with adipose tissue, a decrease in the number of elastic fibers, and an increase in the amount of collagen present in the vasculature. All the changes lead to a decrease in the elastic properties of the arteries, a compromise in the integrity of the vessel walls, and an abnormal dilation of veins that are experiencing elevated pressure, particularly in the lower extremities. Additionally, the accumulation of lipids on the arterial and vessel walls leads to the development of atherosclerosis, a pathological condition that impedes the flow of blood and hinders the pumping action of the heart. This condition prevents the heart from pumping blood effectively. According to Kirkland and Peterson (2009), the consumption of significant quantities of saturated fatty acids in our diet adds to the accumulation of lipids, which is a potentially harmful condition (Figure 8.3).

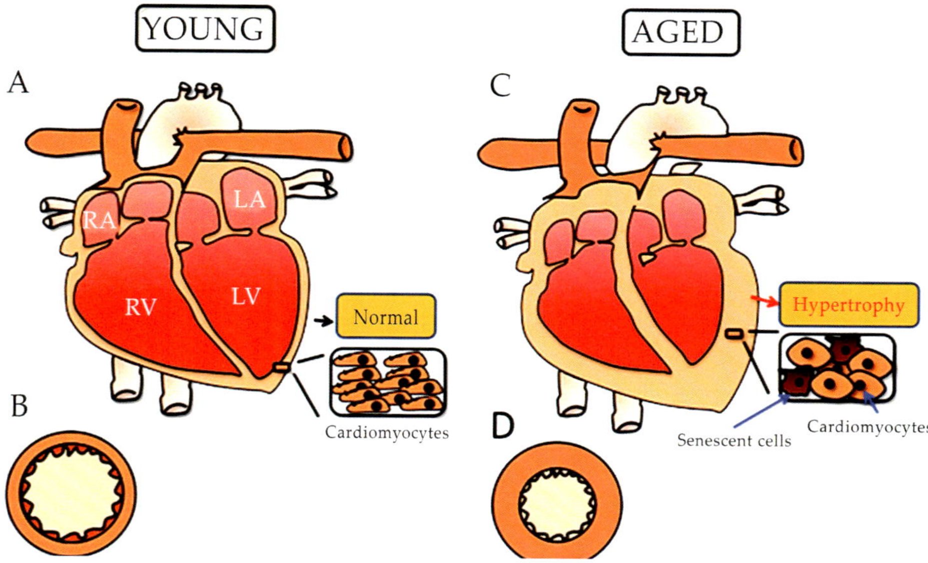

Figure 8.3. *Cardiovascular changes with aging.*

Source: Shaik, S., Wang, Z., Inuzuka, H., Liu, P., & Wei, W. (2013). Endothelium aging and vascular diseases. InTech. doi: 10.5772/53065.

During the natural process of aging, there is a certain degree of elevation in blood pressure that occurs, even in the absence of any indications of cardiovascular pathology. This does not mean that there is no evidence of cardiovascular pathology. Nevertheless, according to Emlet (2006), abnormally high blood pressure is a significant increase. On the contrary, it is associated with an unhealthy eating pattern, obesity, and a sedentary way of life, all of which have effects that are detrimental for a long period of time. According to de Cabo Moreno (2000), the changes that occur in the cardiovascular and respiratory systems lead to a diminished capacity to make efficient use of oxygen. Consequently, this contributes to a reduction in the elderly person's capacity to engage in prolonged physical activity. Despite this, engaging in physical activity can result in a significant reduction in blood pressure as well as an increase in aerobic capacity. It has been observed that the physical training regimen of older master athletes results in a greater decrease in cholesterol levels, a higher oxygen volume, and an increase in lean body weight when compared to their counterparts who engage in sedentary activities (Lefevre et al., 2009).

Nevertheless, it is important to make note of the fact that these results are still lower than those that were observed in younger athletes. Nevertheless, individuals who engage in moderate exercise can still derive certain benefits from their physical activity. According to the findings of the study, the aerobic capacity of older people experiences a significant improvement after participating in a training program that lasts for twenty-four weeks and consists of either low-intensity or high-intensity exercises, such as walking or jogging for thirty minutes. All the discoveries offer a rationale for a positive outlook, which is that alterations in our way of life can improve our physical well-being, even when we are in our octogenarian years.

Nevertheless, it is not possible to eliminate the typical physiological changes that occur with aging and have the potential to be detrimental to our performance (Hayflick, 1994).

8.6. Urinary System

Within the body, the renal system is responsible for filtering blood and urine through a complex network of tubes and capillaries. This system plays a significant role in the maintenance of the body's internal homeostasis. No matter whether there are any underlying pathologies, the glomerular filtration rate is the metric that determines the most significant decline in renal function with age. This decline occurs regardless of whether there are any other underlying pathologies. In the process of regulating fluid concentration and dilution, the renal system experiences a decline in its ability to take in glucose. Elderly people may have a more difficult time tolerating medications that are eliminated through filtration because of this phenomenon, which leads to increased problems with dehydration and a decrease in blood sodium levels (Jacobs, 2007) (Figure 8.4).

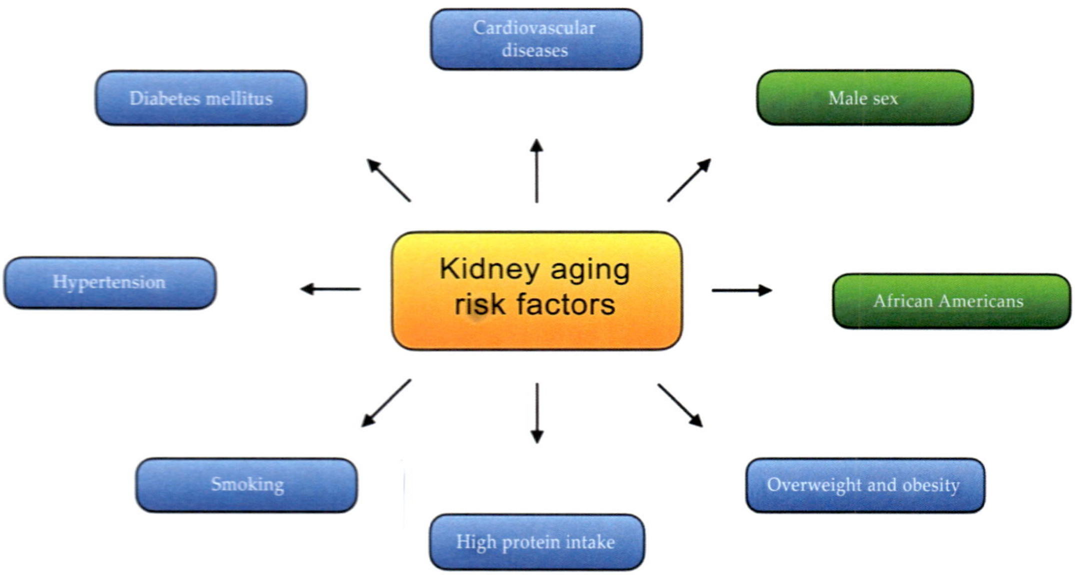

Figure 8.4. *Aging and the kidney.*

Source: Dybiec J, Szlagor M, Młynarska E, Rysz J, Franczyk B. Structural and functional changes in aging kidneys. International Journal of Molecular Sciences. 2022; 23(23):15435. https://doi.org/10.3390/ijms232315435.

There is a possibility that the capacity of the bladder could decrease by as much as fifty percent, and the sensation of the need to urinate could remain delayed. urinary incontinence or urine leakage affects approximately 50% of elderly people who live in their own homes, and a significantly higher percentage of those who are residing in nursing homes. Having the condition of incontinence has the potential to have a significant impact on the social and living circumstances of an individual for that person. According to Schultz et al., (2003), it is frequently the point at which the family's ability to provide care from the comfort of their own home is exceeded, which ultimately results in the individual being placed in a skilled nursing facility.

8.7. Incontinence

Specific situations can lead to certain results, such as the use of drugs, sudden illnesses, or infections in the bladder or urinary tract. These outcomes can be resolved by using antibiotics, as long as the cause is determined. Medical practitioners should assess other physiological factors, such as neurological changes associated with Parkinson's disease and dementia, prostate issues, anemia, diabetes, and various types of cancer (Nelson et al., 2006).

It is crucial to refrain from assuming that incontinence is a permanent condition. Some doctors may suggest using drugs as a treatment, but this often leads to negative side effects. Non-pharmacological approaches to behavior management, such as reducing fluid intake before sleep, engaging in physical activity, using biofeedback, and practicing structured exercises for the pelvic muscles and Kegels to maintain sphincter muscle tone, often produce similar results (Phelan, Anderson, Lacroix, & Larson, 2004). Studies indicate that a substantial percentage of women who seek medical intervention for incontinence observe an amelioration or complete disappearance of their symptoms, with around 80% reporting favorable results. Enhancing their overall quality of life is linked to the improvement of these symptoms. Throughout the entire country, there are support groups that are made available and sponsored by organizations such as the National Association for Incontinence (Specht, 2005).

Unfortunately, because incontinence is often stigmatized, senior citizens and their relatives often lack information about possible treatment options. Many healthcare providers neglect to inquire about bladder issues. The widespread reluctance to acknowledge incontinence can lead to substantial psychological and social repercussions, including social isolation, accidents, bone fractures, and even placement in long-term care institutions (Goode, Burgio, Richter, & Markland, 2010).

8.8. Gastrointestinal System

Changes in the esophagus can result in decreased muscle contractions and an extended duration of the cardiac sphincter, a valve-like structure that helps food move into the stomach. Essentially, this means that the time it takes for food to reach the stomach is prolonged. The result may potentially appear as a feeling of fullness before eating a complete meal. As a result, this can cause a decline in the pleasure derived from eating food and subsequently lead to insufficient nutritional intake. This phenomenon explains why certain elderly individuals tend to eat small amounts during meals, which worries their family members (Dalton et al., 2003).

Individuals over the age of 50 typically experience a decline in the production of digestive juices in the stomach. Older individuals may be more prone to persistent inflammation of the gastric mucosa, which can make them more susceptible to colon and stomach malignancies. Therefore, it is advisable for older individuals who suffer from heartburn or digestive problems to seek medical treatment instead of relying on self-care methods or over-the-counter medications (Brunet-Rossinni & Austad, 2005). Age-related physiological changes in the small intestine result in a decline in enzyme levels and a slower rate of absorption of simple sugars, ultimately leading to reduced efficiency. Changes in the functioning of the colon have been associated with an increased occurrence of chronic constipation. Nevertheless, it is probable that factors related to behavior, such as eating patterns and levels of physical activity, have a more significant impact than changes in anatomy (Margolis et al., 2008) (Figure 8.5).

Main pathogenic mechanisms involved in age-related changes in gastrointestinal system	
Neurological (central)	Impariment in cognitive functions Impariment in swallowing mechanisms
Neurological (peripheral)	Imparied esophageal peristalsis Disturbance in function of lower esophageal sphincter Slowing of gastric emptying Increased colonic transit time
Metabolic	Impaired glucose, lipid and bile acid metabolism Electrolyte disorders
Immunological	Imbalance between anti-inflammatory and pro-inflammatory cytokines Impairment of innate immune system
Microbiome-related	Alterations in composition, diversity and functional features of intestinal microbiota
Drug-induced	Mucosal injury Impaired motility Dysregulation of immune and microbiome homeostasis
Aging-realted fraiiliy	Age-related decline in physiolgical function and adaptive capacity

Figure 8.5. *Main pathogenic mechanisms involved in age-related changes in GI system.*

Source: Gallo A, Pellegrino S, Pero E, Agnitelli MC, Parlangeli C, Landi F, Montalto M. Main disorders of gastrointestinal tract in older people: An overview. Gastrointestinal Disorders. 2024; 6(1):313–336. https://doi.org/10.3390/gidisord6010022.

8.9. Endocrine System

As individuals age, the small intestine experiences functional changes that result in a decrease in enzyme levels and a slowdown in the absorption rate of monosaccharides. This ultimately leads to reduced effectiveness. Physiological changes in the colon have been linked to a higher occurrence of persistent constipation. Behavioral factors, such as dietary patterns and physical activity levels, are likely to have a greater influence than anatomical changes (Starr & Weiner, 1981).

8.10. Immune System

Traditionally, there was a widespread belief that the aging process inevitably causes a decrease in the immune system's effectiveness, leading to immunodeficiency and increased susceptibility to infections and diseases in older people. Moreover, there exists a connection between the altered immune function and age-related conditions such as skin and prostate cancers, as well as cardiovascular disorders (Vincent et al., 2002). Nevertheless, recent research has refuted this assumption. Studies on centenarians, individuals who have reached the age of 100, have shown that their immune responses are significantly more effective compared to certain young-old individuals. Based on the high occurrence of infections as the primary cause of death in individuals aged 80 and above, it can be deduced that their immune system may have become ineffective in these cases (Masoro, 2007).

8.11. Nervous System

The human brain consists of many neurons, also known as nerve cells, which decrease in number as a person ages. It is worth mentioning that the process of neuronal degeneration begins at the age of 30. A slight reduction in the number of neurons does not lead to a noticeable decline in cognitive function. Contrary to common assumptions, a decrease in the number of neurons does not inevitably lead to slight memory loss, as we can still operate effectively with a reduced number of neurons. When it comes to dementia, changes in brain tissue, blood flow, and receptor organs may be more significant than the amount of neuronal loss (Hanlon et al., 2009).

The decrease in brain mass or weight as one gets older is most likely caused by a decline in fluid content. Nevertheless, the difficulties faced in problem-solving, or memory retrieval cannot be solely ascribed to the slight alterations in the size and structure of the brain (Coffey et al., 1998).

Nevertheless, cognitive and motor function may be partially impaired because of neuronal degeneration, changes in neurotransmitters associated with aging, and reduced blood circulation, resulting in a slower reaction time.

Many middle-aged individuals commonly experience concerns about a decline in their reflexes and an increase in the time it takes for them to process information and respond. Elderly individuals may have slower reaction times when performing tasks such as answering a phone call or doorbell, crossing a street, or making decisions compared to younger individuals.

Many elderly individuals adjust to their surroundings and routines by making innovative changes, such as leaving their home an hour before a nearby event, choosing less crowded shopping locations, and avoiding driving during busy traffic times. In summary, the brain has a substantial reserve capacity that compensates for the usual declines associated with aging (Manton, Gu, & Lowrimore, 2008) (Figure 8.6).

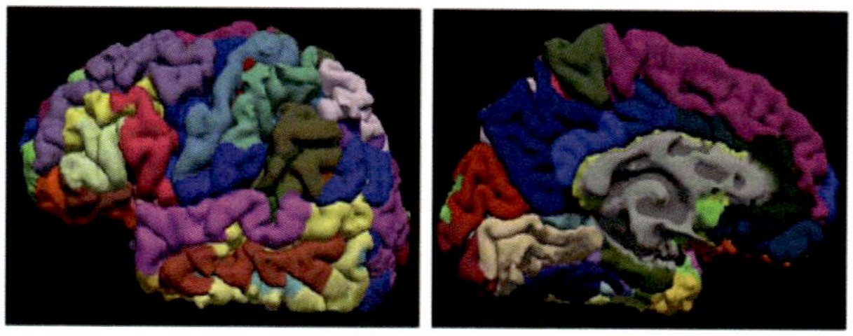

Figure 8.6. *Aging and the brain.*

Source: Gómez-Ramírez J, Fernández-Blázquez MA, González-Rosa JJ. Prediction of chronological age in healthy elderly subjects with machine learning from MRI brain segmentation and cortical parcellation. Brain Sciences. 2022; 12(5):579. https://doi.org/10.3390/brainsci12050579.

8.12. Physiological Changes and Sexuality

There is a common misconception that the physiological changes that come with aging have a negative effect on sexual functioning. Initial studies on sexuality led to the development of certain misunderstandings, as investigations into the sexual behavior of older individuals were rarely carried out or focused solely on the extent of sexual activity. The studies did not consider the subjective or qualitative aspects of sexuality in the elderly population, including the sexual experiences of LGBT individuals (Pearson et al., 2008).

There is no significant correlation between age and changes in the frequency and quality of sexual experiences, whether positive or negative. When sexual activity is broadly defined to encompass actions like hugging, kissing, showing affection, physical closeness, and self-stimulation, it has the capacity to be equally or even more satisfying than in earlier stages of life. The groundbreaking research conducted by Masters and Johnson in 1981 demonstrated that age-related physiological changes do not significantly hinder the capacity to participate in and experience pleasure from sexual activity in older age (Masters & Johnson, 1981). A study conducted by Poindexter and Emlet (2006) found that elderly participants perceived their sexual experiences to be either equal to or better than those they had in their younger years.

Follow-up research has shown that a notable percentage of individuals who are 50 years old and older, including those in their 80s and 90s, participate in sexual activity. People experience a significant degree of sexual satisfaction and arousal, pleasure, and enjoyment. The presence of a partner does not have a significant impact on the sexual frequency of older individuals who continue to engage in sexual activity. Nevertheless, their personal perception may differ from earlier periods of life because of physiological changes linked to the process of aging (Bancroft, 2007).

8.12.1. Women and Age-related Physiological Changes

Menopause is marked by a decrease in estrogen and progesterone levels, which are the main physiological factors that cause changes in women's sexual function and pleasure. Menopause is a natural stage in a woman's life marked by the gradual stoppage of the menstrual cycle as a result of a decrease in reproductive ability (Benyamini, Blumstein, Lusky, & Modan, 2003).

The inevitability of a "menopausal syndrome" cannot be established due to the considerable variation in symptoms and reactions observed among individuals. One may have experienced situations where maternal or ancestral figures have expressed discontentment with hot flashes, which are characterized by a sudden sensation of warmth in the upper body, often accompanied by excessive sweating. These phenomena occur when the nervous system shows an excessive reaction to decreases in hormone levels (Control & Prevention, 2015). This phenomenon affects the hypothalamus, which controls body temperature, causing the expansion or narrowing of blood vessels. Following a stimulus, blood is directed towards the outer layer of the skin, leading to the production of sweat, reddening of the skin, and an increase in both heart rate and body temperature. Hot flashes generally do not hinder a woman's sexual functioning or cause psychological difficulties. The occurrence of hot flashes in certain women while absent in others remains unexplained from a scientific standpoint (Nelson et al., 2006).

Menopause may lead to undesirable symptoms like vaginal wall thinning, but it does not have a physiological effect on an individual's capacity to fully participate in sexual activity. Typically, the sexual response cycle of an older woman includes the same aspects as that of younger women, but with a longer delay in responding to sexual stimulation. Indeed, some women who no longer have worries about getting pregnant have reported experiencing increased levels of sexual satisfaction (Bergman et al., 2007). The sexual behavior of older women is often influenced more by sociocultural norms rather than physiological changes. This can be observed in different forms, including the limited availability of male partners for heterosexual women, the negative societal judgment towards lesbian relationships among older women, and the general perception of older women as lacking sexual appeal (Schriner et al., 2005).

8.12.2. Men and Age-related Physiological Changes

The hormonal rhythms in males have received less attention compared to those of women. Increasing evidence indicates that male menopause, also referred to as micropause, may indeed happen, although it progresses more slowly. The progressive decrease in testosterone levels in men, which occurs at an average rate of approximately 1 percent per year, is less abrupt when compared to the rapid reduction of estrogen in women undergoing menopause. The decline in testosterone levels affects the sexual response of males. The modifications may involve reduced muscle mass and strength, as well as decreased levels of calcium in the skeletal system (Covinsky, Lindquist, Dunlop, & Yelin, 2009).

The study conducted by Lindau et al. (2007) identified two primary health issues: a decline in immune system responsiveness and a variety of psychological symptoms such as fatigue, irritability, indecisiveness, depression, diminished self-esteem, listlessness, reduced appetite, and difficulties with concentration. Although these physiological changes may not directly hinder sexual performance or reduce sexual pleasure, they can potentially alter the nature of the sexual response. According to Lindau et al. (2007), even as men get older, they still find sexual activity to be enjoyable and satisfying.

Although not a universally occurring consequence of aging, erectile dysfunction or impotence, which refers to the inability to achieve and sustain an erection, is the main sexual problem encountered by older males. The factors mentioned above, specifically diseases, age-related deterioration of blood vessels, decreased testosterone levels, and the frequent consumption of tobacco, drugs, or alcohol, are accountable for this condition. It is crucial to provide mature males and their partners with knowledge about the physiological causes of erectile dysfunction, as well as its widespread occurrence and the available treatment options that can be effective (Wierzalis et al., 2006). In recent times, there has been a significant increase in interest in innovative methods for managing erectile dysfunction. The marketing tactics utilized by pharmaceutical companies for different products, such as Viagra and Levitra, can be partially attributed to their acknowledgment of the baby boomer generation's heightened inclination to openly discuss and actively seek sexual satisfaction (Johnson, 2013).

Healthcare professionals may reinforce the idea that sexuality in the elderly population is abnormal. Based on a study, only 38% of men and 22% of women have reported having conversations about sexual health with a medical professional once they turn 50 years old. Healthcare practitioners should routinely inquire about sexual satisfaction, identify possible obstacles and solutions to establishing a satisfying sexual partnership, and address concerns related to sexually transmitted infections and unsafe sexual practices. The older adult sexuality of the LGBT community is affected by a broader range of problems compared to the heterosexual community, primarily due to the existence of homophobia. Research conducted by Connolly et al. (2012) has revealed that the presence of historical social restrictions regarding same-sex relationships negatively impacts the sexual expression of numerous LGBT elders.

8.13. Some Other Physiological Changes

8.13.1. Sleep Patterns

Elderly individuals may potentially manifest discontentment regarding the quality of their sleep. This phenomenon is prevalent among a substantial portion of the elderly population, reaching up to 40%. As people get older, it takes longer for them to fall asleep, and they wake up more often during the night. Older individuals demonstrate a proclivity for shallow sleep, making them more prone to frequent interruptions in their sleep patterns. When individuals try to make up for their lack of sleep by taking more daytime naps, it can disturb their nighttime sleep even more. Patients who inform their primary healthcare provider about their sleep disturbances are often advised to consider pharmacological interventions, such as sedative-hypnotic medications. It is important to acknowledge that pharmacological interventions may not always improve the quality of an individual's sleep cycle (Lesage & Scharf, 2007).

8.13.2. Sensory Functions

As individuals grow older, their sensory faculties, such as vision, hearing, touch, taste, and smell, generally diminish in comparison to younger individuals. Some individuals may have already noticed changes in their sensory perceptions. People typically reach their peak abilities in their twenties, maintain this optimal state for a short time, and then experience a gradual decline, which becomes more pronounced after reaching middle age. Nevertheless, there is considerable variation in the rates at which sensory decline occurs (Swain & Nikolich-Zugich, 2009). Some elderly individuals may have better vision or hearing than their 25-year-old peers, a trait that they may have had since they were young. Elderly individuals exhibit intra-individual variations. The auditory sense may experience early deterioration, while the gustatory and tactile senses tend to remain relatively stable until the later stages of aging. The diminishing sensory capacities can influence the social functioning of aging individuals. As these changes happen gradually, people adapt by using their other senses or changing their behavior (like getting closer to an object to see better) and environment (like choosing quiet restaurants to socialize with friends) (Wolf et al., 1996).

8.13.3. Visual Perception

It is conceivable that people may know others who once had flawless vision throughout their lives, but later in their forties, they may need reading glasses or face difficulties in reading street signs or perceiving variations in color. The incidence of vision impairments increases significantly as individuals age, impacting around 14% of individuals aged 65 and older, and 23% of those aged 85 and older. These impairments can cause challenges in carrying out everyday tasks and even increase the risk of falls and fractures (Berkman, 2006).

The cornea is usually the first part of the eye to undergo changes in the ocular system. The object's surface undergoes a transformation marked by a gradual thickening, a decrease in curvature, and a potential departure from a regular geometric shape. The eye displays a diminished luster and a lower degree of transparency. Occasionally, a deposit rich in lipids may form around the outer edge of the cornea. Nevertheless, this does not have any noticeable impact on visual perception. The pupils' sensitivity to changes in light intensity decreases, causing their aperture to shrink to approximately 66% of its original size (Whitfield & Hayward, 2003). These modifications make it difficult to see in dim lighting or adjust to changes in light levels. Research has shown that older individuals may need lighting that is three times brighter than what younger people need to perform tasks at their best. People may have difficulty perceiving visual stimuli in low light contrast situations, such as driving a vehicle during twilight or in foggy conditions. To adjust, older individuals may choose not to drive in bad weather, heavy traffic, or at night when bright headlights create glare on different surfaces

(Crews & Campbell, 2004). Presbyopia is a prevalent physiological occurrence among the majority of older individuals. It is characterized by changes in the shape and flexibility of the lens, resulting in diminished ability to see objects up close. It is possible that people you know may show the behavior of holding their reading materials far away or needing bifocals and reading guidance. The mentioned physiological changes simultaneously reduce the ability to adjust, thus hindering the perception of objects with clarity when shifting visual attention from close to far distances. This can result in a feeling of being watchful and anxious while driving or walking, as well as challenges with visually scanning tasks like observing a room, going up or down stairs, or writing notes while looking at a chalkboard. The combination of the cornea's irregular flattened surface and its poor light refraction often results in increased sensitivity to glare. The described situation presents difficulties in environments where there is only one source of light that is directed towards a surface that reflects light, such as streetlights on a wet road or a bright incandescent light shining on a linoleum floor (Walford, 1969).

Individuals aged 75 and above, particularly in low-light conditions and without orientation cues, undergo a substantial decrease in their ability to perceive depth and distance. Some examples of these cues include stairs that do not have contrasting colors at the ends, as well as pedestrian ramps or curb cuts that have uneven slopes. Older individuals may be surprised when a fast-moving object like a car or bicycle suddenly appears without warning due to their reduced peripheral vision, which is the ability to see objects on the sides without moving their eyes or head. Older drivers may have trouble perceiving vehicles approaching from the left or right when driving through an intersection or passing another vehicle (Reddy Thavanati, Kanala, De Dios, & Cantu Garza, 2008). As people get older, the clarity of the eye lens decreases, leading to a decrease in the amount of light that passes through. However, some older individuals may experience a more noticeable clouding of the lens in their eyes, which decreases the amount of light that can pass through and leads to vision problems. Cataract is a common medical condition that causes visual impairment in individuals aged 80 and above. Other symptoms that may be present include diplopia (double vision), difficulties with chromatic discrimination (difficulty distinguishing colors), and photophobia (sensitivity to light), which can occur both during the day and at night (Strawbridge, Wallhagen, Shema, & Kaplan, 2000).

If the lens is completely opaque, it is recommended to undergo cataract surgery. Asbell et al. (2005) found that the outpatient surgical procedure frequently performed on older adults carries minimal risk and can improve their daily functioning and overall quality of life. Glaucoma is a condition of the eye that occurs when there is an excessive production of aqueous humor, resulting in elevated pressure within the eye and compression of the optic nerve. When detected in its initial phases, the condition can be efficiently controlled by following a daily routine of applying eye drops. The disease's slow progression and lack of noticeable symptoms can hinder early detection, leading to its development in later stages. As a result, the person may have a limited field of vision, which can hinder their ability to navigate safely. If the condition is severe, surgical intervention or laser therapy may be required to prevent the possibility of vision loss (Asbell et al., 2005).

Macular degeneration is a condition that causes a decrease in sharpness of vision in the central area of the visual field. The condition typically begins with a decrease in visual clarity, followed by a gradual decline in central vision, making activities like reading and driving impractical. When elderly individuals depend on their remaining peripheral vision, they may instinctively focus their eyes on the shoulder area of the person they are talking to, even though they are using their peripheral vision to see the person's face.

The incidence of macular degeneration demonstrates a more significant rise with progressive age in comparison to cataracts. Although a definitive cure for retinal damage has not yet been found, several treatments have been created to reduce its impact by slowing down the advancement of the condition and improving the quality of central vision (Schultz et al., 2003; Schiebinger & Schraudner, 2011).

While it is true that many older individuals experience visual impairment, it is important to highlight that there are various low-tech assistive devices available at a relatively affordable price to enhance their visual acuity and overall quality of life. Multiple aids of this kind are accessible.

- High-wattage light bulbs
- Fluorescent lighting with color correction
- Labels with larger font sizes for prescription bottles, spices, and cooking supplies
- Printed materials with larger font sizes such as newspapers, books, calendars, and phone directories.
- Various assistive devices can aid individuals with visual impairments in performing daily tasks. These devices include books, clocks, playing cards, and magnifying glasses for instances in which large-print substitutes are unavailable. Audiotapes of books, needle threaders for sewing, and appliances with large numbers are also useful.
- Flat-screen computer monitors with large fonts designed to reduce glare and voice-activated computer software can also benefit those with visual impairments.
- Minor modifications can enhance the safety of living and working spaces for elderly individuals experiencing visual impairments.
- Here are several examples.
- It is recommended to distinctly demarcate edges and corners, including but not limited to stairs, walls, doorsills, curbs, and curb cuts, by utilizing texture or colors that are significantly different from each other and lie on the opposite ends of the color spectrum. For instance, red and yellow or green and orange can be employed to enhance depth perception.
- The utilization of contrasting colors and light coding is recommended for demarcating ramps and other alterations in elevation.
- Installing floor coverings that are nonslip and nonglossy is recommended to enhance safety and prevent accidents.
- It is recommended to refrain from utilizing a high-gloss coating on walls or large windows at the terminus of a lengthy, dimly lit corridor, as it may result in excessive glare.
- Increase the number of illumination fixtures and implement dimming functionality.
- Switches are utilized to modify the levels of illumination.
- It is recommended to utilize indirect or task lighting, such as reading and countertop lamps (Bryant & Frankel, 2020).

8.13.4. Hearing

The senses of sight and hearing are the most essential sensory modalities that establish our connection with the outside world. Vision allows us to navigate and engage with the physical surroundings, while hearing facilitates communication. Around 46% of older males and 31% of older females have problems with their hearing, and these rates increase to almost 60% in the oldest age groups. Presbycusis, or age-related hearing loss, is defined by a diminished ability to detect sounds in terms of their volume and range, as well as a possible distortion of perceived sounds. The cochlea, a circular and spiral-shaped organ in the inner ear, undergoes the most pronounced decline in hearing ability as individuals grow older (Chipperfield, 2008). The perception and positioning of sounds, especially at a lower intensity and high pitch, are affected by the oscillation of hair cells in the cochlea. Changes in auditory thresholds can be detected by the age of 30. However, the degradation of hair cells and membranes in the cochlea is usually not observed until a later stage (Agrawal et al., 2008).

Indicators of hearing impairment encompass the subsequent manifestations:

- We experience difficulty discerning high-frequency consonants such as z, s, sh, f, p, k, t, and g, which has a detrimental impact on our comprehension.
- Exhibiting a growing tendency to frequently request individuals to reiterate their previous statements.
- Increasing the audio output of the television or radio or positioning oneself in closer proximity to it
- Engaging in social withdrawal (Dalton et al., 2003)

You may have observed that environmental factors have a substantial impact on the development of hearing loss. Individuals who are consistently exposed to loud and frequent noise over the course of their lives, such as city residents, construction workers, and factory workers, tend to have more hearing problems compared to those who live in quiet rural areas. The prevalence of hearing loss in individuals aged 18–44 is experiencing a substantial rise. Future generations of older individuals will probably experience increased rates of hearing loss that can be attributed to environmental factors they were exposed to earlier in life. This could include listening to loud music on MP3 players during their teenage years and early adulthood (Wingfield et al., 2007).

Older individuals experiencing hearing impairments can reduce negative impacts by implementing behavioral and social interaction modifications using the following strategies:

- Amplifying the sound output of electronic devices like televisions, phones, and radios can improve the ability to hear higher-frequency sounds and significantly enhance the recognition of consonants such as p, t, k, b, d, and g by a margin of 50 to 90 percent.
- It is advisable to listen to music created by instruments that have a lower pitch, such as the organ.
- Look for environments that suppress or reduce visitation.
- Background noises.
- For the best user experience, it is recommended to use telephones that have volume adjusters and illuminated indicators that flash when a call is received.
- Use an auditory assistive device (Kiyak, 1996).

Older individuals may face difficulties in adjusting to the use of hearing aids. Inexpensive assistive devices can only enhance sound, especially background sounds. Modern hearing aids are fitted with small computer chips that can filter sounds to match the specific hearing loss pattern of each user, while also preventing the amplification of background noises. The newer designs demonstrate decreased visibility and enhanced compatibility with the ear canal. However, the costs related to them are roughly double and usually not covered by insurance (Oberdoerffer et al., 2008).

A considerable proportion of elderly individuals display hesitancy in embracing a hearing aid owing to the financial costs involved and unfavorable societal attitudes. After President Clinton, who was in his fifties at the time, received a digital hearing aid in 1997, there was a notable increase in the sales of hearing aids. Based on the research conducted by Crews and Campbell in 2004, only 12% of elderly individuals with hearing loss had chosen to use hearing aids after six years. What other factors could explain why we are less likely to use hearing aids compared to wearing eyeglasses? (Ohayon et al., 2004).

8.13.5. Taste and Smell

While some older individuals may complain about the taste of food, it is improbable that these complaints are caused by age-related changes. Slight decreases in the number of taste buds do not necessarily lead to a decline in taste perception, and there is a considerable amount of variation both within and among individuals. Some elderly individuals may encounter difficulties in discerning varying levels of flavor intensity, such as the bitterness in coffee or the saltiness in food. Nevertheless, they might have an easier time distinguishing different level of sweetness (Hodes, 2006). The sense of smell is also a vital component in the enjoyment of food. The decrease in the sense of smell caused by aging is more noticeable than the decrease in the sense of taste. Among elderly individuals, there is a tendency to increase the amount of salt and sugar in their meals, which goes against the dietary advice given by their healthcare providers. Older individuals demonstrate diminished sensitivity to airborne stimuli, such as the fragrance of a flower, when compared to younger individuals. Research has demonstrated that adding herbs, spices, and color to food can improve the ability of elderly individuals to taste and smell, making the food more enjoyable and increasing their intake of essential nutrients. The absence of the ability to smell and taste is not just a decrease in pleasurable experiences, but it can potentially lead to dangers such as unhealthy eating habits, isolation from social interactions, and the inability to detect dangerous smells like smoke (Markovic et al., 2007).

8.13.6. Touch

The decrease in tactile sensitivity, specifically in the fingertips, palms, and lower limbs, is a result of age-related changes in the skin and a decrease in the number of nerve endings. The modifications affect the performance of everyday tasks that require the sensitivity of the fingertips, such as retrieving medication from a pill container (Forman et al., 2018).

Pain perception is a crucial aspect of tactile sensitivity. With advancing age, older individuals experience a decrease in the efficiency of nerve cells in their skin, resulting in a diminished ability to differentiate between different levels of painful stimuli compared to younger individuals. One negative outcome is that older individuals may experience more serious burns because they react slower to a hot object, which can lead to a delay in receiving timely help (Perreault et al., 2009). Pain tolerance is a subjective perception. There is a portion of the older population that is increasingly showing signs of discomfort, while another group chooses to minimize their pain by not talking about it. Alternatively, some individuals may hold the belief that pain is an affliction that must be endured without any form of remedy. Using spices in cooking can enhance both the sense of smell and taste sensitivity. Underreporting, the act of failing to report signs of a heart attack, can lead to significant negative consequences (Orban et al., 2009).

Elderly individuals have shown the ability to adjust to the physiological changes that come with aging. They often find innovative ways to cope with these changes while still considering themselves to be relatively healthy. Our attention now turns to chronic illnesses, which are not considered to be a normal or inevitable part of aging, but their occurrence does tend to increase as people get older (Palmer et al., 2010).

A Closer Look

Menopause in Aging

Menopause marks a significant physiological milestone in the aging process of women. Typically occurring around the age of 45 to 55, menopause is characterized by the cessation of menstrual periods due to declining ovarian function and hormonal changes. This transition is primarily driven by a decrease in estrogen and progesterone production, leading to various physical and emotional changes.

Physiologically, menopause is associated with symptoms such as hot flashes, night sweats, vaginal dryness, and changes in libido. These symptoms vary in intensity and duration among individuals. Hormonal fluctuations during menopause can also contribute to mood swings, anxiety, and difficulty concentrating, impacting mental well-being.

Beyond its immediate effects, menopause influences long-term health outcomes. Estrogen decline affects bone density, increasing the risk of osteoporosis and fractures. Cardiovascular health also becomes a concern, as estrogen plays a protective role against heart disease before menopause. Managing these risks often involves lifestyle adjustments, including regular exercise, a balanced diet rich in calcium and vitamin D, and sometimes hormone replacement therapy (HRT) to alleviate symptoms and reduce long-term health risks.

Psychologically, menopause can be a time of introspection and adaptation to changes in self-image and identity. Support networks and healthcare guidance are crucial during this phase to address physical symptoms and emotional well-being effectively.

Therefore, menopause represents a complex interplay of biological, psychological, and social factors in the aging process of women. Understanding its implications and providing appropriate support can significantly enhance the quality of life during and after this natural transition.

Summary

- The analysis of physiological changes provides evidence of the gradual aging process. It shows that certain organ systems may start experiencing the effects of aging in the twenties and thirties, while others may progress more rapidly after the age of 70 or 80. Even with a 50% decrease in multiple organ systems, individuals can still preserve their functionality and quality of life by adjusting their activities or environment.
- The rate of deterioration in different bodily organs varies significantly, with the most noticeable decline occurring in complex functions that require the coordination of multiple systems, muscles, and nerves. Various inter-individual variations can result from differences in genetic composition, dietary patterns, levels of physical activity, cultural heritage, and socioeconomic status. Scientists are currently reassessing numerous physiological declines that were previously believed to be permanent in the context of typical aging. Examples of master athletes who continue to engage in competitive physical activities throughout their entire lives illustrate that the declines typically associated with aging are not necessarily severe or inevitable. Adults who begin a regular exercise routine in their later years have observed significant enhancements in their overall well-being.
- The decline in sensory abilities due to aging is a common occurrence, but there are notable differences in how it affects individuals both within and between groups. Age-related visual impairments commonly lead to reduced sensitivity to different light levels, decreased visual clarity in environments with excessive glare, diminished capacity to distinguish between shades of color, and impaired ability to perceive depth and judge distances.
- As individuals age, their peripheral vision and ability to look up and down may become more limited. Older individuals are more prone to ocular conditions like glaucoma, cataracts, and macular degeneration, which, if not treated, can result in total loss of vision. The impaired hearing usually manifests earlier than visual impairments and affects a larger population. Although hearing aids can improve auditory ability, a considerable proportion of older individuals encounter discomfort and social stigma related to their utilization. Therefore, the possible remedies for effectively communicating with elderly individuals who have hearing impairments mainly revolve around adapting to the environment and employing alternative communication strategies. Contrary to the frequent complaints among older individuals about reduced taste sensitivity, research indicates that the changes in taste perception linked to aging are relatively insignificant.
- Although older adults are more prone to chronic illnesses, most of this age group perceive their health status as satisfactory. Health status encompasses an individual's comprehensive physical condition and functional capacity. However, most elderly individuals do not encounter constraints in their daily activities because of chronic ailments. The occurrence and effects of these diseases vary depending on changes in physiology related to age, an individual's ability to adapt, as well as their gender, race, ethnicity, and financial situation.
- The main determinants of death in the elderly population consist of cardiovascular disease, neoplastic tumors, cerebrovascular events, and unintentional injuries. Cardiovascular

diseases are prevalent conditions that primarily impact the heart and blood vessels. Given the strong correlation between hypertension and cardiovascular complications, it is crucial to implement preventive strategies such as maintaining a healthy weight, making dietary adjustments, engaging in appropriate physical activity, and abstaining from smoking. Cancer is the second most common cause of death, and its occurrence increases as people get older. Stroke, also referred to as cerebrovascular accident, ranks as the third most prevalent cause of death. Fortunately, the mortality rates for heart disease, stroke, and cancer are decreasing among the elderly population. The mentioned phenomenon can be ascribed to the implementation of preventive healthcare measures and the timely detection of cancer during the middle stages of life. Similarly, avoidable occurrences, particularly those associated with operating vehicles and slipping, are commonly experienced.

- Arthritis is a common ailment that greatly restricts everyday tasks, especially in older individuals. Osteoporosis is a common condition marked by reduced bone density and heightened fragility. It is primarily seen in older women and can result in fractures. Participating in physical exercise has demonstrated efficacy in diminishing the likelihood of fractures and falls, as well as in managing arthritis. As individuals get older, the occurrence of chronic respiratory problems, particularly emphysema, tends to increase. Diabetes mellitus is a prevalent medical condition that is worrisome because it is often linked to other health issues, such as dementia. Diverticulitis and incontinence are common problems that affect the gastrointestinal and urinary systems.
- The elderly population's utilization of outpatient dental, medical, and mental health services is slightly below the expected level considering their high prevalence of chronic illnesses. The primary goals of health promotion initiatives and biomedical scientists who aim to slow down the aging process are to improve the health of individuals with chronic illnesses associated with old age and enhance their overall quality of life. The progress in medical technology and the growing recognition of environmental stressors, nutritional factors, and physical activity in preventing diseases have resulted in swift changes in treatment methods. To delay the onset of chronic illnesses and decrease disability or loss of functional ability in future generations, it is necessary to widely implement health promotion initiatives and make significant advancements in aging research. However, increases in obesity among younger populations could potentially alter this optimistic prediction.

References

1. Adriaensen, W., Matheï, C., van Pottelbergh, G., Vaes, B., Legrand, D., Wallemacq, P., & Degryse, J. M. (2014). Significance of serum immune markers in identification of global functional impairment in the oldest old: Cross-sectional results from the BELFRAIL study. *Age, 36*, 457–467.
2. Ammar, A., Brach, M., Trabelsi, K., Chtourou, H., Boukhris, O., Masmoudi, L., Bouaziz, B., Bentlage, E., How, D., Ahmed, M., & Glenn, J. M. (2020). Effects of COVID-19 Home Confinement on Eating Behaviour and Physical Activity: Results of the ECLB-COVID19 International Online

Survey. *Nutrients, 12*(6), 1583.

3. Aranyavalai, T., Jalayondeja, C., Jalayondeja, W., Pichaiyongwongdee, S., & Kaewkungwal, J. (2020). Association between walking 5000 step/day and fall incidence over six months in urban community-dwelling older people. *BMC Geriatrics, 20*(1), 194.
4. Baltes, M. M., & Carstensen, L. L. (1996). The process of successful ageing. *Ageing and Society, 16*(4), 397–422.
5. Baron, R. M., & Kenny, D. A. (1986). The moderator-mediator variable distinction in social psychological research: Conceptual, strategic, and statistical considerations. *Journal of Personality and Social Psychology, 51*(6), 1173–1182.
6. Blodgett, J., Theou, O., Kirkland, S., Andreou, P., & Rockwood, K. (2015). The association between sedentary behaviour, moderate–vigorous physical activity and frailty in NHANES cohorts. *Maturitas, 80*(2), 187–191.
7. Brustio, P. R., Magistro, D., Zecca, M., Liubicich, M. E., & Rabaglietti, E. (2018). Fear of falling and activities of daily living function: Mediation effect of dual-task ability. *Aging & Mental Health, 22*(6), 856–861.
8. Bull, F. C., Al-Ansari, S. S., Biddle, S., Borodulin, K., Buman, M. P., Cardon, G., & World Health Organization. (2020). World Health Organization 2020 guidelines on physical activity and sedentary behaviour. *British Journal of Sports Medicine, 54*(24), 1451–1462.
9. Calamia, M., De Vito, A., Bernstein, J. P., Weitzner, D. S., Carmichael, O. T., & Keller, J. N. (2018). Pedometer-assessed steps per day as a predictor of cognitive performance in older adults. *Neuropsychology, 32*(7), 941–949.
10. Canevelli, M., Cesari, M., & van Kan, G. A. (2015). Frailty and cognitive decline: How do they relate? *Current Opinion in Clinical Nutrition & Metabolic Care, 18*(1), 43–50.
11. Cesari, M., Prince, M., Thiyagarajan, J. A., De Carvalho, I. A., Bernabei, R., Chan, P., & Ong, P. (2016). Frailty: An Emerging Public Health Priority. *Journal of the American Medical Directors Association, 17*(3), 188–192.
12. Chen, S., Chen, T., Kishimoto, H., Yatsugi, H., & Kumagai, S. (2020). Associations of objectively measured patterns of sedentary behavior and physical activity with frailty status screened by the frail scale in Japanese community-dwelling older adults. *Journal of Science and Medicine in Sport, 19*(2), 166–174.
13. Clegg, A., Young, J., Iliffe, S., Rikkert, M. O., & Rockwood, K. (2013). Frailty in elderly people. *The Lancet, 381*(9868), 752–762.
14. De Silva, N. A., Gregory, M. A., Venkateshan, S. S., Verschoor, C. P., & Kuspinar, A. (2019). Examining the Association between Life-Space Mobility and Cognitive Function in Older Adults: A Systematic Review. *Journal of Aging Research, 2019*, 3923574.
15. Del Pozo-Cruz, B., Mañas, A., Martín-García, M., Marín-Puyalto, J., García-García, F. J., Rodriguez-Mañas, L., & Ara, I. (2017). Frailty is associated with objectively assessed sedentary behavior patterns in older adults: Evidence from the Toledo Study for Healthy Aging (TSHA). *PLoS ONE, 12*(9), e0183911.
16. Ding, D., Mutrie, N., Bauman, A., Pratt, M., Hallal, P. R. C., & Powell, K. E. (2020). Physical activity guidelines 2020: Comprehensive and inclusive recommendations to activate populations. *The Lancet, 396*(10265), 1780–1782.

17. Dwyer, T., Pezic, A., Sun, C., Cochrane, J., Venn, A., Srikanth, V., & Ortaglia, A. (2015). Objectively measured daily steps and subsequent long term all-cause mortality: The tasped prospective cohort study. *PLoS ONE, 10*(10), e0141274.

18. Feskanich, D., Willett, W., & Colditz, G. (2002). Walking and leisure-time activity and risk of hip fracture in postmenopausal women. *JAMA, 288*(18), 2300–2306.

19. Fried, L. P., Tangen, C. M., Walston, J., Newman, A. B., Hirsch, C., Gottdiener, J., & Burke, G. (2001). Frailty in older adults: Evidence for a phenotype. *The Journals of Gerontology: Series A, 56*(3), M146–M156.

20. Gallucci, A., Trimarchi, P. D., Abbate, C., Tuena, C., Pedroli, E., Lattanzio, F., Stramba-Badiale, M., Cesari, M., & Giunco, F. (2020). ICT technologies as new promising tools for the managing of frailty: A systematic review. *Aging & Clinical Experimental Research, 33*(7), 1453–1464.

21. Gill, T. M., Han, L., Gahbauer, E. A., Leo-Summers, L., & Murphy, T. E. (2020). Risk Factors and Precipitants of Severe Disability Among Community-Living Older Persons. *JAMA, 3*(2), e206021.

22. Gobbens, R. J., van Assen, M. A. L. M., Luijkx, K. G., & Schols, J. M. G. A. (2012). The Predictive Validity of the Tilburg Frailty Indicator: Disability, Health Care Utilization, and Quality of Life in a Population at Risk. *The Gerontologist, 52*(5), 619–631.

23. Gobbens, R. J., van Assen, M. A. L. M., Luijkx, K. G., Wijnen-Sponselee, M. T., & Schols, J. M. G. A. (2010). The Tilburg Frailty Indicator: Psychometric properties. *Journal of the American Medical Directors Association, 11*(5), 344–355.

24. Gregg, E. W., Cauley, J. A., Stone, K., Thompson, T. J., Bauer, D. C., Cummings, S. R., Ensrud, K. E., & Study of Osteoporotic Fractures Research Group. (2003). Relationship of changes in physical activity and mortality among older women. *JAMA, 289*(18), 2379–2386.

25. Hansen, B. H., Dalene, K. E., Ekelund, U., Wang Fagerland, M., Kolle, E., Steene-Johannessen, J., Tarp, J., & Alfred Anderssen, S. (2020). Step by step: Association of device-measured daily steps with all-cause mortality—A prospective cohort Study. *Scandinavian Journal of Medicine & Science in Sports, 30*(9), 1705–1711.

26. Harris, T., Limb, E. S., Hosking, F., Carey, I., DeWilde, S., Furness, C., Wahlich, C., Ahmad, S., Kerry, S., Whincup, P., et al. (2019). Effect of pedometer-based walking interventions on long-term health outcomes: Prospective 4-year follow-up of two randomized controlled trials using routine primary care data. *PLoS Medicine, 16*(12), e1002836.

27. Hashidate, H., Shimada, H., Shiomi, T., Shibata, M., Sawada, K., & Sasamoto, N. (2013). Measuring indoor life-space mobility at home in older adults with difficulty to perform outdoor activities. *Journal of Geriatric Physical Therapy, 36*(3), 109–114.

28. Huisingh-Scheetz, M., Wroblewski, K., Kocherginsky, M., Huang, E., Dale, W., Waite, L., & Schumm, L. P. (2018). The relationship between physical activity and frailty among US older adults based on hourly accelerometry data. *The Journals of Gerontology Series A: Biological Sciences & Medical Sciences, 73*(5), 622–629.

29. Kehler, D. S., & Theou, O. (2019). The impact of physical activity and sedentary behaviors on frailty levels. *Mechanisms of Ageing and Development, 180*, 29–41.

30. Kehler, D. S., Hay, J. L., Stammers, A. N., Hamm, N. C., Kimber, D. E., Schultz, A. S. H., Szwajcer, A., Arora, R. C., Tangri, N., & Duhamel, T. A. (2018). A systematic review of the association between sedentary behaviors with frailty. *Experimental Gerontology, 114*, 1–12.

31. Kempen, G. I., Miedema, I., Ormel, J., & Molenaar, W. (1996). The assessment of disability with the Groningen Activity Restriction Scale. Conceptual framework and psychometric properties. *Social Science & Medicine, 43*(11), 1601–1610.

32. Klimek, M., Peter, R. S., Denkinger, M., Dallmeier, D., Rapp, K., Rothenbacher, D., & Klenk, J. (2022). The relationship of weather with daily physical activity and the time spent out of home in older adults from Germany–the ActiFE study. *European Review of Aging and Physical Activity, 19*, 6.

33. Langhammer, B., Bergland, A., & Rydwik, E. (2018). The Importance of Physical Activity Exercise among Older People. *BioMed Research International, 2018*, 7856823.

34. Lee, I. M., Shiroma, E. J., Lobelo, F., Puska, P., Blair, S. N., Katzmarzyk, P. T., & Lancet Physical Activity Series Working Group. (2012). Effect of physical inactivity on major non-communicable diseases worldwide: An analysis of burden of disease and life expectancy. *The Lancet, 380*(9838), 219–229.

35. Lutz, W., Sanderson, W., & Scherbov, S. (2008). The coming acceleration of global population ageing. *Nature, 451*(7179), 716–719.

36. Magistro, D., Brustio, P. R., Ivaldi, M., Esliger, D. W., Zecca, M., Rainoldi, A., & Boccia, G. (2018). Validation of the ADAMO Care Watch for step counting in older adults. *PLoS ONE, 13*(1), e0190753.

37. Mankowski, R. T., Anton, S. D., Axtell, R., Chen, S. H., Fielding, R. A., Glynn, N. W., & Leeuwenburgh, C. (2017). Device-measured physical activity as a predictor of disability in mobility-limited older adults. *Journal of the American Geriatrics Society, 65*(10), 2251–2256.

38. Miller, M. E., Rejeski, W. J., Reboussin, B. A., Ten Have, T. R., & Ettinger, W. H. (2000). Physical activity, functional limitations, and disability in older adults. *Journal of the American Geriatrics Society, 48*(10), 1264–1272.

39. Mulasso, A., Brustio, P. R., Rainoldi, A., Zia, G., Feletti, L., N'dja, A., & Donini, L. M. (2019). A comparison between an ICT tool and a traditional physical measure for frailty evaluation in older adults. *BMC Geriatrics, 19*(1), 88.

40. Mulasso, A., Roppolo, M., Gobbens, R. J., & Rabaglietti, E. (2016). The Italian Version of the Tilburg Frailty Indicator: Analysis of Psychometric Properties. *Research on Aging, 38*(8), 842–863.

41. Nelson, M. E., Rejeski, W. J., Blair, S. N., Duncan, P. W., Judge, J. O., King, A. C., Macera, C. A., & Castaneda-Sceppa, C. (2007). Physical activity and public health in older adults: Recommendation from the American College of Sports Medicine and the American Heart Association. *Circulation, 116*(9), 1094–1105.

42. Paterson, D. H., & Warburton, D. E. (2010). Physical activity and functional limitations in older adults: A systematic review related to Canada's Physical Activity Guidelines. *International Journal of Behavioral Nutrition and Physical Activity, 7*, 38.

43. Perrig-Chiello, P., Perrig, W. J., Uebelbacher, A., & Stähelin, H. B. (2006). Impact of physical and psychological resources on functional autonomy in old age. *Psychology, Health & Medicine, 11*(4), 470–482.

44. Rejeski, W. J., & Mihalko, S. L. (2001). Physical activity and quality of life in older adults. *The Journals of Gerontology Series A: Biological Sciences & Medical Sciences, 56*(Suppl. 2), 23–35.

45. Robertson, D. A., Savva, G. M., & Kenny, R. A. (2013). Frailty and cognitive impairment—A review of the evidence and causal mechanisms. *Ageing Research Reviews, 12*, 840–851.

46. Soysal, P., Stubbs, B., Lucato, P., Luchini, C., Solmi, M., Peluso, R., Sergi, G., Isik, A. T., Manzato, E., Maggi, S., et al. (2016). Inflammation and frailty in the elderly: A systematic review and meta-analysis. *Ageing Research Reviews, 31*, 1–8.

47. Spiteri, K., Broom, D., Bekhet, A. H., de Caro, J. X., Laventure, B., & Grafton, K. (2019). Barriers and motivators of physical activity participation in middle-aged and older adults—A systematic review. *Journal of Aging and Physical Activity, 27*(6), 929–944.

48. Steen, G., Sonn, U., Börjesson Hanson, A., & Steen, B. (2001). Cognitive function and functional ability. A cross-sectional and longitudinal study at ages 85 and 95 in a non-demented population. *Aging Clinical and Experimental Research, 13*(1), 68–77.

49. Verghese, J., Holtzer, R., Oh-Park, M., Derby, C. A., Lipton, R. B., & Wang, C. (2011). Inflammatory markers and gait speed decline in older adults. *The Journals of Gerontology Series A: Biological Sciences & Medical Sciences, 66*(10), 1083–1089.

50. Watanabe, D., Yoshida, T., Watanabe, Y., Yamada, Y., Kimura, M., & Kyoto-Kameoka Study Group. (2020). Objectively Measured Daily Step Counts and Prevalence of Frailty in 3,616 Older Adults. *Journal of the American Geriatrics Society, 68*(10), 2310–2318.

51. Yuki, A., Otsuka, R., Tange, C., Nishita, Y., Tomida, M., Ando, F., Shimokata, H., & Arai, H. (2019). Daily physical activity predicts frailty development among community-dwelling older Japanese adults. *Journal of the American Medical Directors Association, 20*(8), 1032–1036.

Chapter 9

AGE-RELATED COGNITIVE DECLINE

Contents

Introduction

The study of cognitive function in gerontology is crucial due to its significance as a risk factor for various pathologies in old age, such as physical disability, dependence, depression, and frailty. Early pathological changes in cognitive function are often considered a preclinical state that can progress to dementia, making understanding cognitive aging essential for effective geriatric care (Buckner, 2004).

In this chapter, cognitive functioning is examined in detail, encompassing various dimensions: attention, memory, meta-memory, processing speed, executive functions, visuospatial skills, and language. These dimensions collectively contribute to our understanding of cognitive aging and its impact on individuals as they grow older (Salthouse, 2010).

Age-associated changes in cognitive function are a key focus of this discussion. These changes often termed cognitive decline, are distinguished from those associated with cognitive pathologies, such as mild cognitive impairment and dementia. Understanding these distinctions is crucial for accurate diagnosis and effective intervention strategies (Albert et al., 2011).

To further enhance our understanding, current evidence regarding the conceptualization of cognitive pathologies is examined. This includes an analysis of the diagnostic criteria for mild cognitive impairment and dementia, highlighting the complexities and challenges in distinguishing age-related cognitive decline from pathological cognitive changes (McKhann et al., 2011). Moreover, the chapter examines the identification of risk factors for cognitive functioning in aging, categorizing them into modifiable and nonmodifiable factors. Modifiable factors, such as lifestyle choices and environmental influences, offer opportunities for intervention to potentially mitigate cognitive decline. Nonmodifiable factors, such as genetic predisposition, provide insights into the inherent vulnerabilities that some individuals may face in terms of cognitive aging (Kivipelto et al., 2001).

Orientation and Directional Terms:

Term	Definition	**Illustration**
Cognitive function	The mental processes involved in perception, memory, judgment, reasoning, problem-solving, and language.	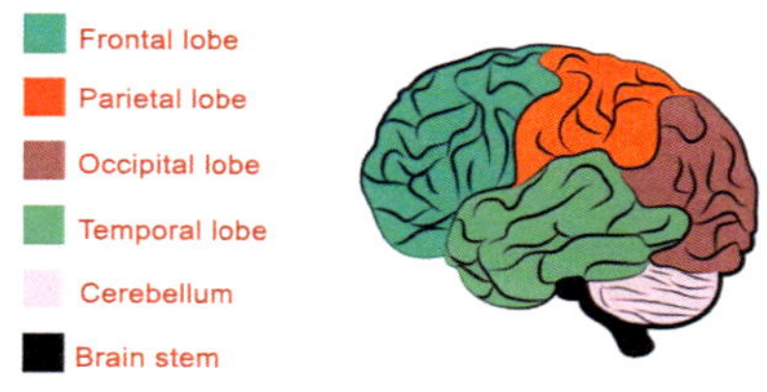
Cognitive aging	The changes in cognitive abilities (such as memory, processing speed, and reasoning) that occur with age.	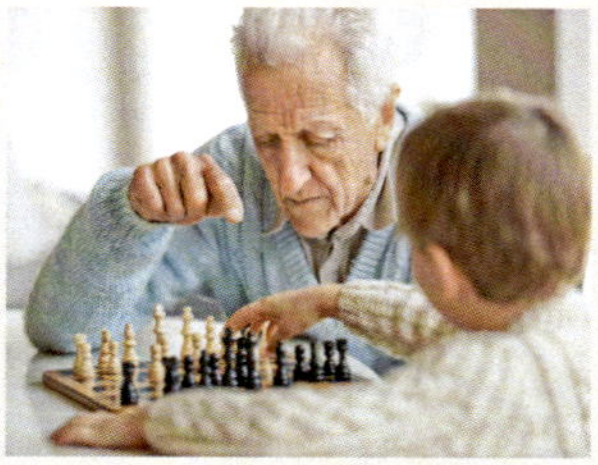
Memory	The mental capacity to retain and recall information, experiences, and past events.	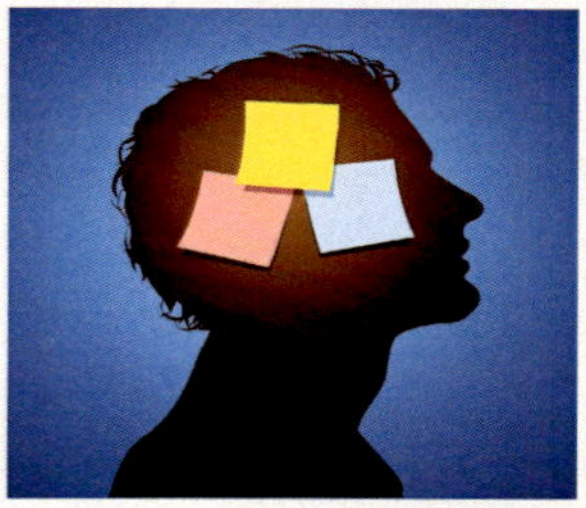
Meta-memory	Awareness of one's own memory processes, including knowledge about when and how to use memory strategies effectively.	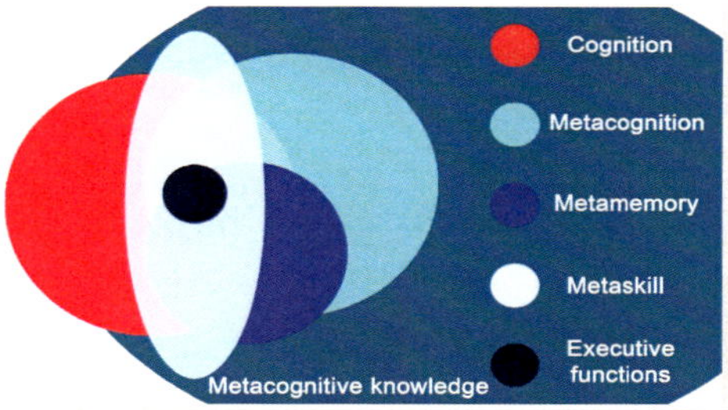
Visuospatial skills	The ability to perceive, analyze, and mentally manipulate visual information in relation to objects and space.	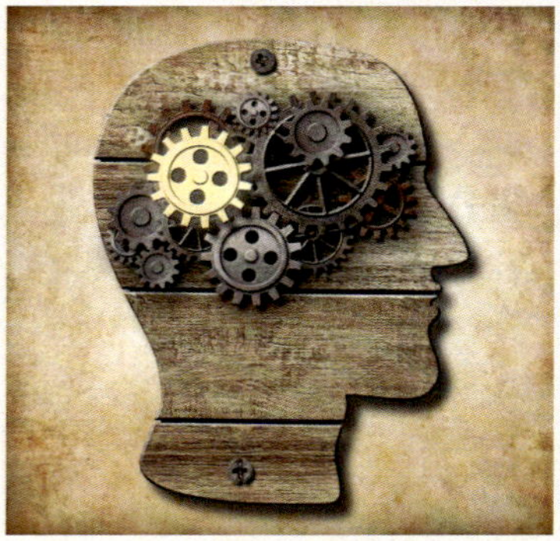

9.1. Fundamentals of Cognitive Aging

Population aging is a global phenomenon characterized by a gradual and inevitable increase in the proportion of elderly individuals within the population. This demographic shift is primarily driven by a combination of factors including low birth rates, decreased mortality rates, and advancements in healthcare leading to increased life expectancy. However, aging is not just a demographic trend; it is also a deeply personal experience marked by significant changes at biological, psychological, and social levels.

In psychology, aging is associated with a variety of changes in domains such as personality, affectivity, emotions, emotional regulation, and interpersonal relationships. Of particular interest to gerontology is the study of cognitive aging, given its potential implications, especially in its most severe form, dementia.

The study of cognitive functions has a rich history, dating back to the works of ancient philosophers and early neuroscientists. For example, Galen proposed that consciousness resided in the brain's ventricles, encompassing various capacities like perception, intellect, and memory. Descartes later advanced a neurophysiological theory linking mental functions to the brain's ventricles and the pineal gland.

The 19th century saw significant progress in understanding the relationship between brain structures and cognitive functions. Scholars like Flourens argued that all neural tissues were involved in cognitive functions, while Gall's phrenology theory attempted to map cognitive functions to specific skull areas. This era also marked the beginnings of neuropsychology, with pioneers like Luria, Vygotsky, and Leontiev focusing on the relationship between brain organization and behavior, emphasizing the role of social and cultural factors. Neuropsychology, as a discipline, provides an integrative view of cognitive functioning, emphasizing its development in the context of sociocultural factors. It considers cognitive functions as dynamic processes that interact with the environment, shaping both the nervous system and behavior over time.

Various conceptualizations of cognitive functioning exist. It can be viewed as an evolutionary process, starting from conception and ending with death, involving continuous changes in both the organism and the nervous system. Alternatively, cognitive functions can be seen as functional interactions within distributed cortical networks, encompassing processes such as memory, attention, perception, language, and intelligence.

From a psychopedagogical perspective, complex cognitive functions involve planning, multitasking, cognitive flexibility, context-based responses, resistance to distraction, and inhibition of inappropriate behaviors. Piaget's theory emphasizes the constructive nature of cognitive development, rejecting both empiricist and innatist theories.

The structural cognitive modifiability theory categorizes cognitive functions into perceptual thinking, strategic, analogical, and reflexive, based on the constructivist paradigm. Lastly, from a neuropsychological standpoint, cognitive functions are viewed as abilities developed by brain structures to process information acquired from the environment, categorized into basic functions (sensation, perception, memory, attention, concentration) and higher cognitive functions (thought, language, intelligence). (Mirra et al., 1999)

9.2. Age-associated Changes

Over the past few decades, significant scientific efforts have been directed toward understanding the processes of normal cognitive aging. Despite this, there remain both agreements and discrepancies in the field, largely stemming from differences in research methodologies and the challenge of controlling variables closely linked to cognitive functioning. One of the key challenges in this area is distinguishing between normal cognitive aging and cognitive impairment associated with pathology, as the diagnostic boundaries are often imprecise. This task is further complicated by the influence of variables such as age, education, and other population differences.

The concept of cognitive functioning in normal aging is often described as the adaptation or alteration of the cognitive system, which can either lead to regression or successful management of daily life functions in older adults. Understanding the changes that occur in cognitive domains involves considering both physiological and social aspects.

Research on the human brain using techniques such as brain mapping, electroencephalography (EEG), and magnetic resonance imaging (MRI) has suggested that successful cognitive aging may be linked to the preservation of hippocampal function combined with high responsiveness in the frontal area. EEG studies have indicated a reduction in age-dependent cerebral electrical power in cortical areas like the parietal, temporal, and occipital lobes, leading to declines in memory, attention, visuospatial skills, and processing speed. This decline is attributed to the loss of synaptic contacts and neuronal apoptosis, impacting sensory aspects, processing, motor performance, and some cognitive functions.

Additionally, studies like that by Steffener et al. have linked cognitive changes in normal aging to a gradual decrease in cerebral blood flow and gray matter volume, particularly in areas such as the prefrontal cortex and temporal convolutions of the putamen and occipital regions. Social aspects, as identified in longitudinal studies, play a role in cognitive functioning changes in older adults and include factors like education, good health, social participation, lifestyle, and genetic factors.

Socioenvironmental variables can influence an individual's cerebral aging and modify their cognitive and behavioral profile. While some factors may negatively impact cognitive function, precipitating deterioration in normal aging, others may mitigate or even slow these effects.

Identifying which cognitive functions typically decline in older adults and when these declines occur is challenging. However, research indicates that attention, verbal memory, visuospatial and visuoconstructive skills, processing speed, and some executive functions such as inhibition, working memory, and mental flexibility are generally affected. Functions like semantic memory and language tend to be preserved and may even improve with age.

Attention, a complex and hierarchical system, plays a crucial role in processing information and selecting relevant stimuli for various activities. Cognitive changes related to attention, particularly difficulties in tasks involving orientation among elements or switching between testing options, may stem from a decrease in selective visual attention, partly due to sensory processing degradation. Furthermore, attention control is intertwined with other cognitive functions, such as processing speed, suggesting that older adults may be less adept at tasks requiring anticipatory attentional resources due to slower reaction times associated with aging.

Age-related changes in cognitive functioning have been extensively studied across various domains. Memory, for instance, plays a crucial role in recording, encoding, consolidating, retaining, storing, retrieving, and evoking information. The memory process involves three types: sensory, short-term (a transient and fragile storage susceptible to interference), and long-term memory (responsible for more permanent storage through consolidation). Each type operates uniquely but collaborates in the memorization process, representing three necessary steps in forming lasting memories. Human memory comprises three main processes: encoding, storage, and recall (retrieval).

Memory is among the most studied cognitive domains due to its frequent complaints by older adults during normal aging. Research, such as that by Kral since 1962, has identified a gradual memory loss characterized by difficulties in recalling relatively unimportant aspects of past experiences. The impact on acquisition, consolidation, and spontaneous recall processes is related to cerebral biological functioning, influenced by factors like quality of life.

Different types of memory are affected by aging. Immediate and episodic memory decline more than semantic memory, while evocation is more affected than consolidation. Aging also impacts the encoding of new information, particularly when strategic processing is necessary.

Perception, another cognitive function, integrates and recognizes information through our senses, allowing us to create knowledge patterns. Spatial and constructional skills, involving the ability to integrate elements into an organized whole, can be challenging to dissociate. Changes in these functions during aging are attributed to declines in visual acuity and processing, leading to issues with illumination sensitivity, vision in dimly lit places, color distinction, focusing at varying distances, and deficits in spatial perception.

Executive functions, responsible for planning and supervising cognitive processes, involve high-level operations that sequence and control basic operations, making decisions in choosing alternatives. Evaluating executive functions is complex due to their interconnection with other cognitive functions. Tasks involving executive functions include working memory and tasks requiring goal establishment, operation implementation and follow-up, and final purpose fulfillment. In normal aging, changes in executive functions are mainly observed in working memory, inhibition, and mental flexibility.

Processing speed, defined as reaction time affecting cognition globally, declines with normal aging and is associated with cognitive changes in other domains like attention and executive functioning. Older adults may lack the necessary mental resources for complex cognitive tasks due to slower cognitive functioning, impacting task completion. Studies comparing young and older adults have shown lower performance in inhibitory control, abstraction, and working memory among older adults.

Subjective perception of cognitive functioning, known as meta-memory, significantly influences activities of daily living during aging. A recent study found that a third of the population evaluated reported memory problems, thinking skills, and reasoning abilities, all associated with overall health (Petrou et al., 2015).

Importantly, cognitive changes in normal aging are typically mild and do not interfere significantly with independence. Any significant changes should raise suspicion of cognitive deterioration or pathology-related cognitive changes.

9.3. Mild Cognitive Impairment and Dementia

In the context of cognitive aging, a normal decline is observed. Certain cognitive functions exhibit stability while others experience a decline as a natural part of the aging process. These age-related cognitive changes occur in individuals without any memory or cognitive impairments, and they do not hinder their ability to engage in daily activities. Nevertheless, the cognitive alterations that occur with aging can vary greatly, ranging from typical changes to pathological changes, with a range of intermediate changes in between. The term used to describe this transitional state is Mild Cognitive Impairment (MCI).

Mild Cognitive Impairment (MCI) is widely utilized globally, both in clinical and research contexts, to delineate the intermediate stage between normal cognitive functioning and clinical impairment. The MCI aims to recognize the intermediate phase of cognitive impairment, which is frequently, though not always, a transitional stage between normal age-related cognitive changes and the cognitive decline typically observed in dementia. In this context, MCI is regarded as a pre-dementia syndrome.

In 2013, the American Psychiatric Association (APA) introduced new guidelines for diagnosing dementia in the fifth edition of the Diagnostic and Statistical Manual for Mental Disorders (DSM-5). These guidelines also acknowledge the early stage of cognitive impairment that precedes dementia. The condition, exhibiting several characteristics of MCI, is referred to as mild neurocognitive disorder (NCD). Mild Neurocognitive Disorder (NCD) identifies subtle characteristics of cognitive decline that are distinct from the natural aging process but do not indicate the presence of dementia. In addition, mild neurocognitive disorder (NCD) specifically targets the early stages of cognitive impairments and comes before major NCD, which is similar to the previous diagnosis of dementia.

There are multiple subtypes of Mild Cognitive Impairment (MCI), each characterized by varying types and degrees of cognitive impairment. The most prevalent subtype is amnesic MCI, which primarily affects memory function. In contrast, nonamnesic MCI does not significantly impact memory operations. Similarly, if only one aspect of cognitive functioning is impacted, it is referred to as Domain Cognitive Impairment (DCL). If multiple cognitive abilities such as memory, reasoning, and executive functions are affected, it is called Multidomain Cognitive Impairment. The various subtypes of MCI are typically associated with distinct pathological mechanisms. For instance, individuals with amnestic DCL have a higher likelihood of transitioning to Alzheimer's disease (AD), whereas those with nonamnestic MCI are more prone to developing Lewy Body Dementia (Braak and Braak, 1987; Braak and Braak, 1991; Braak et al., 2003; Braak et al., 2006).

Based on this definition, MCI is measured and defined using clinical data that assess changes in cognitive abilities. Objective cognitive measures, such as neuropsychological test batteries, are necessary to verify the subjective cognitive complaint. Objective cognitive impairment refers to a subpar performance in one or more cognitive assessments, indicating deficiencies in one or more cognitive areas or domains. There is currently no universally accepted benchmark to determine which neuropsychological test battery should be used. However, it is crucial to assess all the primary cognitive domains. Generally, executive functions, attention, language, memory, and visuospatial skills are considered. Functional abilities are assessed through a comprehensive interview with the individual and their close family members. The results are recorded using scales that measure activities of daily living (ADL) and instrumental activities of daily living (IADL) (Figure 9.1).

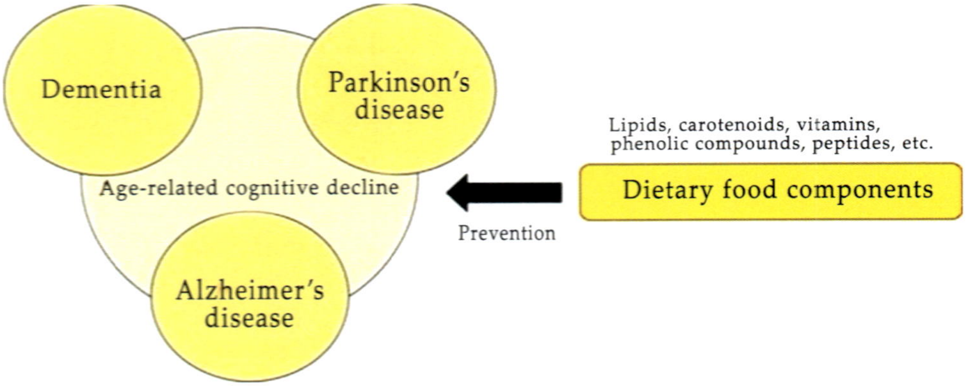

Figure 9.1. *Comparison of the different diagnostic criteria in normal aging, mild cognitive impairment and dementia (according to DSM-IV and DSM-5).*

Source: Ozawa H, Miyazawa T, Miyazawa T. Effects of dietary food components on cognitive functions in older adults. Nutrients. 2021; 13(8):2804. https://doi.org/10.3390/nu13082804.

Research has demonstrated that a substantial portion of individuals with Mild Cognitive Impairment (MCI) experience a transition to dementia within 1–2 years, and around 50% of them develop dementia within a 5-year timeframe. Dementia is a non-communicable disease (NCD) that typically starts slowly and worsens over time. The progression of cognitive impairment can be unpredictable, and there is typically a significant time gap between the initial manifestation of symptoms and the point at which they satisfy the diagnostic criteria for dementia. In 2013, the American Psychiatric Association (APA) replaced the term "dementia" with "Major neurocognitive disorder." This new term refers to a significant decline in mental ability that hinders independence and daily functioning. Nevertheless, not all care professionals and organizations will probably adopt the new terminology. Presently, the Alzheimer's Association, for example, employs the term dementia in lieu of neurocognitive disorder.

Worldwide, approximately 47 million individuals suffer from dementia, with nearly 60% residing in low- and middle-income nations. Each year, there are 9.9 million new cases reported. Alzheimer's disease is the primary cause of dementia, accounting for 60–70% of cases. The prevalence of dementia in the general population aged 60 years and over is estimated to be between 5 and 8 percent. By 2030, the global population of individuals with dementia is expected to approach 75 million, and it is predicted to nearly triple by 2050, reaching 132 million. The majority of this rise can be attributed to the growing population of individuals with dementia residing in low- and middle-income nations. Alzheimer's disease and vascular dementia (VD) are the prevailing types of dementia.

9.4. Risk Factors for Mild Cognitive Impairment and Dementia

Research has gradually revealed which risk factors (RF) for mild cognitive impairment and dementia can currently be taken into consideration. The prevention of these pathological processes is significantly aided by the knowledge of radiofrequency (RF) for these processes. In a perfect world, prevention strategies would focus on individuals who are not even exhibiting any symptoms. The prevention of dementia is a priority for the public health system.

In the field of health sciences, a risk factor (RF) refers to the likelihood of experiencing a particular disease, developing a complication, or passing away. In this section, we will discuss some of the most well-known RF, categorizing them according to their origins in social, biological, and psychological contexts, as well as their nature, which can be classified as either modifiable or nonmodifiable (see the Table for more information) (Table 9.1).

Table 9.1. Comparison of Classical ad and ARCD Based on Clinical Course and Risk Factors. When Examining the Background and Clinical Course of Classical Ad and Ard, it Becomes Clear that they Describe Entirely Different Disease Processes that Should be Considered Separately. PSEN—Presenilin. App—Amyloid Precursor Protein

	Early-Onset (Classical) Alzheimer's Disease	**Age-Related Dementia**
Age of Onset	30–60 years	>60 years
Genetics	Monogenic/familial: PSEN1, PSEN2, APP. ~40–50% of mutations are sporadic.	Polygenic. Most significant risk gene (ApoE) contributes ~5% of total risk and is variably penetrant based on context and environment.
Clinical Course	Homogeneous	Heterogeneous
Effect of Environment	Minimal, or poorly described.	Substantial. Education, diet, exercise, cardiovascular and metabolic health, history of trauma, sleep, stress, pollutants, smoking, and alcohol all have a documented role.
Prevalence	~1% of all AD cases and decreasing (previously estimated to represent 5% of all AD).	~10% of individuals >65 and increasing (projected to double by 2050). ~99% of all AD cases.

Source: Turknett J, Wood TR. Demand coupling drives neurodegeneration: A model of age-related cognitive decline and dementia. Cells. 2022; 11(18):2789. https://doi.org/10.3390/cells11182789.

9.4.1. Biological Factors

9.4.1.1. Vascular Disorders

Both hypertension and hypotension have been associated with cognitive impairment and dementia. The significance of vascular structure and function in brain health is emphasized by the involvement of cerebral blood vessels in various pathologies that contribute to cognitive impairment. The exact biological processes that explain the connection between blood pressure (BP) and cognitive function are not well understood. However, reduced blood flow and the gradual breakdown of nerve cells have been identified as possible underlying mechanisms. The findings of a longitudinal study conducted as part of the Kungsholmen Project revealed that individuals with low diastolic pressure had a higher likelihood of developing dementia in advanced age. During the study, there was a significant reduction in blood pressure for about 3 years before the onset of clinically detectable dementia syndrome.

Conversely, cohort studies have indicated that higher blood pressure levels during middle age may raise the likelihood of developing dementia in later stages of life. Consequently, being exposed to four risk factors associated with blood pressure, namely smoking, hypertension, high cholesterol, and diabetes, during middle age, increases the likelihood of developing dementia in old age, compared to having only one of these risk factors. The association between blood pressure and the likelihood of developing dementia may be influenced by the age at which blood pressure is measured, as well as the time gap between blood pressure assessment and dementia evaluation (Newman et al., 2005; Ogrodowczyk et al., 2016; Panza et al., 2019).

9.4.1.2. Metabolic Disorders: Diabetes Mellitus

Older adults in the community who have diabetes mellitus (DM) are at a 1.5–2.5 times higher risk of developing dementia. Dementia is a notable contributing factor not just for vascular dementia but also for Alzheimer's disease. The precise mechanisms underlying this association remain uncertain, but they are likely to be multifactorial in nature. Possible factors include cardiovascular risk factors, glucose toxicity, alterations in insulin metabolism, and inflammation.

Both elevated blood sugar levels (hyperglycemia) and excessive insulin levels (hyperinsulinemia) contribute to the development of type 2 diabetes (DM2) and are linked to cognitive impairment and stroke-related dementia. This is frequently accompanied by comorbidities of cognitive impairments, such as depression or anxiety. An epidemiological study found that the rate of hospitalization for VD in adults aged 70 years and older was twice as high in patients with DM2 compared to those without the condition.

9.4.1.3. Genetic Factors Play a Role

The influence of genetics in Alzheimer's disease (AD) is evident, impacting both early and late-onset cases. Early-onset Alzheimer's disease (AD), which occurs before the age of 65, can be attributed to one of over 200 genetic mutations in the beta-amyloid precursor protein, presenilin 1 (PSEN1), or presenilin 2 (PSEN2). Although there is a consistent genetic foundation for Alzheimer's disease (AD), there is considerable variation in the age at which it occurs. This indicates that environmental factors or genetic modifiers play a significant role in determining the age of onset. The occurrence of late-onset Alzheimer's disease (AD) is significantly impacted by genetic factors, although the specific pattern of inheritance following Mendelian principles is frequently uncertain. Various factors may account for this phenomenon, even in the presence of causal mutations. Late-onset Alzheimer's disease (AD) is a multifaceted condition, and apolipoprotein E is the sole genetic risk factor that is universally acknowledged to contribute to its development. Advanced genetic technologies have revealed several genes associated with AD, but numerous other genes remain unidentified.

About this, an extensive study examining the Genealogical Index of Familiarity up to 14 generations revealed a significant correlation between individuals with familial connections who passed away due to AD. The risk of Alzheimer's disease (AD) death among the relatives of individuals who died of AD increased significantly for both close and distant relatives.

9.4.1.4. Earlier Instances of Brain Trauma

An emerging field of study focuses on comprehending the impact of head trauma on the behavior and cognitive functions of brain aging. This matter assumes greater significance as the geriatric demographic expands.

Traumatic brain injury (TBI) is a type of injury that can have severe and long-lasting effects on cognitive function. Over 70% of individuals with TBI experience memory impairments. Contact sports are a frequent cause of TBI. A study found that athletes who experienced their last concussion during early adulthood, more than 30 years before the examination, exhibited lower performance in episodic memory and response inhibition. Additionally, these athletes demonstrated significantly slower movement speeds in neuropsychological tests compared to athletes of the same age who had no history of concussion. Concerning cognitive aging, the evidence indicates that young adults who have experienced severe TBI exhibit cognitive difficulties that resemble the attention deficit and poor working memory commonly observed in elderly individuals without any neurological conditions. There is evidence suggesting that TBI can cause a reduction in cognitive reserve, which in turn can expedite the normal cognitive decline process, resulting in premature aging and potentially raising the likelihood of developing dementia.

9.4.2. Psychological Determinants

- **Depression:** Depression can impact cognitive functions and can mimic cognitive impairment. Comorbidity, a prodromal factor, or a consequence of vascular cognitive impairment, can be regarded as opposed to being a factor that directly affects vascular physiology or neural health, resulting in cognitive impairment. Several studies have found a connection between depressive symptoms and cognitive impairment. However, more research is needed to understand the specific mechanisms that link these two prevalent conditions. The relationship between cognitive impairment over time and depression is uncertain, as it remains unclear whether the impairment is a result of depression or an early indication of dementia.

9.4.3. Social Factors

9.4.3.1. Age and Sex

Research findings have indicated that age and sex are significant risk factors for mild cognitive impairment and dementia. Several studies have indicated that the occurrence of dementia rises exponentially in correlation with age, and it doubles every 5 years after reaching the age of 65. Multiple studies have demonstrated a rising occurrence among the elderly population. The prevalence of this condition among individuals over 65 years old in higher-income countries is estimated to be between 5% and 10%. Sex-related studies have shown that women have a higher prevalence of dementia compared to men. A plausible rationale for this phenomenon is that females have a greater life expectancy compared to males. However, a cohort study revealed that men had a higher prevalence and incidence compared to other groups.

9.4.3.2. Education and Intellectual Commitment

Dr. James A. Mortimer was among the pioneers who suggested a correlation between the number of years spent in formal education and the likelihood of developing dementia. He proposed that education can serve as a safeguard against dementia, augmenting the level of "intellectual reserve." In relation to this matter, a comprehensive analysis of the existing research on the correlation between education and dementia over the past 25 years determined that lower levels of education were linked to a higher likelihood of developing dementia in numerous studies, although not in all of them.

The relationship between education and the risk of dementia varied across different populations, and the impact of years of education on reducing the risk of dementia was not consistent. It appears that a stronger correlation between dementia and education was observed when the level of education aligned with cognitive ability. This suggests that the impact of education on the risk of dementia can be more accurately evaluated within the framework of a life development model.

Moreover, engaging in occupations that did not involve intricate cognitive tasks or stimulating activities during one's lifetime appears to be linked to a higher likelihood of developing dementia. For instance, in a study involving a cohort of nuns with an average age of 54, a significant correlation was observed between lower levels of education and occupation and the occurrence of dementia. Participants with low educational attainment, lack of professional training, and no experience in leadership positions had a higher risk of developing dementia. These findings corroborate the hypothesis that possessing a cognitive reserve capacity can provide advantages in mitigating the effects of brain diseases. According to the report, individuals who underwent university preparation had a lower likelihood of developing dementia compared to those in five other categories. Among these categories, illiterates had the highest proportion of individuals with dementia, while university students had the lowest proportion.

9.5. Intervention in Cognitive Aging

In general, studies on cognitive aging indicate a gradual decrease in cognitive abilities, which may or may not be considered normal, and is linked to age and previously identified factors that increase the risk. The transition from a state of normalcy to a state of pathology is a significant concern within the health sciences field, as it carries adverse consequences for individuals' lives, particularly in terms of mild cognitive impairment and dementia.

Gerontology has prioritized the examination of nonpharmacological intervention methods that enhance or sustain cognitive functioning at a level that enables individuals to live functional and disability-free lives linked to cognitive disorders. The primary theoretical foundation for nonpharmacological intervention on cognitive functioning in aging primarily revolves around the principles of brain plasticity, brain reserve, and cognitive reserve.

In the past 25 years, evidence has emerged to support the concept of brain plasticity, which suggests that the brain is more adaptable in both its structure and function than previously thought. Brain plasticity, also known as neuroplasticity, is the remarkable capacity of the brain to alter its own structure and function in response to internal or external changes. While its strength is most pronounced in childhood, the brain's fundamental and significant property persists throughout the aging process. Brain plasticity is involved in cognitive abilities and has a crucial function in neurodegenerative brain disorders. Recent research indicates that the development of Alzheimer's disease is linked to a decline in the brain's ability to change and adapt, known as plasticity.

Brain reserve is associated with neurobiological factors and takes a more passive stance, as it pertains to the quantity and size of neurons an individual possesses following a brain injury.

The cognitive reserve refers to the brain's ability to adapt to an injury by utilizing existing cognitive processing resources or compensation resources through the activation of neural networks. Cognitive reserve enables individuals to withstand the impact of dementia-related diseases, allowing for a higher threshold of neuropathological changes before exhibiting symptoms of the disease. Cognitive reserve has an impact on how cognitive impairment symptoms are shown and to some extent, on the progression towards dementia. Individuals with Mild Cognitive Impairment (MCI) and low cognitive reserves experience a more rapid decline in the early stages of deterioration, in contrast to those with high cognitive reserves who exhibit this significant decline towards the end of the deterioration process. This discrepancy can be attributed to the protective function of cognitive reserves.

The intervention for optimizing cognitive functions is grounded in these principles to implement nonpharmacological therapies, to address the cognitive challenges associated with aging, preventing conditions like MCI and dementia, and, if necessary, mitigating their impacts.

The British Psychological Society states that there are several nonpharmacological treatments and interventions available to help individuals maintain optimal mental health, particularly following a diagnosis of MCI or dementia. Psychosocial interventions can aid in the diagnosis of dementia by reducing stress, improving mood (such as anxiety or depression), enhancing and preserving cognitive functioning, and promoting overall quality of life. More precisely, the treatments aimed at enhancing and preserving cognitive abilities in older individuals include Cognitive Training, Cognitive Stimulation Therapy, and Cognitive Rehabilitation. These interventions differ significantly in terms of their objectives, intended recipients, duration, and administration.

Cognitive training, also known as brain training, focuses on improving targeted aspects of memory and other cognitive abilities. Activities such as crosswords, Sudoku, games, or computer exercises that are not specifically designed for an individual can also be considered as cognitive training. Cognitive training is suitable for individuals seeking to maintain mental agility and derive pleasure from engaging in brain training activities and puzzles, including those affected by dementia. The purpose of exercises is to enhance and develop specific cognitive functions, such as word memory, logical and analytical thinking, attention, problem-solving, and mathematical skills. Training is a recurring and ongoing activity that can be self-directed.

Cognitive Stimulation Therapy (CST) is a form of group therapy aimed at enhancing personal communication skills, cognitive abilities, and memory. CST groups typically consist of a finite number of sessions, usually ranging from 12 to 14, with one or two sessions per week. In addition, the maintenance cognitive stimulation therapy (MCST) groups have an ongoing duration and are designed to sustain the advantages offered by CST groups. Cognitive Stimulation Therapy (CST) and Multicomponent Cognitive Stimulation Therapy (MCST) are appropriate for individuals who have been diagnosed with mild cognitive impairment or dementia in the mild-to-moderate stages. A typical Cognitive Stimulation Therapy (CST) session has a duration of 1 hour and encompasses activities such as games, singing, applying reminiscence therapies, sharing stories, discussing current events, practicing arts, and making crafts. Cognitive

Stimulation Therapy (CST) has demonstrated positive effects on cognitive function and overall quality of life, while also proving to be a cost-effective intervention. Moreover, when CST is accompanied by MCST, it presents a notable enhancement in cognitive function, resulting in enduring advantages.

Cognitive rehabilitation is a method used to address the effects of cognitive impairments, such as difficulties with memory and thinking that arise from dementia. Its purpose is to help individuals manage these challenges in their daily activities. It is advisable for individuals experiencing early-onset dementia. Cognitive rehabilitation focuses on acquiring strategies to compensate for or improve the management of thinking and memory difficulties associated with dementia, rather than aiming to cure or reduce these difficulties. Several cognitive rehabilitation programs may incorporate the participation of families and caregivers. Typically, gerontologists, occupational therapists, clinical psychologists, or clinical neuropsychologists are the ones who implement it. Cognitive rehabilitation primarily centers on identifying and addressing individual needs and goals, which may necessitate the use of strategies for absorbing new information or compensatory techniques like memory aids. It has shown initial indications of its potential advantages in enhancing everyday activities in individuals with mild Alzheimer's disease.

For any cognitive intervention to be effective, it is essential to have a prior diagnosis, which should include two types of assessment. The initial step involves a screening process, typically utilizing the Mini-Mental State Examination. The subsequent step entails a comprehensive evaluation, employing standardized tests that consider the sociocultural context, age, and educational background of the individual. This evaluation assesses the individual's cognitive abilities across various tasks. Based on the diagnosis results, if an individual demonstrates "normal" or preserved cognitive performance, it means that they maintain their cognitive functions at the expected level for their age and education in their specific context. On the other hand, if they exhibit a significantly lower performance, it can be categorized as mild cognitive impairment and may indicate the presence of suspected dementia. Prior assessment is essential to determine whether an intervention is warranted and what specific type is required, which aspects should be focused on, and which capacities should be fostered.

The goals of intervention programs that utilize training and/or cognitive stimulation are typically defined as "enhancing, preserving, fortifying, and reinstating." In cognitive rehabilitation programs, the objectives are defined in terms of "compensation."

After selecting the type and purpose of the treatment, it is important to consider basic methodological aspects during the planning of the cognitive intervention. This will help to systematize the steps involved in the process. The guidelines encompass the following: (1) A methodical arrangement of the session and its activities, (2) a gradual progression, commencing with simple tasks and advancing to more challenging ones, (3) an appropriate and adjusted level of intensity, maintaining a suitable pace, (4) a coherent and logical structure, ensuring meaningful and sequential order. (5) The activities should be engaging and captivating. (6) They should stimulate motivation, curiosity, and a strong desire to learn. (7) The activities should be rewarding and satisfying. (8) Personal and emotional engagement is crucial, as the components of the process should evoke positive emotions. (9) The components of the process should foster interpersonal connections between individuals and their surroundings. During intervention work, it is advisable to follow a structured session routine as a basic guideline. As part of the training and cognitive stimulation, a session plan is suggested. It includes the following elements, not necessarily in this order: (Table 9.2).

1. Reality orientation (personal, spatial and temporal).
2. Attention/concentration technique.
3. Relaxation technique.
4. Psycho-educational techniques, knowledge and theoretical information promote the improvement of the perception of memory.
5. Practical training in the use of mnemonic strategies adapted to the needs of the person.
6. Feedback and closure. Always ask: How does this help me in everyday life?

Table 9.2. Environmental and Lifestyle Exposures and Stimuli Associated with Reduced Risk of Age-Related Dementia, All of Which are Likely to Provide a Significant Proportion of their Benefit Through Cognitive Demand

Intervention/ Exposure	Evidence
Exercise	1. Dose-dependent increase in cognitive function with minimal effective dose around 25 or 15 min of moderate or vigorous physical activity, respectively, per day. 2. Increased hippocampal volume in older adults with walking intervention. 3. Increased cognitive function in older adults after resistance training intervention. 4. Greater benefit from coordinative exercise such as dance, likely due to greater cognitive demand.
Language	1. Improved cognitive function in older adults learning a language. 2. Protective effect of bilingualism on the age of onset of AD. 3. Lifelong bilingualism maintains white matter integrity in older adults.

Music	1. Decreased biological brain age in musicians, with greater benefit in amateur musicians, likely due to greater demand. 2. Lifelong musicianship associated with greater white matter integrity. 3. Playing a musical instrument associated with reduced risk of dementia. 4. Older adults who played a musical instrument demonstrated higher processing speed, attention, learning, episodic memory, working memory, and executive functions.
Brain Training	1. Structured cognitive training results in improved structural and functional brain connectivity, as well as improvements in executive function and memory.
Social Connection	1. Increased dementia risk with lack of social support. 2. Loneliness associated with lower brain volume and up to 3-fold increase in dementia risk.
Sensory Input	1. Increased AD risk in those with cataracts, which is reversed with cataract removal. 2. Increased risk of cognitive decline with loss of sense of smell—COVID as a recent example. 3. Peripheral nerve impairments associated with higher risk of dementia after adjustment for age and other health factors. 4. Hearing loss associated with a doubling of dementia risk in those age 45–65, which may be reversible with hearing aids.

Source: Turknett J, Wood TR. Demand coupling drives neurodegeneration: A model of age-related cognitive decline and dementia. Cells. 2022; 11(18):2789. https://doi.org/10.3390/cells11182789.

Mnemonic strategies are utilized to enhance memory processes and, as a result, ensuring that essential information is conveniently accessible whenever it is required in our day-to-day lives. There is a distinction that can be made between memory strategies based on their origin, in particular, whether they are internal or external. When it comes to remembering things, the first method involves the utilization of aids that are external to our bodies. On the other hand, internal strategies are mental activities that engage the individual in the process of remembering information. Both of these types of strategies are effective ways of learning and remembering information, and they are frequently utilized as components of training and cognitive stimulation programs in the process of aging.

On the other hand, interventions that are based on cognitive rehabilitation and are designed for people who have mild to severe dementia should be highly personalized to fulfill the requirements regarding both the potential and the deterioration of the person. Because of this, it is difficult to design sessions that adhere to rigid schemes. In spite of this, it is not the case that the work should not be organized systematically (Wharton et al., 2023).

A Closer Look

Cognitive Aging

Cognitive aging refers to the changes that occur in cognitive abilities as individuals grow older. These changes can affect various aspects of cognition, such as memory, processing speed, decision-making, and attention. Consider a senior executive who has decades of experience in a fast-paced corporate environment. Over the years, this executive has been known for sharp decision-making, effective multitasking, and precise memory recall of key business data. However, as they approach their late sixties, subtle changes begin to manifest. They may find it slightly harder to recall names and details in meetings that they once effortlessly remembered. Processing complex information or adapting quickly to new technologies or market trends might become more challenging.

In practical terms, this could mean that the executive takes longer to process information during critical negotiations or strategic planning sessions. They might rely more on notes or aides to recall details that were previously ingrained. This cognitive shift can impact leadership effectiveness and decision-making speed, potentially influencing organizational outcomes.

To mitigate these effects, organizations often implement strategies such as mentoring programs where older executives pass on their knowledge and skills to younger colleagues. They may also provide cognitive training programs or adapt workplaces to be more age-friendly, supporting ongoing cognitive health and performance.

Understanding cognitive aging is crucial not only for personal well-being but also for designing inclusive workplaces and societal structures that support individuals as they age, ensuring continued productivity and quality of life in an aging workforce.

Summary

- The cognitive changes that occur with aging can vary in severity, but those that are typical of normal aging are generally mild and do not hinder one's ability to engage in regular daily activities. Conversely, cognitive pathologies, such as dementia, impair an individual's capacity to live autonomously and can be extremely burdensome for the families of those affected. Families can experience significant stress due to physical, emotional, and economic pressures. To cope with these challenges, families need to receive support from various systems such as health, social, financial, and legal systems. Mild cognitive impairment is a condition that lies between these two extremes. In the context of Mild Cognitive Impairment (MCI), the cognitive alterations are more significant compared to the typical cognitive changes associated with normal aging, yet they do not reach a level of severity that would result in disability. Both MCI and dementia are pathological conditions resulting from underlying brain disorders or conditions that are not associated with the typical aging process.
- The investigation of age-related alterations has revealed decreases in memory, attention, perception, processing speed, and certain executive functions. Nevertheless, there is a significant lack of consistency in the findings. An analysis of the limitations of the studies is necessary to identify any biases related to the methodology, variations in assessment tools, and diagnostic and performance criteria. To effectively study the decline in cognitive function associated with aging, it is best to conduct a long-term analysis of aging groups within the general population. Nevertheless, studying cognitive decline in normal aging remains highly pertinent in the field of gerontology, as it may potentially mirror a less severe yet comparable process observed in dementia. Furthermore, since a decrease in cognitive abilities and the beginning of dementia are linked to advanced age, it is imperative to investigate the social, environmental, and individual factors that contribute to these conditions.
- Assessing the extent of the disease and the portion of it caused by the primary risk factors of mild cognitive impairment and dementia enables the implementation of effective preventive measures, particularly targeting those risk factors that can be modified and are strongly influenced by lifestyle choices. Adopting a healthy diet, engaging in regular physical exercise, and effectively managing therapy can reduce the risk of cardiovascular disease and type 2 diabetes. Additionally, engaging in lifelong cognitive training and intellectually challenging leisure activities can reduce the likelihood of cognitive impairment. Furthermore, effective treatment for depression symptoms can also be achieved.
- In addition to examining cognitive changes that occur with aging, the field of gerontology focuses on understanding the development of diseases and risk factors associated with aging. Furthermore, it aims to address the challenge of creating effective intervention programs that promote cognitive health in older adults. Research has demonstrated that cognitive decline can be partially prevented and controlled through cognitive stimulation and rehabilitation strategies. Although there is a wide range of interventions and outcomes, which limits the ability to apply the findings to a broader population, nonpharmacological

interventions aimed at MCI show promise and most studies have found a positive effect from the intervention.

- Population aging is closely linked to other concurrent and interconnected global trends that are influencing our shared future, particularly about epidemiological transitions. Over the past decades, there has been a significant shift in the types of diseases that are the main contributors to disability and death. Currently, chronic, noncommunicable diseases are the primary contributors to mortality and morbidity, and their prevalence is increasing. Most elderly individuals suffer from chronic ailments, with a significant number experiencing multiple conditions concurrently. There is currently a strong focus on mental disorders that affect cognitive abilities, particularly dementia, which is regarded as a top priority in public health. The profound consequences of cognitive aging, including mild cognitive impairment and dementia, are reverberating across society. The economic ramifications of these diseases affect families, healthcare systems, businesses, and social frameworks. The cognitive pathologies that occur with aging have a significant impact on individuals, their families, and the formal support networks that provide assistance. These pathologies result in emotional, psychological, and physical burdens.
- The challenge in the field of Gerontology involves reevaluating the trajectory of one's life to transform the process

References

1. Aisen, P. S., Cummings, J., Doody, R., Kramer, L., Salloway, S., Selkoe, D. J., Sims, J., Sperling, R. A., & Vellas, B. (2020). The Future of Anti-Amyloid Trials. *Journal of Prevention of Alzheimer's Disease, 7*(3), 146–151.
2. Alafuzoff, I., & Libard, S. (2020). Mixed Brain Pathology Is the Most Common Cause of Cognitive Impairment in the Elderly. *Journal of Alzheimer's Disease, 78*(2), 453–465.
3. Alafuzoff, I., Ince, P. G., Arzberger, T., Al-Sarraj, S., Bell, J., Bodi, I., Bogdanovic, N., Bugiani, O., Ferrer, I., Gelpi, E., et al. (2009). Staging/typing of Lewy body related α-synuclein pathology: A study of the BrainNet Europe Consortium. *Acta Neuropathologica, 117*(6), 635–652.
4. Alafuzoff, I., Thal, D. R., Arzberger, T., Bogdanovic, N., Al-Sarraj, S., Bodi, I., Boluda, S., Bugiani, O., Duyckaerts, C., Gelpi, E., et al. (2009). Assessment of beta-amyloid deposits in human brain: A study of the BrainNet Europe Consortium. *Acta Neuropathologica, 117*(4), 309–320.
5. Andrés-Benito, P., Fernández-Dueñas, V., Carmona, M., Escobar, L. A., Torrejón-Escribano, B., Aso, E., Ciruela, F., & Ferrer, I. (2017). Locus coeruleus at asymptomatic early and middle Braak stages of neurofibrillary tangle pathology. *Neuropathology and Applied Neurobiology, 43*(4), 373–392.
6. Beardmore, R., Hou, R., Darekar, A., Holmes, C., & Boche, D. (2021). The locus coeruleus in aging and Alzheimer's disease: A postmortem and brain imaging review. *Journal of Alzheimer's Disease, 83*(1), 5–22.
7. Bennett, S., & Thomas, A. J. (2014). Depression and dementia: Cause, consequence or coincidence? *Maturitas, 79*, 184–190.
8. Berridge, C. W., Stellick, R. L., & Schmeichel, B. E. (2005). Wake-promoting actions of medial basal forebrain beta2 receptor stimulation. *Behavioral Neuroscience, 119*(3), 743–751.

9. Braak, H., & Braak, E. (1987). Argyrophilic grains: Characteristic pathology of cerebral cortex in cases of adult onset dementia without Alzheimer changes. *Neuroscience Letters, 76*(1), 124–127.

10. Braak, H., & Braak, E. (1991). Neuropathological staging of Alzheimer-related changes. *Acta Neuropathologica., 82*(3), 239–259.

11. Braak, H., & Tredici, K. D. (2011). Alzheimer's pathogenesis: Is there neuron-to-neuron propagation? *Acta Neuropathologica, 121*(5), 589–595.

12. Braak, H., Alafuzoff, I., Arzberger, T., Kretzschmar, H., & Del Tredici, K. (2006). Staging of Alzheimer disease-associated neurofibrillary pathology using paraffin sections and immunocytochemistry. *Acta Neuropathologica, 112*(4), 389–404.

13. Braak, H., Del Tredici, K., Rüb, U., de Vos, R. A., Steur, E. N. J., & Braak, E. (2003). Staging of brain pathology related to sporadic Parkinson's disease. *Neurobiology of Aging, 24*(2), 197–211.

14. Braak, H., Thal, D. R., Ghebremedhin, E., & Del Tredici, K. (2011). Stages of the pathologic process in Alzheimer disease: Age categories from 1 to 100 years. *Journal of Neuropathology & Experimental Neurology, 70*(11), 960–969.

15. Brunnström, H., & Englund, E. (2009). Clinicopathological Concordance in Dementia Diagnostics. *The American Journal of Geriatric Psychiatry, 17*(8), 664–670.

16. Buratti, E., Dörk, T., Zuccato, E., Pagani, F., Romano, M., & Baralle, F. E. (2001). Nuclear factor TDP-43 and SR proteins promote in vitro and in vivo CFTR exon 9 skipping. *The EMBO Journal, 20*(7), 1774–1784.

17. Crary, J. F., Trojanowski, J. Q., Schneider, J. A., Abisambra, J. F., Abner, E. L., Alafuzoff, I., Arnold, S. E., Attems, J., Beach, T. G., Bigio, E. H., et al. (2014). Primary age-related tauopathy (PART): A common pathology associated with human aging. *Acta Neuropathologica., 128*(6), 755–766.

18. Duyckaerts, C., Braak, H., Brion, J. -P., Buée, L., Del Tredici, K., Goedert, M., Halliday, G., Neumann, M., Spillantini, M. G., Tolnay, M., et al. (2015). PART is part of Alzheimer disease. *Acta Neuropathologica., 129*(5), 749–756.

19. Forbes, J. M., & Cooper, M. E. (2013). Mechanisms of Diabetic Complications. *Physiological Reviews, 93*(1), 137–188.

20. Friberg, N., Ljungberg, O., Berglund, E., Berglund, D., Ljungberg, R., Alafuzoff, I., & Englund, E. (2019). Cause of death and significant disease found at autopsy. *Virchows Archiv., 475*(6), 781–788.

21. Gale, S. A., Acar, D., & Daffner, K. R. (2018). Dementia. *American Journal of Medicine, 131*(10), 1161–1169.

22. Galgani, A., & Giorgi, F. S. (2023). Exploring the Role of Locus Coeruleus in Alzheimer's Disease: A Comprehensive Update on MRI Studies and Implications. *Current Neurology and Neuroscience Reports, 23*(3), 925–936.

23. Ganguli, M., Snitz, B. E., Saxton, J. A., Chang, C. C. H., Lee, C. W., Bilt, J. V., Hughes, T. F., Loewenstein, D. A., Unverzagt, F. W., & Petersen, R. C. (2011). Outcomes of mild cognitive impairment by definition: A population study. *Archives of Neurology, 68*(6), 761–767.

24. Gauthreaux, K., Bonnett, T. A., Besser, L. M., Brenowitz, W. D., Teylan, M., Mock, C., Chen, Y. -C., Chan, K. C. G., Keene, C. D., Zhou, X. -H., et al. (2020). Concordance of Clinical Alzheimer

Diagnosis and Neuropathological Features at Autopsy. *Journal of Neuropathology & Experimental Neurology, 79*(5), 465–473.

25. Ghosh, A., Torraville, S. E., Mukherjee, B., Walling, S. G., Martin, G. M., Harley, C. W., & Yuan, Q. (2019). An experimental model of Braak's pretangle proposal for the origin of Alzheimer's disease: The role of locus coeruleus in early symptom development. *Alzheimer's Research & Therapy, 11*(1), 59.
26. Glass, C. K., Saijo, K., Winner, B., Marchetto, M. C., & Gage, F. H. (2010). Mechanisms underlying inflammation in neurodegeneration. *Cell, 140*(6), 918–934.
27. Grossman, M., Seeley, W. W., Boxer, A. L., Hillis, A. E., Knopman, D. S., Ljubenov, P. A., Miller, B., Piguet, O., Rademakers, R., & Whitwell, J. L., et al. (2023). Frontotemporal lobar degeneration. *Nature Reviews Disease Primers, 9*(1), 40.
28. Grudzien, A., Shaw, P., Weintraub, S., Bigio, E., Mash, D. C., & Mesulam, M. M. (2007). Locus coeruleus neurofibrillary degeneration in aging, mild cognitive impairment and early Alzheimer's disease. *Neurobiology of Aging, 28*(3), 327–335.
29. Hobson, J. A., McCarley, R. W., & Wyzinski, P. W. (1975). Sleep Cycle Oscillation: Reciprocal Discharge by Two Brainstem Neuronal Groups. *Science, 189*(4196), 55–58.
30. Hyman, B. T., Phelps, C. H., Beach, T. G., Bigio, E. H., Cairns, N. J., Carrillo, M. C., Dickson, D. W., Duyckaerts, C., Frosch, M. P., Masliah, E., et al. (2012). National Institute on Aging-Alzheimer's Association guidelines for the neuropathologic assessment of Alzheimer's disease. *Alzheimer's & Dementia, 8*(1), 1–13.
31. Jellinger, K. A., & Bancher, C. (1998). Senile dementia with tangles (tangle predominant form of senile dementia). *Brain Pathology, 8*(2), 367–376.
32. Josephs, K. A., Murray, M. E., Whitwell, J. L., Parisi, J. E., Petrucelli, L., Jack, C. R., Petersen, R. C., & Dickson, D. W. (2013). Staging TDP-43 pathology in Alzheimer's disease. *Acta Neuropathologica., 127*(3), 441–450.
33. Josephs, K. A., Murray, M. E., Whitwell, J. L., Tosakulwong, N., Weigand, S. D., Petrucelli, L., Liesinger, A. M., Petersen, R. C., Parisi, J. E., & Dickson, D. W. (2016). Updated TDP-43 in Alzheimer's disease staging scheme. *Acta Neuropathologica., 131*(4), 571–585.
34. Josephs, K. A., Whitwell, J. L., Weigand, S. D., Murray, M. E., Tosakulwong, N., Liesinger, A. M., Petrucelli, L., Senjem, M. L., Knopman, D. S., Boeve, B. F., et al. (2014). TDP-43 is a key player in the clinical features associated with Alzheimer's disease. *Acta Neuropathologica., 127*(6), 811–824.
35. Kaalund, S. S., Passamonti, L., Allinson, K. S. J., Murley, A. G., Robbins, T. W., Spillantini, M. G., & Rowe, J. B. (2020). Locus coeruleus pathology in progressive supranuclear palsy, and its relation to disease severity. *Acta Neuropathologica. Communications, 8*(1), 11.
36. Kaufman, S. K., Del Tredici, K., Thomas, T. L., Braak, H., & Diamond, M. I. (2018). Tau seeding activity begins in the transentorhinal/entorhinal regions and anticipates phospho-tau pathology in Alzheimer's disease and PART. *Acta Neuropathologica., 136*(1), 57–67.
37. Killinger, B. A., Madaj, Z., Sikora, J. W., Rey, N., Haas, A. J., Vepa, Y., Lindqvist, D., Chen, H., Thomas, P. M., Brundin, P., et al. (2018). The vermiform appendix impacts the risk of developing Parkinson's disease. *Science Translational Medicine, 10*(465), eaar5280.
38. Klimek, V., Stockmeier, C., Overholser, J., Meltzer, H. Y., Kalka, S., Dilley, G., & Ordway, G. A.

(1997). Reduced Levels of Norepinephrine Transporters in the Locus Coeruleus in Major Depression. *Journal of Neuroscience, 17*(21), 8451–8458.

39. Kovacs, G. G., Alafuzoff, I., Al-Sarraj, S., Arzberger, T., Bogdanovic, N., Capellari, S., Ferrer, I., Gelpi, E., Kövari, V., Kretzschmar, H., et al. (2008). Mixed Brain Pathologies in Dementia: The BrainNet Europe Consortium Experience. *Dementia and Geriatric Cognitive Disorders, 26*(4), 343–350.
40. Kovacs, G. G., Ferrer, I., Grinberg, L. T., Alafuzoff, I., Attems, J., Budka, H., Cairns, N. J., Crary, J. F., Duyckaerts, C., Ghetti, B., et al. (2015). Aging-related tau astrogliopathy (ARTAG): Harmonized evaluation strategy. *Acta Neuropathologica, 131*(1), 87–102.
41. Leino, M., Popova, S. N., & Alafuzoff, I. (2017). Transactive DNA Binding Protein 43 Rather Than Other Misfolded Proteins in the Brain is Associated with Islet Amyloid Polypeptide in Pancreas in Aged Subjects with Diabetes Mellitus. *Journal of Alzheimer's Disease, 59*(1), 43–56.
42. Lu, H. -T., Shen, Q. -Y., Xie, D., Zhao, Q. -Z., & Xu, Y. -M. (2019). Lack of association between appendectomy and Parkinson's disease: A systematic review and meta-analysis. *Aging Clinical and Experimental Research, 32*(11), 2201–2209.
43. Mackenzie, I. R., Neumann, M., Baborie, A., Sampathu, D. M., Plessis, D. D., Jaros, E., Perry, R. H., Trojanowski, J. Q., Mann, D. M. A., & Lee, V. M. Y. (2011). A harmonized classification system for FTLD-TDP pathology. *Acta Neuropathologica., 122*(1), 111–113.
44. Madonna, R., Balistreri, C. R., Geng, Y. -J., & De Caterina, R. (2017). Diabetic microangiopathy: Pathogenetic insights and novel therapeutic approaches. *Vascular Pharmacology, 90*, 1–7.
45. Marković, M., Milošević, J., Wang, W., & Cao, Y. (2023). Passive Immunotherapies Targeting Amyloid-β in Alzheimer's Disease: A Quantitative Systems Pharmacology Perspective. *Molecular Pharmacology, 105*(1), 1–13.
46. Martínez-Hernández, A. (2000). The autopsy in crisis. *Revista Medica de Chile, 128*(4), 457–459.
47. McAleese, K. E., Colloby, S. J., Thomas, A. J., Al-Sarraj, S., Ansorge, O., Neal, J., Roncaroli, F., Love, S., Francis, P. T., & Attems, J. (2021). Concomitant neurodegenerative pathologies contribute to the transition from mild cognitive impairment to dementia. *Alzheimer's & Dementia, 17*(7), 1121–1133.
48. McAleese, K. E., Walker, L., Erskine, D., Johnson, M., Koss, D., Thomas, A. J., & Attems, J. (2020). Concomitant LATE-NC in Alzheimer's disease is not associated with increased tau or amyloid-β pathological burden. *Neuropathology and Applied Neurobiology, 46*(8), 722–734.
49. McAleese, K. E., Walker, L., Erskine, D., Thomas, A. J., McKeith, I. G., & Attems, J. (2017). TDP-43 pathology in Alzheimer's disease, dementia with Lewy bodies and ageing. *Brain Pathology, 27*(4), 472–479.
50. McKeith, I. G., Galasko, D., Kosaka, K., Perry, E. K., Dickson, D. W., Hansen, L. A., Salmon, D. P., Lowe, J., Mirra, S. S., & Byrne, E. J., et al. (1996). Consensus guidelines for the clinical and pathologic diagnosis of dementia with Lewy bodies (DLB): Report of the consortium on DLB international workshop. *Neurology, 47*(5), 1113–1124.
51. Messerli, F. H., Williams, B., & Ritz, E. (2007). Essential hypertension. *The Lancet, 370*(9587), 591–603.
52. Mirra, S. S., Heyman, A., McKeel, D., Sumi, S. M., Crain, B. J., Brownlee, L. M., Vogel, F. S., Hughes, J. P., van Belle, G., & Berg, L. (1991). The Consortium to Establish a Registry for

Alzheimer's Disease (CERAD). Part II. Standardization of the neuropathologic assessment of Alzheimer's disease. *Neurology, 41*(4), 479–486.

53. Montine, T. J., Cholerton, B. A., Corrada, M. M., Edland, S. D., Flanagan, M. E., Hemmy, L. S., Kawas, C. H., & White, L. R. (2019). Concepts for brain aging: Resistance, resilience, reserve, and compensation. *Alzheimer's Research & Therapy, 11*(1), 1–3.
54. Montine, T. J., Phelps, C. H., Beach, T. G., Bigio, E. H., Cairns, N. J., Dickson, D. W., Duyckaerts, C., Frosch, M. P., Masliah, E., Mirra, S. S., et al. (2012). National Institute on Aging–Alzheimer's Association guidelines for the neuropathologic assessment of Alzheimer's disease: A practical approach. *Acta Neuropathologica, 123*(1), 1–11.
55. Nelson, P. T., Lee, E. B., Cykowski, M. D., Alafuzoff, I., Arfanakis, K., Attems, J., Brayne, C., Corrada, M. M., Dugger, B. N., Flanagan, M. E., et al. (2022). LATE-NC staging in routine neuropathologic diagnosis: An update. *Acta Neuropathologica, 145*(1), 159–173.
56. Newman, A. B., Fitzpatrick, A. L., Lopez, O., Jackson, S., Lyketsos, C., Jagust, W., Ives, D., DeKosky, S. T., & Kuller, L. H. (2005). Dementia and Alzheimer's disease incidence in relationship to cardiovascular disease in the Cardiovascular Health Study cohort. *Journal of the American Geriatrics Society, 53*(7), 1101–1107.
57. Ogrodowczyk, M., Dettlaff, K., & Jelinska, A. (2016). Beta-Blockers: Current State of Knowledge and Perspectives. *Mini Reviews in Medicinal Chemistry, 16*(1), 40–54.
58. Panza, F., Lozupone, M., Logroscino, G., & Imbimbo, B. P. (2019). A critical appraisal of amyloid-β-targeting therapies for Alzheimer disease. *Nature Reviews Neurology, 15*(2), 73–88.
59. Petrou, M., Dwamena, B. A., Foerster, B. R., MacEachern, M. P., Bohnen, N. I., Müller, M. L., Albin, R. L., & Frey, K. A. (2015). Amyloid deposition in Parkinson's disease and cognitive impairment: A systematic review. *Movement Disorders, 30*(7), 928–935.
60. Rabin, J. S., Schultz, A. P., Hedden, T., Viswanathan, A., Marshall, G. A., Kilpatrick, E., Klein, H., Buckley, R. F., Yang, H. -S., Properzi, M., et al. (2018). Interactive Associations of Vascular Risk and β-Amyloid Burden with Cognitive Decline in Clinically Normal Elderly Individuals: Findings from the Harvard Aging Brain Study. *JAMA Neurology, 75*(9), 1124–1131.
61. Rösler, T. W., Marvian, A. T., Brendel, M., Nykänen, N. -P., Höllerhage, M., Schwarz, S. C., Hopfner, F., Koeglsperger, T., Respondek, G., Schweyer, K., et al. (2019). Four-repeat tauopathies. *Progress in Neurobiology, 180*, 101644.
62. Roy, S., Trudeau, K., Behl, Y., Dhar, S., & Chronopoulos, A. (2009). New insights into hyperglycemia-induced molecular changes in microvascular cells. *Journal of Dental Research, 89*(2), 116–127.
63. Schneider, J. A., Arvanitakis, Z., Bang, W., & Bennett, D. A. (2007). Mixed brain pathologies account for most dementia cases in community-dwelling older persons. *Neurology, 69*(22), 2197–2204.
64. Shi, Y., & Vanhoutte, P. M. (2017). Macro- and microvascular endothelial dysfunction in diabetes. *Journal of Diabetes, 9*(5), 434–449.
65. Skrobot, O. A., Attems, J., Esiri, M., Hortobágyi, T., Ironside, J. W., Kalaria, R. N., King, A., Lammie, G. A., Mann, D., Neal, J., et al. (2016). Vascular cognitive impairment neuropathology guidelines (VCING): The contribution of cerebrovascular pathology to cognitive impairment. *Brain, 139*(9), 2957–2969.

66. Spires-Jones, T. L., Attems, J., & Thal, D. R. (2017). Interactions of pathological proteins in neurodegenerative diseases. *Acta Neuropathologica., 134*(2), 187–205.

67. Tamsen, F., & Alafuzoff, I. (2023). When is a postmortem examination carried out? A retrospective analysis of all Swedish deaths 1999–2018. *Virchows Archiv., 482*(5), 721–727.

68. Thal, D. R., Rüb, U., Orantes, M., & Braak, H. (2002). Phases of A beta-deposition in the human brain and its relevance for the development of AD. *Neurology, 58*(12), 1791–1800.

69. van Arendonk, J., Neitzel, J., Steketee, R. M. E., van Assema, D. M. E., Vrooman, H. A., Segbers, M., Ikram, M. A., & Vernooij, M. W. (2023). Diabetes and hypertension are related to amyloid-beta burden in the population-based Rotterdam Study. *Brain, 146*(1), 337–348.

70. Vitek, G. E., Decourt, B., & Sabbagh, M. N. (2023). Lecanemab (BAN2401): An anti–beta-amyloid monoclonal antibody for the treatment of Alzheimer's disease. *Expert Opinion on Investigational Drugs, 32*(1), 89–94.

71. Wharton, S. B., Simpson, J. E., Ince, P. G., Richardson, C. D., Merrick, R., Matthews, F. E., & Brayne, C. (2023). Insights into the pathological basis of dementia from population-based neuropathology studies. *Neuropathology and Applied Neurobiology, 49*(4), e12923.

INDEX

FSC
www.fsc.org
MIX
Papier | Fördert gute Waldnutzung
FSC® C083411

Kolibri 360 GmbH
Ferdinand-Jühlke-Straße 7
99095 Erfurt, Deutschland
produktsicherheit@kolibri360.de